"Behavioural scientists have recently developed interesting new ways of thinking about and responding to addiction, but these are largely unknown to the general public and even to many specialists in the addiction field. This book admirably fills that gap, especially in relation to the ancient concept of '*akrasia*' and its role in making sense of addiction. I recommend it for anyone with a serious interest in the enduring puzzle of addiction, especially those who are dissatisfied with narrow biomedical formulations."

—**Nick Heather**, *Emeritus Professor of Alcohol and Other Drug Studies in the Department of Psychology at Northumbria University, UK*

"... a wonderfully clear and engaging book, which connects social, psychological and neuroscience factors influencing the use and abuse of alcohol and other drugs. Reinout Wiers helps answer important questions. Is addiction a choice or a brain disease? What therapy programs work best to help people recover? Where do behavioral addictions fit in? Wiers gives us an illuminating analysis of the nature of addiction and drug abuse that will be helpful and informative to anyone concerned with these issues."

—**Kent C. Berridge**, *James Olds Distinguished University Professor of Psychology and Neuroscience, University of Michigan*

"Professor Wiers places *akrasia*—the distorted but deliberate decision making that leads us to do what we know is not good for us—centre stage in the addiction arena. In support of this approach, he draws on comprehensive research findings, spanning the developmental spectrum. He skilfully probes scientific fields as diverse as molecular biology, cognitive bias modification and mindfulness practice in an effort to understand and help overcome our quintessentially human tendency towards akrasia. Throughout he maintains a humane, humorous and reflective tone that makes this book a joy to read."

—**Dr Frank Ryan**, *Honorary Clinical Senior Lecturer, Imperial College London*

"Finally an intelligent answer to the question of whether addicts are addicted by choice. A delight to read."

—**Prof. Wim van den Brink**, *emeritus professor addiction treatment, UMC-Amsterdam*

"...full of fascinating insights about addiction."

—**Laura Molenaar**, *Trouw, National Newspaper, The Netherlands*

"...an excellent overview of the state of the art in the science of addiction written by a leading expert in the field. The book achieves that delicate balance between accessibility and scientific accuracy that characterizes the best popular science writing. I highly recommend it to anyone who is interested in the facts about addiction."

—**Denny Borsboom**, *Professor of Psychological Methods, University of Amsterdam*

A New Approach to Addiction and Choice

This engaging book provides a novel examination of the nature of addiction, suggesting that by exploring *akrasia*—the tendency to act against one's better judgement—we can better understand our addictive behaviors. It offers an alternative to the dominant biomedical model of addiction as a chronic brain disease by looking at the nature of how we make decisions and proposing the idea that biased choice is central to addiction.

The book looks at both classic substance use disorders and newer "addictions" to smartphones, meat and fossil fuels. It discusses current perspectives on free will in philosophy, psychology and neuroscience, and the questions surrounding free will versus determinism, including our ability to steer our behaviors guided by the promise of future outcomes. Different perspectives on addiction and choice are presented in an eloquent style, and illustrated by personal stories.

Through a lively discussion of the key scientific and philosophical issues surrounding addiction, this book is valuable for students in psychology, criminology, sociology and social work, as well as health care professionals and general readers interested in the nature of our free will.

Reinout W. Wiers is Professor of Developmental Psychopathology, at the University of Amsterdam, where he leads the Addiction Development and Psychopathology (ADAPT) Lab and he is (co)director of the University of Amsterdam's interdisciplinary Centre for Urban Mental Health. He is internationally known for his work on assessing and changing implicit cognitive processes in addiction. In addition to his primary work as researcher, he has been trained as a cognitive behavior therapist.

A New Approach to Addiction and Choice

Akrasia and the Nature of Free Will

Reinout W. Wiers

Routledge
Taylor & Francis Group
LONDON AND NEW YORK

Designed cover image: Print Collector/Hulton Archive via Getty Images

First published 2025
by Routledge
4 Park Square, Milton Park, Abingdon, Oxon OX14 4RN

and by Routledge
605 Third Avenue, New York, NY 10158

Routledge is an imprint of the Taylor & Francis Group, an informa business

British Library Cataloguing-in-Publication Data
A catalogue record for this book is available from the British Library

ISBN: 978-1-032-63453-1 (hbk)
ISBN: 978-1-032-63161-5 (pbk)
ISBN: 978-1-032-63454-8 (ebk)

DOI: 10.4324/9781032634548

Typeset in Times New Roman
by MPS Limited, Dehradun

Contents

Acknowledgments

A number of people have been kind enough to read and comment on an earlier version of this book: Arno Ambrosius, Lieke Asma, Wim van den Brink, Annemie Ploeger, Steven Pont, Annelies van der Meij, Richard Ridderinkhof, Tim Schoenmakers, Tom Ter Bogt, Peter Vonk and Jochem Wiers. Several international friends and colleagues have read (part of) the English draft and given additional useful feedback—many thanks for that to Kent Berridge, Ron Dahl, Mike Le Pelley, Frank Ryan and Spencer Weisbroth. Remaining errors are of course entirely my responsibility. Needless to say, not every proofreader necessarily agrees with all my statements.

The ideas I describe in this book were formed over a long period of time, from the reading club with Paul Verschure and others in the early 1990s to recent discussions with the same Paul and other colleagues, such as Lieke Asma, Denny Borsboom, Ron Dahl, Wilhelm Hofmann, Bernhard Hommel, Jan de Houwer, Thomas Gladwin, Peter de Jong, Catalina Köpetz, Mike Le Pelley, Han van der Maas, Colin MacLeod, Richard Ridderinkhof, Mike Rinck, Ken Sher, Alan Stacy, Pieter Van Dessel, Simon Van Gaal and Sanne de Wit. In translating the work into clinical applications, I learned a lot from Maarten Merkx, Elske Salemink, Eni Becker and Johannes Lindenmeyer. In addition, I have drawn much inspiration from interactions with students and PhD students I have supervised and colleagues from home and abroad with whom I have collaborated in relation to the central theme of this book, especially Nick Heather and Matt Field. Finally, I would like to thank Emke and my children for their patience when I went back to work on *that book*.

1 Introduction

About twenty years ago, I received a letter at my then work address—a handwritten letter on thin airmail paper, sent from a Florida prison. Someone, let's call him Jim, was sharing his thoughts with me on what his alcohol addiction from age 15 had done to his brain. He wrote that my research had shown how his frontal cortex had become less effective, and how he had been controlled by his automatic impulses; how he had lost his capacity to make conscious decisions or plans. This had resulted in two life sentences after a conflict got out of hand ("self-defense against gays") in a fit of "intermittent insanity". He did not give further details; however, he did make an appeal to support his claim that he could no longer make decisions and could therefore not be held responsible for his intoxicated deeds.

From my corner office in the new psychology building at Maastricht University, I looked out over the beautiful hills of Limburg, the most southerly province of the Netherlands, closer to Brussels and Germany than to Amsterdam. Was it true what this man wrote, I thought, that his long history of alcohol addiction that had started at a young age, had turned him into an automaton, that he could no longer decide for himself, and therefore was less accountable? And what was I to make of the fact that he was using my research as his evidence? His alcohol addiction had undoubtedly got him into trouble, and could well have played a role in the crimes for which he had been convicted. By his own account, he had now decided to turn his life around. He was training as an Alcoholics Anonymous (AA) coach, and had taken the initiative to write me a letter. Returning my gaze to the letter still in my hand, I mused, writing this letter is hardly the behavior of an automaton; he appeared to still have some capability to decide left in him after sobriety.

Addiction as chronic brain disease affecting free will

In the last decade of the twentieth century, addiction was defined as a chronic brain disease, in a widely cited article in one of the leading

DOI: 10.4324/9781032634548-1

scientific journals *Science*, with the telling title *Addiction is a Brain Disease and it Mattters.*[1] The piece was written by Alan Leshner, at the time (1997) the director of NIDA (the US National Institute on Drug Abuse), the world's largest addiction research fund.

Not surprisingly, in recent decades, the vast majority of money spent on addiction research went to research aimed at unraveling this "chronic brain disease", and its underlying genetic and neurobiological mechanisms.[2] The idea that addiction is a chronic brain disease was reiterated by Leshner's successor as NIDA director, Nora Volkow, who spoke in public speeches and blogs about the loss of free will in addiction.[3,4] In doing so, she presented the latest scientific findings from neuroscience and combined them with her personal story about her addicted grandfather to conclude that addiction leads to a loss of free will and that awareness of this would reduce the stigma surrounding addiction. While people had long condemned addicted people[i] as morally weak individuals who were themselves to blame for their addiction (the moral model of addiction), the view of addiction as a chronic brain disease should lead to more empathy and decrease in stigma. This should ultimately result in the humane treatment of addicted people instead of exclusion and incarceration.[5]

Most people would likely agree that this is a laudable goal, but the question is to what extent the brain disease view actually led to decreased stigma. As we will see in Chapter 4, research has shown that the notion of a chronic brain disease can sometimes have the opposite effect and lead to *increased* stigma. The idea that addiction is a chronic brain disease also reduces confidence in the possibility of lasting change, among both the addict themselves and the therapist, which has also been found with other mental health problems when they were defined as chronic brain disease, such as depression.[6]

It has also been argued that the notion of addiction as a chronic brain disease has fueled the "War on Drugs", both in the US, where many Americans (particularly African Americans) suffered, and internationally (e.g., the state-sponsored killing of many thousands of addicted people in the Philippines).[7–9] Prisons in the US are disproportionately full of young men of color arrested for addiction-related offenses (in most cases, possession of prohibited substances). This has been related to the difficult conditions in which many youth of color grow up (poor neighborhoods), which is compounded by US laws that punish possession of addictive

i Note that I speak of "addicted people" which is sometimes perceived as stigmatizing and politically incorrect. The reason is that the alternative is to speak of "people who suffer from a substance use disorder or other addictive behavior," which does not improve readability. So please forgive this boorishness.

substances in the form popular among Black youth (*crack*) more severely than when it is in the form popular among the White population (*cocaine*), as Carl Hart has pointed out in papers and books.[10]

Regardless of the potentially negative consequences of the notion that addiction is a chronic brain disease, it may of course be scientifically true. Sometimes the current scientific view has potentially unfavorable social consequences, which in itself is not a good reason to deny it. However, it *is* a good reason to critically consider the evidence. Much research has been done that shows that the brain does indeed change under the influence of addictive substances, and to some extent under the influence of addictive activities, or even more broadly, under the influence of all rewarding and repeated activities. However, changes in the brain by themselves do not say much: when we learn something, our brain changes, as is the case when we fall in love, and may suddenly remember a whisper of a loved one, decades later. The question is the extent to which such changes are unique to addiction and contribute to the maintenance of addiction, as well as the extent to which these adaptations in the brain are still flexible (i.e., can normalize again after a person has successfully recovered from addiction).[11] I summarize the current state of scientific support for the idea that addiction is a chronic brain disease in Chapter 3.

But free will was declared dead, wasn't it?

There is another curious thing about Leshner and Volkow's contention that neuroscience research has conclusively shown that addiction undermines free will, namely that at the same time, the notion of "free will" was declared dead by prominent scholars in philosophy, psychology and neuroscience. Around the same time that Leshner's *Science* article appeared, the late Harvard psychologist Daniel Wegner published a book and related article demonstrating that free will sometimes turns out to be an illusion.[12,13] This idea was based on a series of ingenious experiments. For example, he showed that when something is whispered into a person's ear at the right time, when they perform related actions moments later, they perceive their action as being "self-willed", even though it was actually directed by the whisperer. In the experiment, two participants sat opposite one another, both controlling the same computer mouse: one of these participants was a "real" subject, whereas the other was an accomplice of the researchers. They each wore headphones through which words sounded. On the screen, a variety of objects appeared, and occasionally the participants would click on an object together. When a word was heard in the subject's headphones (e.g., "bucket") and the accomplice then moved the cursor to the bucket and clicked on it, the subject would later report having sent the cursor to the bucket herself, with no awareness of its relation to the word heard or the accomplice's movements. The conclusion was that we apparently infer that we willed something that caused our action if we thought about it shortly before, even in cases where that is demonstrably not true. Hence, free will is an illusion, or in Wegner's words: "the mind's best trick".[13]

One might question the extent to which this sweeping conclusion is justified on the basis of this sort of (rather specific) experiment. For example, while the experiment was ingeniously designed to create the illusion of a connection between what was in the subject's mind (the named object) and an action visible on the screen, normally you don't control a mouse together with someone else—and when you control a mouse alone, you are also much more certain whether or not you did something yourself. In the experiment, subjects reported being 62% sure that they had moved the mouse to the object in question, whereas normally (when you control the mouse alone) this would be close to 100%.[14,15] So the experiment showed that we can fool our sense of control over an action, but it does not prove that this is what normally happens.

In another famous series of experiments, psychologists had shown that people often misjudge the actual predictors of their own choices. For example, when they pick out a pack of cookies and are then asked the reasons for their choice, they invariably mention motives such as price, quality and previous experience rather than other factors like position on the shelf, even though the latter turns out to be the strongest predictor.[16] The authors (Nisbett and Wilson from the University of Michigan) continued the description of the study with one of the finest sentences I have come across in a scientific publication: "And, when asked directly about a possible effect of the position of the article, virtually all subjects denied it, usually with a worried glance at the interviewer suggesting that they felt either that they had misunderstood the question or were dealing with a madman" (p. 244). Their research has shown that when people make everyday choices, they are sometimes influenced by factors of which they are unaware, but the conclusion that we therefore in general only make something up when asked for reasons after the fact is arguably taking things too far. Many of the reasons people come up with in this situation—such as previous positive or negative experiences, or price, may well normally have influenced their choices (there is plenty of evidence for both), but there are also influences that we overlook. This is partly why it makes sense to examine motives in human actions, not only in the lab and in an Agatha Christie whodunnit (and why), but also in justice.[17]

These experiments, and popular science books written about them since, have undermined the belief in free will, at least among the relatively small group of people who read such books and take their message seriously. At the same time, you could also say that the belief in free will still stands proudly in society (I discuss this in Chapter 2). So, on the one hand, an influential movement in psychology and neuroscience has argued that free will is just an illusion and, on the other hand, influential scientists in the field of addiction have argued that free will disappears when a person becomes addicted. Obviously, the two viewpoints are incompatible, because if both are true then the person who gets addicted loses only an illusion![18] And that seems illogical, given the misery addictions cause, for the individual, their immediate environment and for society as a whole: addictions are one of the most common and costly of all mental and brain disorders.[19,20] Hence, there seems to be more going on than just an illusion of losing control.

In addictions, changes take place in the brain that affect the will. Total loss is an extreme outcome, but that the will is influenced is evident and closely related to the early conceptions of addiction in the nineteenth century. The English word "addiction" is derived from the Latin word *addicere*, which meant "to enslave", and represents the idea a person becomes "enslaved" to an addictive substance or habit, apparently losing something we can describe as "will". As explained in Chapter 2, I agree that it makes sense to speak of some degree of "free will" and thus that something could be impaired as someone becomes addicted. At the same time, the loss of free will is not complete, and some capacity for choice typically remains even in severe cases of addiction, as I discuss in Chapter 4. For the vast majority of people with addiction problems, addiction limits, rather than obliterates, freedom of choice (which is always constrained to some extent). And it is an important question to what extent it can grow again after successful abstinence.

My journey to addiction research

Jim, the prisoner writing me a letter, had taken my research as the reason he thought he was an "automaton". In his eyes, my research had shown that he had snorted and drunk away his frontal cortex. This was surprising, as at the time when I received the letter—some twenty years ago—I had conducted psychological research on relatively automatic or implicit processes in addiction (explained later), but I had not yet done any research directly assessing the brains of addicted people, for example by using an electroencephalogram (EEG) or imaging techniques (fMRI). I did get involved in those techniques later, in collaboration with experts in human neuroscience field. After my graduation at the University of Amsterdam, I was hired by Maastricht University, and I was busy setting up new addiction research, combining my old love of questions about conscious and unconscious thought processes and the relationship between brain and mind with the new knowledge I had gained during my PhD studies on risk factors for addiction.

I had been on a long quest to find my niche to study questions concerning the relationship between brain and mind. After high school, I started studying chemistry at the University of Amsterdam, with the goal of discovering how the brain could produce the mind through biochemistry, probably a surprising choice of study with this goal in mind, but I had talked to a number of people about my desire to study the mind and its relation to the brain, and this was what came out of these conversations: in the brain, biochemistry rules—so the advice was to start my studies there. In practice, the biochemistry route was even more indirect than anticipated, as the study of chemistry consisted largely of mathematics and physics, which was based on a similar reasoning: if you want to understand chemistry, you have to understand mathematics and physics. So that was what I did, but I wanted to investigate the mind.

In my first year of college, I became acquainted with a psychology student who lived right above me, in the same dorm. I met her at a house party. She asked me, "who are those folks who were loudly singing along with U2 every so often?" "Ah," I said, slightly embarrassed, "that's me and my mate." U2 had just released the album *The Unforgettable Fire*, and we were belting it out before going out for a run or a party. She laughed and later told me about her studies in *psychonomics*, the more mathematical and neurobiological approach to psychology.[ii] The more I heard, the more it seemed like she did exactly what I wanted to do: study the relationship between brain and behavior. Later that evening, she showed me some of her textbooks, which I could borrow for a while, if I promised to take singing lessons. And maybe I should go talk to some of her psychology professors. I did it all.

One of them was Professor Frijda, an internationally renowned emotion researcher, who was kind enough to speak to this roaming chemistry student. We spoke about the importance of psychological processes, which he felt could not be meaningfully reduced to a description of neural activity or even further to biochemical processes, because what matters in thought is the associated meaning and importance to the individual. Who joined the resistance under the Nazi occupation of the Netherlands, and who collaborated or did nothing? Did I really believe I would find this out by studying biochemistry? It turned out he had hidden as a Jewish teenager during the occupation. He maintained that our relevant decisions are made at

ii I later learned the term was a bit of a pun, stating that psychonomics related to psychology like astronomy to astrology, obviously not considered funny by the rest of psychology.

the psychological level; the rest was implementation of these processes. I was persuaded, and switched to psychology. Several years later, I became his research assistant. One day, I asked him about our meeting years earlier; he couldn't remember that conversation at all! Looking back now as a busy professor myself, I appreciate even more that he took the time to speak with me. His kindness is one of the things I keep in the back of my mind: I try to make time for roaming students with big questions. Some are like me at the time, obsessed with the mind–body problem, most with the effects of marijuana or psychedelics on their mind, brain and life.

It was only later, after my studies in psychology (bachelor's and master's were combined at the time), that I developed an interest in studying addiction. My master's thesis, which was written under supervision of philosopher of science Jaap van Heerden, was about the concept of representation in psychology and neuroscience. It was awarded the Nico Frijda Prize,[iii] for the best psychology thesis, and as a result I was approached by Prof. Sergeant to do a PhD on risk factors in children of alcoholics. At the time, I had virtually no knowledge about addiction, and had not given the subject of children of addicted people any thought. But, after some further consideration … wasn't addiction one of the most concrete instances of the mind–body problem? How was it possible for people to self-destruct and continue with their addiction when the negative consequences were becoming more and more apparent? And what would be the effect of an addicted parent on the ideas and intentions of growing children? I began to get curious.

I read a bit about it, became more interested, and decided to accept the offer to do my PhD research on risk factors for addiction in children of alcoholics. This returns in Chapter 6, including a recent conversation with one of the participants at the time. While I was working on this book, I received an email from a former participant, let's call her Chantal, who had participated in my research some 25 years before, and wanted to have coffee and a chat about the impact of our research on her subsequent life—in particular how she had been affected by the feedback she had received about her enhanced risk for addiction. She had been a participant in the group of children of alcoholics, who were compared with children of parents without an addiction problem, and her parents had received personalized feedback about her development, which they shared with her in a brief summary: watch out with alcohol and other substances, or you'll be just like your mom. What had this warning done to her?

iii Named after Prof. Frijda following his retirement.

Unconscious processes in addiction

But my PhD research is not what Jim (the prisoner) was referring to when he wrote to me—instead he wrote about a new line of research that I had started after I had joined the faculty at Maastricht University's new school of psychology and neuroscience. In one of our first studies in this new direction, we had shown that students who drank heavily had strong *negative* associations with alcohol, which did not differ from their more moderately drinking peers. This was a surprise! If they had strong negative associations, much stronger than their positive associations, why did they drink so much? It was so surprising that we checked the results several times before submitting the article for publication.

We found that the same students did differ in their associations between alcohol and arousal: these were significantly stronger than those of light drinkers.[21,22] Their alcohol associations were measured with a reaction time task, a variant of the Implicit Association Test (IAT), originally developed by Tony Greenwald and colleagues[23] from the University of Washington, that we had adapted to measure alcohol associations. Participants were asked to categorize words that appeared in the center of a computer screen as quickly as possible to the left or right, using two buttons (see Figure 1.1). Heavy drinkers, like light drinkers, were much faster in their responses when alcohol and negative words shared the same response key (as did soft drinks and positive words) than when alcohol and positive words shared the same response key (as did soft drinks and negative words). This was interpreted as an indication of relatively strong negative alcohol associations. In contrast, only the heavy drinkers sorted alcohol words more quickly when combined with "active" words[iv] (e.g., "energetic," "lively," and "funny"), than with "passive" words ("sleepy," "quiet"). And that pattern was related to the amount of alcohol they consumed.

We had decided to measure alcohol associations in two dimensions, the same as those that had also emerged as the two most general dimensions in emotion research: valence (positive-negative) and arousal (active-passive). Note that since these findings, there has been much discussion about the precise interpretation of the results obtained with variants of the IAT,[24–26] and most researchers now agree that these associations should not be regarded as unconscious and that it is better to speak instead of automatically activated associations.[27,28]

Prisoner Jim had concluded, based on this and related research by Alan Stacy into automatic alcohol associations,[29,30] that addicted people

iv We used "active" in Dutch, as there is no word for "arousal" without a sexual connotation.

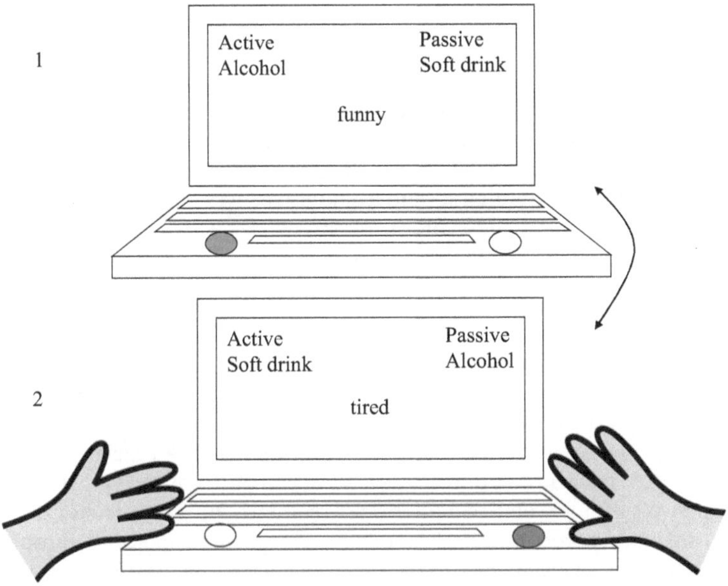

Figure 1.1 An example of the Implicit Association Test (IAT) applied to alcohol and the "active" dimension (active versus passive). In one combination stage (1), participants' task is to sort alcohol words (e.g., "beer") with active words, using one response key (here the left button) and soft drink words (e.g., "coke") with passive words (using the right button). In another combination phase (2), soft drink words are combined with active words (left button) and alcohol with passive words (right button). When a person is faster with one of the combinations it is interpreted as an association between the concepts involved (here, alcohol-active), which was found in heavier drinkers only.

can only react like automatons when confronted with their drug of choice. That was clearly an exaggerated conclusion, since we had reported *relatively* strong associations between alcohol and arousal in heavy drinking students who were otherwise still functioning well, not in people suffering from alcoholism. And in these students, the amount they drank was predicted to some extent by these relatively automatic associations, but to a larger extent by their motives for drinking, measured using a questionnaire. For example, those who drink to a greater extent to have fun or temporarily forget about their problems drank more. While our research and that of others indeed could be interpreted to indicate that some psychological processes involved in addiction could be set in motion automatically, it would be a major leap (or two) to conclude from this study that addicted people no longer have free will. That might be true if these alcohol-associations inevitably determined behavior, but there is no evidence for that. Indeed, some of Carl Hart's research from the same era has shown that even severely addicted people can refuse their drug of choice if they want to, in order to choose an alternative reward, such as a meal voucher.[31] Note that there are influential addiction researchers who argue that addictive behavior becomes automatic and compulsive over time,[32,33] but that conclusion has come under fire in recent years.[34] I discuss the current state of support for this theory in Chapter 4.

Quitting with AA

Letter writer Jim further referred to his training as an AA coach. Alcoholics Anonymous (AA) is a successful worldwide movement with its origins and center of gravity in the US. Its central aim is to change the lives of people suffering from alcoholism for the good. A crucial element in the AA method is to recognize that you are powerless over the addictive substance and therefore must renounce drinking alcohol once and for all,[35] a perspective close to that of the contemporary "chronic brain disease", which comes to the same conclusion that abstinence is the only way to deal with the chronic disease, which does not fit the epidemiological data, as we will see in Chapter 4: most people who meet criteria for an alcohol use disorder at some point in their lives reduce or stop without formal help.[36,37]

AA's historical roots can be traced back to the nineteenth-century *temperance movement*, which from Christian conviction strove to moderate alcohol consumption—especially spirits—and from the end of the nineteenth century advocated for complete prohibition.[38] The temperance movement was an emancipatory movement that sought to offer workers an alternative to the pub, where many turned in their meager wages right after receipt—resulting in immense poverty for the depending families. Cynically, the pub was often owned by the employer, creating a means to reclaim employees' wages right after they had been paid out. Many English towns still have a Temperance Hall, the nineteenth-century alternative sober place for celebration or relaxation after work.[39]

AA was founded in 1935 by Bill Wilson and Robert Smith ("Dr. Bob"). At that time, alcohol addiction was still often seen as a moral failing. People who became addicted were thought to have weak character, a lack of spirituality and a weakly developed conscience—based on the Puritan idea that one chooses whether or not to sin.[38] Until the eighteenth century, excessive drinking was considered a habitual sin (intemperance): a person who drank a lot and was often drunk apparently liked liquor very much and was therefore responsible for the excess, reasoning in line with what was later called the moral model of addiction. In the late eighteenth century, the disease concept of (alcohol) addiction was introduced by the influential medical professor Benjamin Rush, one of the signers of the Declaration of Independence and close friend of second president John Adams. He described several cases of "drunkards" who had lost control over their drinking and described alcoholism as a disease of the will, quoting a chronic drunkard: "Were a keg of rum in one corner of a room, and were a cannon constantly discharging balls between me and it, I could not refrain from passing before that cannon, in order to get at the rum." The chronic drunkard could be saved only by total abstinence, the essence of the disease model of addiction.[38] Tragically, after describing addiction as a progressive disease, one of his own sons was plagued with addiction and mental health issues, as described in a captivating recent book by Carl Eric Fisher on the (American) history of addiction.[40]

Bill Wilson suffered from a severe alcohol problem and attended meetings of the Christian Oxford Group, a society that emerged from the *temperance movement* in the 1920s and aimed to help people overcome their alcohol addiction. The Oxford Group's mottoes capture the essence: all people are sinners; all sinners can change; confession is a prerequisite for change; the changed person has direct access to God; miracles are possible and the changed person must help others change.[41] Wilson initially felt helped by the Oxford Group meetings, yet this did not prevent him from relapsing several times. This pattern was broken only when he was convinced of the need for total abstinence, or teetotalism, by Dr. Bob, a recovered member of the Oxford Group himself. Wilson had been treated by a doctor who was convinced that alcohol addiction was a disease and that the addict's ego had to be broken down before it could be rebuilt—the basis of the confrontational addiction treatment that was dominant well into the last century. Furthermore, Wilson received the then-popular Belladonna treatment, which involved administering hallucinogenic substances, an approach which has seen renewed recent popularity as alternative medication for addiction and other mental health problems,[42] that may have contributed to his sensations. Whether under the influence or not, Wilson reported to have literally seen the light and ecstatically experienced a new serenity in which he was able to renounce alcohol once and for all. The notion that alcoholism and other addictions are a spiritual disease has remained at the core of the AA movement and related therapeutic interventions, and is also important in contemporary approaches to recovery that emphasize that recovery is not only about reducing or completely stopping alcohol or drug use, but also about improving mental health, social functioning and well-being.[37]

Wilson and Dr. Bob joined forces and developed the twelve-step program to help people overcome their alcohol addiction. Many of the Oxford Group's principles remained intact: spiritual surrender was a prerequisite for recovery, clients acknowledge their powerlessness and surrender to a higher power. Unlike the Oxford Group, however, this was more freely interpreted than the Christian God only: you direct your prayers to whichever higher power or God is relevant to you. Previous sins were to be confessed and those who had suffered as a result were to be asked for forgiveness and compensated, as far as possible. Another original core idea is still characteristic of AA's approach: that part of recovery involves volunteer work to help other people overcome their addiction. This has contributed to the success of the organization characterized by motivated volunteers. Wilson and Smith tried to get money for the further development of their movement and payment for AA helpers from the businessman and philanthropist John Rockefeller, but he refused because paying AA helpers could destroy the volunteer-based core of the movement, which indeed proved to be one of its great strengths.

The AA model combines features of the moral model of addiction (which involves sins that must be confessed and repaired) with the model of chronic illness: alcohol has become stronger than you, you always remain vulnerable for relapse, and therefore total abstinence is the only remedy. This combination goes back to the common source, Benjamin Rush's disease model.[38] However, the effectiveness of treatment based on the AA principles is subject to debate, as we will see in Chapter 7.

Akrasia

The final topic of this introduction concerns that ancient Greek word in this book's subtitle: *akrasia*. This is a concept from Greek philosophy that goes back to Socrates. Plato, in his book *Protagoras*, wrote about his teacher Socrates, who left no writings of his own. In this dialogue, among other things, he describes Socrates asking whether someone who is convinced that a certain action is the best thing to do can do something else. Socrates believed that this *not* to be the case, as we will see in Chapter 2: man cannot act against one's own judgement. In other words, when people do something, the reasons for doing this must have been stronger than the reasons against doing this, at the moment of acting. Hence, at the lunch counter, when you take a slice of pepperoni pizza instead of a salad, even though you resolved to lose weight and to reduce meat consumption, you must have had stronger reasons to take the pizza at that moment, otherwise it would be a case of *akrasia*. Same thing when you order a nice glass of wine at a restaurant, even though you resolved to not drink alcohol anymore on weekdays.

It should come as no surprise that there is a relationship between the concept of *akrasia* and addiction: maybe you take the wine because you have an overwhelming craving for it, when you see it on another table, or when you just imagine drinking a glass. Maybe you're just a social drinker who likes to drink wine with a nice meal. If you view the choice to drink alcohol as rational behavior, even in alcohol addiction, you logically come to the conclusion that the drinker apparently really likes alcohol and is willing to accept the negative consequences, in line with the moral model and descriptions of addictive behaviors before the eighteenth century.[38] The alternative is that addiction is a disease that has impaired the will, so that the drinker can no longer make rational choices and can therefore be held less responsible for choosing to drink again. In that case *akrasia* is real and a manifestation of a (brain) disease, chronic or not.

These questions go back to the classics, when the concept of *akrasia* was coined. Even further back in history, Homer describes how Odysseus figured out a way to achieve ecstasy without perishing from it, in this case from the singing of the Sirens, demi-goddesses with beautiful voices long before YouTube. This was an irresistible lure that led to the downfall of those who became enchanted by it. Warned by the witch of Circe, Odysseus took accurate precautions: he instructed his crew to tie him to the mast of his ship and to block their ears with beeswax. He further ordered them to ignore his orders as long as the singing continued and the Sirens were still in sight. In this way, Odysseus could enjoy the sirens' divine temptations without succumbing to them. Nowadays, in the spirit of Odysseus, some young people try to enjoy new psychoactive substances while minimizing the associated risks. Cultural anthropologist Anita Hardon investigated these practices in her project *Chemical Youth*, diving with her team into the youth culture of experimenting with new substances. She described how, during an experimentation session, the group was well organized, including a "designated driver" role of one of the team members, who stayed sober to be able to call emergency services if necessary.[43]

In Chapter 2, I address the philosophical and psychological questions surrounding *akrasia*: can we do things we don't want to, when we've gone over all the arguments? And if we appear to do things that we don't want to, does that mean that we actually (unconsciously) wanted to do those things anyway? Or does that notion take us back to untestable Freudian notions, that fueled behaviorism in the history of psychology? And what are we to think of free will in times when it has been declared dead by influential scholars? And how does that relate to addiction?

In Chapter 3, I summarize the current biomedical story of addiction as a chronic brain disease. This is followed by criticisms of that biomedical account (Chapter 4), and then in Chapter 5 by a synthesis that boils down to my current view that addiction implies biased or compromised choice, which is fundamentally different from the view that there is no more choice left because of a chronic brain disease, as well as from the view that choice in addiction is like choice in any other domain, and therefore the addicted person is immoral or has a weak character. Chapter 6 examines the development of addiction versus resilience: what we can learn from people who develop in a healthy way despite adversities. This leads to questions about the current ideas on the best ways to promote resilience and healthy development. The next two chapters deal with treating addictions: Chapter 7 on traditional treatments (medication and psychotherapy) and Chapter 8 on new treatment methods that aim to directly target decision making in addiction.

In Chapter 9, I broaden the perspective to other putative addictions, such as those to meat, sex, smartphones and fossil fuels, to the extent that these can be called addictions. If not addictions, they are at least *akrasia* problems that affect us all; we as a species are in danger of going down and taking many other species with us. For example, most people know that it is better, both for our own health and for the future of the earth, to eat little or no meat, and yet the smell of grilled chicken is almost irresistible. Most people know that it is bad for the environment to fly, and yet again we stand in long lines at our local airport to go enjoy our well-deserved vacation. Perhaps we can draw general conclusions and learn lessons about the pressing *akrasia* problems that characterize our time. I give my start to this in Chapter 10.

This book can be seen as a somewhat belated response to prisoner Jim. I had to ponder on the answer first.

References

1. Leshner AI. Addiction is a brain disease, and it matters. Sci New Ser. 1997;278:45–7.
2. Hall W, Carter A, Forlini C. The brain disease model of addiction: Is it supported by the evidence and has it delivered on its promises? The Lancet Psychiatry [Internet]. 2015;2:105–10. Available from: http://dx.doi.org/10.1016/S2215-0366(14)00126-6
3. Volkow ND, Koob GF, McLellan AT. Neurobiologic advances from the brain disease model of addiction. N Engl J Med [Internet]. 2016;374:363–71. Available from: www.nejm.org/doi/10.1056/NEJMra1511480
4. Volkow ND. Addiction is a disease of free will [Internet]. National Institute on Drug Abuse Blog. 2015. Available from: www.drugabuse.gov/about-nida/noras-blog/2015/06/addiction-disease-free-will
5. Heather N, Segal G. Understanding addiction: Donald Davidson and the problem of akrasia. Addict Res Theory. 2013;21:445–52.
6. Barnett AI, Hall W, Fry CL, Dilkes-Frayne E, Carter A. Drug and alcohol treatment providers' views about the disease model of addiction and its impact on clinical practice: a systematic review. Drug Alcohol Rev. 2018; 37:697–720.

7. Hart CL. Viewing addiction as a brain disease promotes social injustice. Nat Hum Behav [Internet]. 2017;1:1. Available from: http://dx.doi.org/10.1038/s41562-017-0055
8. Hart CL, Hart MZ. Opioid crisis: another mechanism used to perpetuate American racism. Cult Divers Ethn Minor Psychol. 2019;25:6–11.
9. Hart CL. Exaggerating harmful drug effects on the brain is killing Black people. Neuron [Internet]. 2020;107:215–8. Available from: https://doi.org/10.1016/j.neuron.2020.06.019
10. Hart CL. High price: drugs, neuroscience and discovering myself. London: Penguin; 2013.
11. Heather N, Best D, Kawalek A, Field M, Lewis M, Rotgers F, et al. Challenging the brain disease model of addiction: European launch of the addiction theory network. Addict Res Theory [Internet]. 2018;26:249–55. Available from: https://doi.org/10.1080/16066359.2017.1399659
12. Wegner DM, Wheatley T. Apparent mental causation: sources of the experience of will. Am Psychol. 1999;54:480–92.
13. Wegner DM. The mind's best trick: how we experience free will. Trends Cogn Sci. 2003;7:65–9.
14. Asma L. Mijn intenties en ik. Filosofie van de vrije wil. Amsterdam: Boom; 2021.
15. Shepherd J. Scientific challenges to free will and moral responsibility. Philos Compass.
16. Nisbett RE, Wilson TD. Telling more than we can know: verbal reports on mental processes. Psychol Rev. 1977;84:231–59.
17. Sandis C. Verbal reports and "real" reasons: confabulation and conflation. Ethical Theory Moral Pract. 2015;18:267–80.
18. Wiers RW, Field M, Stacy AW. Passion's slave? In: Sher KJ, editor. The Oxford handbook of substance use and substance use disorders [Internet]. Oxford: Oxford University Press; 2014. pp. 311–50. Available from: http://oxfordhandbooks.com/view/10.1093/oxfordhb/9780199381678.001.0001/oxfordhb-9780199381678-e-009
19. Effertz T, Mann K. The burden and cost of disorders of the brain in Europe with the inclusion of harmful alcohol use and nicotine addiction. Eur Neuropsychopharmacol [Internet]. 2013;23:742–8. Available from: http://dx.doi.org/10.1016/j.euroneuro.2012.07.010
20. World Health Organization (WHO). Global status report on alcohol and health 2018. World Health Organization; 2019.
21. Wiers RW, Van Woerden N, Smulders FTY, De Jong PJ. Implicit and explicit alcohol-related cognitions in heavy and light drinkers. J Abnorm Psychol [Internet]. 2002 [cited 2013 Mar 12];111:648–58. Available from: http://doi.apa.org/getdoi.cfm?doi=10.1037/0021-843X.111.4.648
22. Houben K, Wiers RW. Assessing implicit alcohol associations with the Implicit Association Test: fact or artifact? Addict Behav [Internet]. 2006 [cited 2013 Mar 28];31:1346–62. Available from: www.sciencedirect.com/science/article/pii/S0306460305002674
23. Greenwald AG, Mcghee DE, Schwartz JLK. Measuring individual differences in implicit cognition: the Implicit Association Test. J Pers Soc Psychol. 1998;74:1464–80.
24. Rothermund K, Wentura D. Underlying processes in the implicit association test: dissociating salience from associations. J Exp Psychol Gen. 2004;133:139–65.

25. De Houwer J, Geldof T, De Bruycker E. The implicit association test as a general measure of similarity. Can J Exp Psychol. 2005;59:228–39.
26. Greenwald AG, Poehlman TA, Uhlmann EL, Banaji MR. Understanding and using the Implicit Association Test: III. Meta-analysis of predictive validity. J Pers Soc Psychol. 2009;97:17–41.
27. Gawronski B, Hofmann W, Wilbur CJ. Are "implicit" attitudes unconscious? Conscious Cogn. 2006;15:485–99.
28. Wiers RW, Gladwin TE. Reflective and impulsive processes in addiction and the role of motivation. In: R Deutsch, B Gawronski, W Hofmann (Eds.), Reflective and impulsive determinants of human behavior. Abingdon: Routledge; 2016. pp. 173–88.
29. Stacy AW. Memory activation and expectancy as prospective predictors of alcohol and marijuana use. J Abnorm Psychol. 1997;106:61–73.
30. Wiers RW, Stacy AW, Ames SL, Noll J a, Sayette M a, Zack M, et al. Implicit and explicit alcohol-related cognitions. Alcohol Clin Exp Res [Internet]. 2002;26:129–37. Available from: www.ncbi.nlm.nih.gov/pubmed/11821663
31. Hart CL, Haney M, Foltin RW, Fischman MW. Alternative reinforcers differentially modify cocaine self-administration by humans. Behav Pharmacol. 2000;11:87–91.
32. Everitt BJ, Robbins TW. Neural systems of reinforcement for drug addiction: from actions to habits to compulsion. Nat Neurosci. 2005;8:1481–9.
33. Everitt BJ, Robbins TW. Drug addiction: updating actions to habits to compulsions ten years on. Annu Rev Psychol [Internet]. 2016;67: 150807174122003. Available from: www.annualreviews.org/doi/abs/10.1146/annurev-psych-122414-033457
34. Hogarth L. Addiction is driven by excessive goal-directed drug choice under negative affect: translational critique of habit and compulsion theory. Neuropsychopharmacol. 2020;45:720–35. Available from: http://dx.doi.org/10.1038/s41386-020-0600-8
35. What A.A. owes to its antecedents. Markings. [Internet]. 2004. Available from: www.aa.org/newsletters/en_US/f-151-markings_mar-april04.pdf
36. Heyman GM. Addiction: a disorder of choice. Harvard University Press; 2010.
37. Tucker JA, Chandler SD, Witkiewitz K. Epidemiology of recovery from alcohol use disorder. Alcohol Res Curr Rev. 2020;40.
38. Levine HG. The discovery of addiction: changing conceptions of habitual drunkenness in America. J Stud Alcohol. 1978;39:143–74.
39. In our time podcast. Temperance movement. [Internet]. Available from: www.bbc.co.uk/sounds/play/m0013zl8
40. Fisher CE. The urge. Our history of addiction. London: Penguin; 2022.
41. History of Alcoholics Anonymous. Wikipedia. 2021. [Internet]. Available from: https://en.wikipedia.org/wiki/History_of_Alcoholics_Anonymous
42. Bogenschutz MP, Ross S, Bhatt S, Baron T, Forcehimes AA, Laska E, et al. Percentage of heavy drinking days following psilocybin-assisted psychotherapy vs placebo in the treatment of adult patients with alcohol use disorder: a randomized clinical trial. 2023;10016.
43. Hardon A. Chemical youth: navigating uncertainty in search of the good life. Springer Nature; 2021.

2 *Akrasia*, free will and addiction

As already briefly introduced, *akrasia* is a concept from classical Greek philosophy that stands for acting against one's better judgment. Plato first describes it in a dialogue between the sophist Protagoras and Socrates. The dialogue starts with a discussion on the origins of virtue. Protagoras was a wise man who taught moral lessons and was even paid for doing so, which was unusual in the Greek classical world. Socrates asked him in his characteristic "Socratic" way whether virtue can be taught. That, according to Protagoras, was certainly the case and the reason why we raise children. Just as it makes no sense to ask who taught them Greek, it also makes no sense to ask from whom they learned to do good, because that is what we all teach together. It also took a village to raise a child in the ancient world. At some point the state would take over the education and punish criminals, for example, to set a good example, so that others could learn from it and not do the same.

Socrates disagreed with this and argued that the origins of virtue are innate. He questioned Protagoras whether virtue should be seen as a single entity, or whether it involves multiple aspects, that could be taught separately. Protagoras argued for the latter, with virtue being like a face consisting of different parts with different functions, which together form a whole. As the discussion continued, they came to the conclusion that positive qualities like courage and wisdom are somewhat different from sheer goodness, because sometimes you have to do something painful or dangerous to achieve the good and sometimes you have to refrain from something pleasant to do good. Sometimes you have to go to war to achieve the good, which may result in sacrificing your life. Or you should not drink too much of the delicious wine when you have to teach the next day or have a discussion with Socrates. Thus, virtues like courage and wisdom are not only about what brings about the most pleasant feelings *now*, but also about future consequences.

DOI: 10.4324/9781032634548-2

According to Socrates, man naturally knows what is good or bad without having to be taught. This idea was also at the root of his Socratic method: with his interrogations, he aimed to uncover universal truths. On this account, the only reason someone can do evil is ignorance of the negative consequences; once those become apparent, any person will choose to do the good. In contrast, Protagoras, and later Aristotle, both emphasized that virtue must be learned and that people are fallible when it comes to making wise choices.

Akrasia and addiction

The central issue of *akrasia* is whether you can do anything other than what you think is best to do, once you have carefully considered and weighed all the consequences. In the Bible, Paul wrote in his letters that sometimes he did not understand his own actions: in such cases he did not do what he wanted, but rather exactly what he did *not* want.[1] Thus, Paul was describing suffering from *akrasia*, exactly what happens to many of us when we snack on junk food in the evening, while we are on a diet. Or when we have another beer, when we had resolved to take it easy tonight in order to wake up fresh tomorrow. Why do we succumb to such temptations so easily? And isn't it obvious that at such times there is *akrasia*? If not with bad habits such as snacking, then surely with addictions?

Every adult smoker knows that smoking greatly increases the risk of fatal diseases, and many are aware of the fact that about half of smokers die from smoking-related illnesses. Assuming that the smoker, like other people, would prefer to live a long and happy life, it appears to be plain irrational to smoke, hence smoking must be an example of *akrasia*. In fact, most current smokers wish to quit.[2] However, upon further prompting … maybe not right now, but some other time soon, when they are less busy or stressed.[i] Importantly, from the *akrasia* perspective, what ultimately matter in decision making are the *considerations of the smoker at the time the decision is made*. How does the smoker weigh the long-term health information versus expected short-term benefits, which may outweigh the long-term disadvantages, even if these include an increased risk of disease and death? Long-term health effects involve probabilities (which are notoriously difficult for people who do not specialize in statistics),[3] while perceived positive effects such as

i To illustrate this, consider a big online smoking cessation study we did, where over 2,000 smokers signed up for free help with a smoking cessation method. A research assistant phoned them all, to check that they were ready to start a quit attempt with the program *in the next couple of weeks*—and at that point, over 75% of the participants dropped out of the study.[86]

sociability or relaxation are within reach. So, the decision to smoke might reflect an internal trade-off, in which the expected short-term benefits at the moment of lighting the cigarette outweigh the long-term health consequences—in which case smoking would fall short of constituting *akrasia*. To count as a true case of *akrasia*, the successful ex-smoker (to rule out withdrawal effects on the decision-making process), should, *after having carefully weighed all the pros and cons and having come to the conclusion that it is much better to refrain from smoking*, subsequently light up a cigarette. Is that possible?

Let's make the example concrete. Martin, a smoker friend, regularly throws parties at his home with his wife Janet. He loves making music and jamming with his guests, which creates the special atmosphere of a unique shared experience. At the end of one such special evening, Martin is offered a cigarette by two old friends with whom he sits outside, in the courtyard garden he has just renovated. It's a beautiful evening; this is what he did it all for, this long and tiresome renovation: sitting outside with friends on a summer evening and chatting some more after the conversation in music. Want a cigarette? Martin is aware of the alternative—politely decline, since he's quit for a year—and also of the fact that this alternative is better for his health, for his relationship (Janet has also quit successfully, his daughter has asthma), for his reputation (many friends have admired him over the past year because of his successful quit attempt), and he knows he can say "no" just fine (he's done so many times). He also spots an alternative: a carrot on a tray with a bowl of hummus next to it. He can hold that in his hand like a cigarette, as if he's smoking. And yet … the cigarette lures, the pungent smell of burning tobacco. A sense of unease scratches at the door. The cheerfully smiling friends, smoking in their cool way, as they used to do together when they were young, without worries about the future. If Martin now takes the cigarette and smokes it, it could be an example of *akrasia*. The next day, or maybe that very night, he would tell himself and his wife: how could I have been so stupid? I accepted the cigarette, knowing I do not want to smoke anymore, knowing what I was doing!

First- and second-order desires and dual process models

Conceptually similar solutions to this problem have been found in philosophy on the one hand and in psychology and neuroscience on the other. In philosophy, Harry Frankfurt, a Princeton emeritus professor and one of the most influential American philosophers of the twentieth century,[ii] argued that it is important to distinguish

ii also known outside the field of philosophy for his bestseller *Bullsh!t*.

between first- and second-order desires, which can contradict each other.[1] A first-order desire is directly linked to an action; it involves the lure of the cigarette whispering: "Smoke me!" Second-order desires are about *what we would like to desire* (and thus indirectly about what we would like to do). While a lion eats an antelope because he's hungry and it's been caught, we can decide to not eat meat anymore, out of animal welfare considerations or as a small contribution to prevent climate change. Hence, second-order desires are linked to ideas about the future and to one's values—in the case of Martin, to ideals about finally renouncing the cigarette because of his own health and that of his daughter. Perhaps his self-image also plays a role: he has now proven that he is someone who is stronger than his impulses. The tricky thing, of course, is that the context (two old friends at the end of a uniting party) activates yet another self-ideal: that of Martin as a social guy who is socializing with his friends like in the good old days, after a couple of beers—an image accompanied by an increased attraction to smoking.[4] The question is which force prevails here: the primary desire to smoke the cigarette, activated by the smell of burning tobacco, reinforced by the activated goal of renewed social *bonding* and perhaps having a moment's indifference to the rest of the world and all of its responsibilities—what matters is the here and now with friends—or the second-order desires related to the will to be a good and sensible man, good for his future self and for his family, stronger than his addiction.

Similar ideas have been developed in psychology and neuroscience in the form of so-called dual process models. These assume that our behavior is guided by both impulsive and reflective processes and their interplay.[iii] These models have become widely known through the work of the recently deceased Nobel prize winner Daniel Kahneman.[5,6] According to dual process models, impulsive or associative processes are evolutionarily old and operate quickly and often unconsciously, while reflective processes originated later in evolution, operate slowly with limited capacity, but allow for further thinking about the future. Much of our behavior can be controlled "on autopilot", but when that mechanism bogs down, we need to bring our attention to it. Sometimes you don't realize that the autopilot is sending you in the wrong direction. That is what happens in cases of misconceptions or cognitive biases that were investigated by Daniel Kahneman and his late colleague Amos Tversky. To illustrate,

iii Different theorists have labelled the different processes differently, e.g., Type 1 and Type 2; reflexive and reflective, with roughly similar distinctions (for a review, see Smith and DeCoster).[87] I will use impulsive and reflective, following the influential dual process models by German psychologists Strack and Deutsch.[88]

consider the following, simple riddle: "A baseball bat and a ball together cost $11. The bat costs $10 more than the ball—how much does the ball cost?"[iv] This riddle demonstrates how we tend to jump to conclusions, when the answer seems obvious, based on automatically activated associations, built on previous experience. However, once we realize that simple process has led us astray, we can reflect further to find the right answer.

The dual process models of Kahneman and other scientists involve a general description of human thought processes to explain our behavior. With my American colleague Alan Stacy, I applied this thinking to addiction, to which the inmate letter writer Jim from the introduction referred.[7,8] According to dual process models of addiction, the impulsive processes become stronger as addiction develops, while the reflective processes lose their grip on the impulse to use, even when there are good reasons to stop.[8–11] This can lead to *akrasia*: while the addicted person knows that it is better not to use (anymore), he continues to use anyway, driven by impulsive processes (or first-order desires).

Dual process models in psychology correspond conceptually to models from neuroscience, where specific neural structures or circuits are associated with these processes.[9,12–15] One influential model developed by Rita Goldstein from the Mount Sinai School of Medicine in New York and Nora Volkow from NIDA, emphasizes two important factors. First, abnormal salience attribution in addiction refers to the idea that addiction-related cues become very salient, while everyday motivating stimuli become less salient. Second, impaired inhibition refers to the idea that the temptation created by these (salient) cues to addiction becomes more difficult to resist. We will revisit this model and the underlying brain changes in the next chapter. Neuroscientific dual process models often distinguish between subcortical circuits, with evolutionarily ancient structures such as the amygdala and the *striatum*, containing the *nucleus accumbens* that is important in addiction. A neural circuit in which these structures play a major role responds strongly to signals announcing a possible reward. The impulse activated thereby to perform the associated action (e.g., accept and light the cigarette), must then be restrained by an evolutionarily more recent circuit, from the familiar frontal cortex, as inmate Jim already referred to. This model resembles MacLean's old model from the 1960s that is still often cited in popular science. The bottom line is that deep in our brains, there is a "reptilian brain", which must be kept in check by the more recently evolved mammalian brain containing the capacity for

iv The solution that immediately comes to people's minds is $1, but it's actually $0.50 (and the bat is $10.50).

impulse control. This simple model has a lot of appeal, but is wrong. Neuroscience has since clearly demonstrated that the human brain is a highly integrated system in which no separate "reptilian brain" can be distinguished.[16,17] Hence, popular simplistic versions of dual process models are outdated, but modern varieties of these models distinguish different integrated brain networks and then the interaction between these networks gets impaired in addiction.[18]

Another problem of this type of model is that it does not explain where the reflective system (the "mammalian brain") derives its wisdom from and how the decision is made to opt for a short-term reward versus a long-term benefit.[19] As my mentor Nico Frijda pointed out in the preface to my first popular science book on addiction,[20] there is a homunculus in the statement that the reflective system keeps the impulsive system in check. How does the decision process work in the reflective system? Is there another reflective system in there who makes the smart decisions (think of the Russian dolls in which there is always a smaller doll)? This leads to an ever-repeating question, or a homunculus problem.

The idea of impulsive processes that must be kept in check by a rational system is intuitively appealing and goes back to classical antiquity (the discussions of *akrasia*) and to medieval descriptions of struggles between passion and reason.[21] Basing ourselves on those ancient mythological images, some colleagues and I depicted the struggle as that of a rider having to restrain a wild horse, with the wild horse representing the impulsive processes enhanced by addiction and the rider representing the weakened reflective processes.[20,22] While the model may be helpful in explaining addiction to people dealing with it, we have to acknowledge that scientifically it is an over-simplification.[16,19,23] Just because we can experience an inner struggle in situations like the one Martin faces after his party, does not mean that this is an accurate representation of what is happening in the brain. In Chapter 5, I discuss the current view of the neurocognitive processes underlying such internal struggle.

Free will and addiction

What can we say about free will in relation to addiction? As noted in the introduction, the term "addiction" incorporates lack of freedom: the addict has enslaved himself to the drug, how can this come about? According to dual process models, it happens through changes in the brain that reinforce impulsive or automatic responses to the drug and weaken reflective processes (focused on long-term interests);[20] which could be described as a gradual loss of free will.[20,24] But in order to lose something, you must first have something, and had free will not been declared dead by influential psychologists and neuroscientists? What is left of free will after the various subversions from psychology and neuroscience in recent years?

Let us first establish what we mean by free will. Contemporary philosopher Lieke Asma, in her recent book *My Intentions and Me*, arrives at the following definition: *free will is the ability to act for a reason.*[25] Those reasons operate at the level of the person—hence the title. By making decisions and performing actions, we influence the person we are and want to be. In doing so, an image of the future and of the person we would like to be is important (an idea that we will return to when we talk about change). This is also the basis of our justice system: for example, someone who has consciously planned a crime is punished more severely than one who does the exact same thing without consciousness, for example, in a reflex or while sleepwalking.[26]

In recent years, many influential books have appeared arguing that free will does not exist and is merely an illusion, for example those by Sam Harris,[28] Dan Wegner[29] and Dick Swaab.[30],[v] They adhere to variants of the philosophical position described as "hard determinism". According to this view, our behavior is determined by our brain, which is a physical system that, like other physical systems, is fully determined by nature's laws. From that idea, it is not logically possible that a person, given the state of the brain at the time, could have done anything other than what he or she was doing at the time. The brain does provide a subjective sense of free will, but in reality that is necessarily an illusion.[28,29]

One of the most influential studies that cast doubt on the widely held idea that our conscious considerations determine our behavior is that of UCSF neurophysiologist Benjamin Libet from the 1980s. He showed that brain activity can consistently be observed before a person makes a conscious decision.[31] His research contributed greatly to the notion that people are driven by unconscious brain processes when making decisions and that they make up stories afterwards to explain their behaviors (so called confabulations[32]). Libet gave his participants were given a simple task: "Make a finger movement at a self-selected time." Meanwhile, their brain activity was measured and they watched a clock, allowing them to pinpoint exactly when they made their decision to move. This was about 150 milliseconds before the visible movement. Crucially, systematic brain activity (the so-called readiness potential) could be observed about a second earlier, which could be related to the impending decision. This was interpreted as evidence that the conscious consideration itself could not be

v As one proofreader noted: all white men! Would they have particular problems with free will?

the cause of the behavior: the brain would have already reached a decision before the person in question had consciously made a decision.[28,33,34]

These Libet-type experiments were very influential in the neuroscience-based claims that free will does not exist, but have since been challenged on several grounds.[25,26,35] First, one can question the setup of the specific experiment. For example, the instruction to make a spontaneous movement is paradoxical—if the movement is instructed and planned, it can't be spontaneous—so one can question to what extent such an experimental setup can tell us anything about decision-making in real life.[36,37] A related argument is that free will is not tested at all in these experiments: in fact, it is not the person who decides that the subject should make a certain movement at a given moment, but the experimenter who designed the task.[25,38] As we saw, in everyday life, free will refers to actions that are done for reasons, related to one's wishes, desires, moral beliefs, anticipated consequences of the act, and so on. In the Libet experiment, the participant is instructed to act spontaneously at a certain moment, with a very restricted repertoire (a finger tap). In later varieties, "free won't" experiments,[vi] the participant is further asked to subsequently inhibit the urge to move on about half of the occasions, *without pre-planning*. In this experimental setup, the normal reasons to act or to refrain from acting are all excluded. Compare this with the real world, where I would normally grab a cup of coffee in the morning (because I like drinking coffee at breakfast) or refrain from drinking coffee in the afternoon (because I found out doing so has a negative impact on my sleep later). By contrast, in the Libet-type experiments all that is left of "free will" is acting on a "spontaneous urge" that is instructed by the experimenter: in everyday life, most people do not spontaneously experience any urge to start tapping their fingers, without appropriate background music. Hence, these experiments are about "spontaneous urges" in a very specific unnatural context and therefore tell us little about the effects of free will (as understood in everyday life as reasoned action) on behaviour.[38]

A second line of argument is more methodological in nature: in the original analysis of Libet and later scientists in this line of research, the assumption is that the brain signal ("readiness potential") that is observed prior to the movement and before the moment people are aware of their decision to act, is *the cause* of the action. However, recent research has undermined this assumption.[37,39,40] Aaron Schurger, working in Paris with the famous consciousness researcher Stanislas Dehaene has demonstrated that, when you calculate back from a moment of action, a *readiness*

vi I was involved in one of those "free won't" experiments in healthy volunteers, where we also tested to what extent drinking alcohol would influence the processes involved (both the neural correlates and the subjective decision; neither was confirmed).[89]

potential can be seen, by definition, based on reaching a threshold in a complex system with spontaneous fluctuations. As an analogy, when the buildup of electricity in a cloud exceeds a certain threshold and a discharge occurs "spontaneously" in the form of lightning.[41] But just as the readiness potential of a cloud does not reflect a decision by a cloud to discharge at that moment and send a lightning bolt to earth, the readiness potential of the brain does not reflect the decision of the participant in the experiment to move *at that specific moment.*

The researchers based their conclusion on a series of ingenious experiments in which subjects were given a simple task: they had to look at dots moving randomly on a screen and indicate when these were moving in one direction. Some of the participants could skip the current trial when a dot on the screen changed color, while others could decide themselves to skip a trial.[37,40] Under both conditions, a readiness potential could be calculated by counting backward from the time the task was skipped. Yet an interesting difference was observed: in the people who decided to skip the trial themselves, a unique brain signal could be observed that distinguished the internally generated decision to *skip* from the externally indicated skip of the task, and this was observed about 150 milliseconds before the action and thus coincided with the conscious decision. Thus, the idea that the brain has already made a decision before one is aware of it oneself appears to be an artifact of the method used to provide the readiness potential.[37,39,40] Thus, contrary to the claims of many psychologists and neuroscientists, the Libet experiment did not prove that the brain has already decided before our conscious considerations come into play, nor does it prove the non-existence of free will.

About the same time as Libet's experiment, brain researcher Michael Gazzaniga wrote about research with so-called *split-brain patients.*[32] In a number of patients with severe epilepsy, the connection between the brain hemispheres had been surgically severed, with the aim to protect them from the spread of epileptic seizures to other brain regions. These patients were put into a special research setup, in which both hemispheres received different information: the left field of view (which connects to the right hemisphere) was shown different information than the right field of view (connected to the left hemisphere, where language resides in most people). For example, the left hemisphere of the brain saw a chicken claw and the right hemisphere saw a snowy landscape. Then the participant had to choose a picture that matched the images seen. The left hand (controlled by the right hemisphere that had seen the snowy landscape) chose a shovel. When asked to explain this choice, the participant indicated that a shovel was useful for cleaning the chicken run. In short, the linguistic left hemisphere used the information available to it (the chicken claw, and the fact that a shovel had been selected) and tried to come up with a logical explanation for that choice, while the real explanation (a shovel to shovel away snow) was unavailable. From such experiments, Gazzaniga concluded that our linguistic consciousness constantly confabulates, or makes up an explanation after the fact to explain our behavior.[42,43] This system gives rise to the feeling of living in a single subjective reality, while behind the scenes all sorts of automatic processes determine behavior. As the psychologist Daniel Wegner so eloquently put it in his book on the illusion of the will: just as a compass does not steer a boat, consciousness does not guide man's actions.[29]

What this kind of research has shown is that our self-reports about reasons behind our decisions are not always correct, as was also evident from the classical research by Nisbett and Wilson on everyday decision making in the supermarket, which we encountered in the introduction. As elegant and surprising as such experiments often are, they do not logically lead to the conclusion that our stories about why we do what we do are *always* incorrect, that we are just making up reasons after the fact to explain our unconscious choices. As one of the authors of the original article on in-store choices remarked a few years later, "If we're so dumb, how come we made it to the moon?"[44] In other words, why should evolution have provided a complex and high energy-demanding system by which we can communicate, reason and decide, if it only brings us an illusion, and no way to influence behavior with long-term goals in mind?[45]

In alternative models that are currently important in cognitive neuroscience, the brain is primarily focused on constantly predicting the immediate future: "whatever's next", as Andy Clark summarized this basic function of our brain.[46] Thereby, the idea is that this prediction machine does influence behavior and thus does not just provide an interpretation after the fact in automatically directed behavior. When we can imagine the consequences of an action, and also of an alternative action, there is something to choose from. I will return to this in Chapter 5.

Philosophical views on free will and determinism

There are three broad views of free will currently distinguished in philosophy. The first is hard determinism, which boils down to the idea that free will is an illusion because the feeling of possessing free will stems from the brain—a physical system in which the state of that system is in principle entirely predictable from background (genes, environment and experience) and thus also the "output" of the system, including the so-called free choice (and the illusion that that choice was free).[28] "We are our brains", as the Dutch neuroscientist Dick Swaab put it. The problem here is that our subjective experiences take place at a different level of description than the world of neurons and neurotransmitters and cannot be reduced to this level (the so-called "hard problem": the relationship between mind and brain).

There are different issues with this position. First, not all physical systems are deterministic: chaos theory has shown that complex systems are fundamentally unpredictable, because minimal differences in initial values can lead to completely different outcomes proverbial butterfly in Brazil that could cause a hurricane in Texas.[47] Complex systems are networks of interconnected elements that exhibit emergent behavior. Importantly, this cannot be fully understood by studying the elements in isolation, as the emergent behavior depends on nonlinear dynamics, feedback loops and self-organization. Although complex systems such as the human brain cannot be understood in a deterministic way, this does not prove free will, it merely emphasizes the impossibility of a deterministic prediction of behavior, based on the state of the brain measured at a given time, if that were even possible, let alone make predictions on the slightly longer term. But based on long-term unpredictability alone, we cannot attribute free will to the brain, or to weather systems for that matter.

The other extreme in the spectrum of thinking about free will is the so-called "libertarian position", which assumes free will. Historically, this position has often been linked to dualism: the brain obeys the physical laws of this world, while the mind operates in a different dimension. The classic problem with this position, going back to Descartes, is how the mind should then affect the material world (from which it is separate). The essence of the libertarian position is that we do have complete control over our actions, or—to quote Sartre—that we are "condemned to freedom",[45] but this makes subjective experience and perceived will very difficult to link to the brain or other physical systems. A recent variant of libertarianism argues that quantum uncertainty leaves room for free will, but it is not clear why principled unpredictability at the level of elementary particles should lead to free will or to free action.[28]

The third position is so-called "compatibilism", which holds that our behavior and choices are determined by our (material) brains, while at the same time there is some degree of conscious choice and free will. This view is defended in contemporary philosophy by Daniel Dennett among others,[48,49] with historical roots going back to Hume and Hobbes.[50] How does compatibilism unite these two seemingly mutually exclusive positions, determinism and free will?

According to compatibilists, we have little or no control over our thoughts, but some degree of control over our actions. This premise is consistent with ideas that are also important in cognitive behavioral therapy: people sometimes fear thoughts (e.g., I sometimes feel an urge to jump in front of a train when I see one coming), or sometimes feel ashamed of thoughts (e.g., I secretly love my teacher). The therapist will teach the client that there is no reason to be ashamed of your thoughts, as long as you have control over your actions: it is what you do that matters, not what you think. As Hume stated, "By freedom, then, we can understand only the power to do, or not to do, an act according to the decision of the will; that is, if we choose to remain inactive, we do so, and if we choose to proceed to action, we can do so. Well, this hypothetical freedom possesses, by common sense, everyone who is not a prisoner in chains.[50–53] The idea that our perceived freedom is only an illusion, produced by deterministic brains, is poorly reconciled with the strong motivation people experience to counter perceived restrictions on freedom, whether actual restrictions on freedom or the idea of being manipulated.[45] Of course a hard determinist can reason this away as the product of a deterministic brain.

Regarding the relationship between determinism and free will, Lieke Asma, inspired by the British analytic philosopher Elisabeth Anscombe, makes an important observation: determinism is focused on explaining how things happened (a look at the past), while free will is future-oriented. Free will is related to images of possible futures and the expected consequences of intentional actions. Why did Lee Harvey Oswald shoot John F. Kennedy? We can look back to his childhood, his character, the time shortly before the assassination, how he got into crime, etc. You could write many books about it and create plenty of movies as well, all working toward that one fatal moment in an attempt at arriving at a deterministic story. In contrast, zooming in on the choice he had at the time of the shooting, involves considerations that could have influenced the action at the time. Oswald could have imagined a scenario in which he hits, escapes and is rewarded (or not punished, if he acted under threat as some have argued). Perhaps he could have also envisioned a scenario in which he would be caught by the police after his deed, and later sentenced to death. He could also have chosen to *not fire* or to deliberately misfire, perhaps imagining scenarios featuring those who threatened him, likely a variety a death penalty). Free will involves looking forward and the imagined effects of our behavior, determinism involves explanations of how someone got somewhere.

Ultimately, issues of determinism and free will revolve around the hypothetical question of whether or not someone with exactly the same genetic background and learning history would always do the same thing in exactly the same circumstances. The determinist will answer this with a resounding yes, the libertarian with an equally resounding no. The compatibilist will probably come up with a "sometimes yes" or "mostly no" answer: free will has evolved to influence our choices with our forward-looking imagination, but we must have the time and take the time to do so.

Free will, imagination and working memory

In my opinion, what free will is all about is being able to be aware in the moment of the consequences of one choice (e.g., accepting the cigarette) and of the other choice (politely thanking and persisting in not smoking). People have the ability to do this, described by the term "working memory", which allows them to keep information active so that it can be used in thought processes.[54] Working memory develops in childhood and forms the basis of our ability to reason. It is strongly related to intelligence, control of attention and being able to exercise self-control, or influencing your own behavior in accordance with your goals.[55–57] This ability is often seen as one of the distinguishing characteristics of humans from other animals,[45] which explains why it now appears strange to us to take animals to court, while this was done in the Middle Ages, for example, when a horse had run wild that led to an accident.[58] In humans, the capacity for self-control is something that develops and in which individual differences can be found, which have proven to be good predictors of a happy, healthy and successful later life, as we will see in Chapter 6.

Language and imagination are important factors in human development, something the Israeli historian Yuval Harari writes convincingly about in his widely read books *Homo Sapiens* and *Homo Deus*.[59,60] He argues that humans have been able to develop their all-powerful (if not overly powerful) role on earth because of language and imagination, which allow us to influence many more people than those immediately around us and to build on each other's knowledge (see also Henrich's *the secret of our success*[61]). Whereas chimpanzees and early human species could only cooperate in groups of up to about a hundred individuals whom they knew personally and could trust, in humans that ability has been greatly expanded with the help of our imagination. As a result, we can work with thousands of people to build a pyramid, cathedral, or with billions to fall under the spell of a game like soccer. Based on a system of shared ideas, we could travel to the moon, as well as enslave animals (the vast majority of all other mammals are now our slaves).

This same powerful imagination can also be used to influence our own behavior, for example, by imagining a different life, for example a life without drugs. This is an important ingredient in psychotherapy, especially in a technique called "motivational interviewing", which will be discussed in Chapter 7. Since this type of therapy helps at least some people change their addictive behavior, it seems clear that our ability to imagine the future indeed influences our behavior. The ability to make a choice between different options, which moreover we can imagine the consequences of, is a psychological reality created in our brain.

Rats and people with imagination

One of the founders of cognitive psychology was American psychologist Edward Tolman. He had been trained in early twentieth century behaviorism, the dominant movement in psychology in the US at the time, which aimed to create an objective psychology, by refraining from speculating about processes in the "black box" between stimulus and response. A stimulus elicits a response if it has been rewarded in the past, and so a whole series of behaviors can be elicited. According to behaviorism, a rat in a maze should take a certain path only if it leads to a reward. What Tolman observed, however, was that the rats would also explore a maze without any reward. This turned out to be advantageous if a reward could be obtained later or a punishment could be avoided (for example, provoked by fox scent): they had created a mental map of the maze and therefore could immediately find the fastest way out.

Things got even wilder (from the behaviorist perspective): Tolman put rats on a platform from which they could jump down into one of two rooms: one with a white door and one with a dark door. Behind one of the doors, say the dark one, there was always a reward to be found. Once the rat had jumped to a given door and found out whether or not it hid the reward, it could not return to its starting platform—and had to wait to be returned by the experimenter. Tolman described that the rats sometimes paused on the starting platform and looked back and forth for a while before taking a leap towards one of the doors, as if they were weighing their options before taking a decision. What reinforced that impression was the finding that this looking back and forth was actually predictive of the animal's learning rate. Rats that looked back and forth more quickly learned which type of door to jump to for the reward more readily.

This observation was initially ridiculed by behaviorists (Tolman's rat would remain deep in thought, sitting on the platform in the pose of Rodin's thinker), but eventually formed one of the pillars of the "cognitive revolution" in psychology.[52,62] This centered on the idea that humans and many animals actively map their surroundings, creating "mental maps" of the environment, which help to predict future events. Recent neuroscience research has made it plausible that Tolman was right, and that the rats actively saw a simulation of the consequences of the two choice options as they looked back and forth.[52,63] Based on these simulations, the rat chose the optimal choice that would or would not lead to a reward, and so the laboratory animal learned behind which door the reward was to be found. Apparently, not only humans have imagination that helps them choose, but so do rats.

This is the essence of conscious choice: being able to imagine different outcomes and making a choice based on them. Denying this reality because the brain itself conforms to the laws of physics is, in the words of philosopher Daniel Dennett, similar to denying the existence of everyday concepts such as colors, promises, countries or money.[64] These exist at the level of psychology and are influenced by culture. Of course, on some level, a $100 bill is nothing more than a piece of paper: a toddler or a dog can look at it that way and shred or eat it. But to anyone with an awareness of economic significance, the real value of the bill is clear. These are agreements between people, with real-world consequences (people are being shot for those "pieces of paper"). That cannot be explained if you do not include the psychological meaning of those "pieces of paper". Hence, the psychological meaning cannot be reduced to the neurological (or atomic) level, because then the meaning is lost, just like the value of a shredded banknote, in line with Nico Frijda's argument that convinced me to switch studies from chemistry to psychology.

Beliefs and desires (psychological concepts) are important tools for describing and predicting behavior of others and of ourselves, and they cannot be meaningfully reduced to brain processes, although they derive from them. You can make a comparison to driving a car. When you take driving lessons, you learn the functions of the accelerator and brake pedals and how to operate them optimally in a complex environment. You don't learn how fuel is converted into forward power by the engine; for that you have to study automotive engineering, which is not relevant to driving a car. That knowledge only becomes relevant when your car breaks down and you need to venture inside the engine to see what's going on. As long as you are driving, it is more important to have an idea of what other road users are possibly planning to do. Is that car in front of me suddenly slowing down because an exit is coming up? Or is something else going on? We cannot navigate socially without having ideas about the beliefs and desires of others, which is therefore an important psychological reality.[65]

My choice

This image of choosing based on simulations brings me back to the difficult choice I faced in quitting chemistry. I had passed the first year with flying colors, and fellow students and the student advisor declared me crazy when I considered switching to another study, especially to something vague like philosophy or psychology. Trading a study that would provide a secure job for one that would surely lead to unemployment! I cycled at night along Amsterdam's beautiful canals, constantly wondering which course of action would be best, and looking back, I see myself now back as the little rat on Tolman's platform: should I jump left or right? Embark on the unknown adventure, which I could not yet properly imagine, or continue on the path that I could better estimate and which had so far been rather disappointing? Meanwhile, I had also become intrigued by the question of how you actually make such a choice, which may have contributed to the switch.

When I look back on this choice, I still have a strong memory of the difficult process of making such a drastic choice. How rational was my consideration? What if I had not met that nice and clever psychology student studying *psychonomics*, but had met a floaty type representing psychology? What if Prof. Frijda had not taken the time to speak to a searching chemistry student? I will be the last to claim that we choose only on rational grounds, but at the same time I am convinced that we can choose when we can imagine the consequences of different choices. How we imagine the future is something in which we are influenced by our personal history and upbringing.

Tolman came from an evangelical Christian family in which pacifism was seen as of great value. He developed into an opponent of the First World War and then (and perhaps partly because of it) was independent enough to oppose the dominant scientific stream in his field: behaviorism. Our learning history influences what we see in our simulations of the consequences of our possible choices, on the basis of which we choose and act (more in Chapter 5). Furthermore, there are factors that influence the extent to which we are able to imagine the consequences of different choices when comparing people with each other (related to differences in working memory capacity), but also within a person: if you are tired and tipsy, you will be less able to imagine all the possible consequences of your actions. But within those limitations, we can choose.

The usefulness of conscious thought

What does consciousness add to our thinking and decision making? There is both a theoretical evolutionary argument and an empirical argument that conscious thought can influences behavior. The evolutionary explanation is that conscious thought costs us a lot of energy and therefore it is extremely unlikely that it would have evolved if it did not bring benefits.[55,56] An important benefit attributed to conscious thought and imagination is the integration of information. Our brains are made up of a variety of evolutionarily formed modules with specific functions, such as quickly detecting danger, food or a possible mate. Different modules can signal opposite courses of action, for example, when one module indicates that we should flee while another indicates that we should go after a *once-in-a-lifetime opportunity* of ultimate sex. "Houston, we have a problem", as is said, as we have only a single body to act with and cannot split ourselves, with one part of our body fleeing while another part chases the rare opportunity. Therefore, there must be a common language in which the subsystems can communicate and come to a solution. Contemporary neuroscientist Ezequiel Morsella argued that this internal communication between brain modules is at the heart of consciousness.[66] Precisely because we must come to a decision as an integrated organism, there had to be an internal language for the different parts of the brain to communicate with each other. The brain integrates all input into a picture, and creates a simulation of the expected state that will result from an action. And when we are aware of a choice, there is also another picture of the possible future, and like Tolman's rat, we look from left to right before jumping.

Consciousness has many aspects, and this might be mainly the function of a fairly basic form of consciousness that we share with many other animals. But in humans (and probably to some extent in some other species) conscious thought has expanded further and we can weigh pros and cons against each other and reason about possible consequences of a choice, and sometimes perhaps, like Socrates, reason our opponent into a corner. Here, language—and therefore culture—plays an important role, and this in turn has had a great influence on the evolutionary success of humans.[55,56] Of course, this success also has a negative downside, manifested, for example, in the climate crisis caused by our unbridled growth and domination of other species. This is where the so-called "Fermi paradox" is relevant, named after the Italian physicist Enrico Fermi, Nobel Prize winner and part of Oppenheimer's secret Project Y in the Second World War, which led to the development of the atomic bomb. The Fermi paradox concerns the question of why we still have not found other intelligent life in the universe, even though it is likely that there are billions of planets where conditions allow the emergence of life. One of the possible answers is that life did arise in many places, but it is doomed to self-destruct: when one species begins to dominate the others to such an extent that the balance is upset, life destroys itself again. Hopefully this resolution of the paradox is not predictive of life on Earth, although the omens of an irreversible point in climate change are alarming, as the international IPCC reports have shown (about which more in Chapter 9).[67] Thus, given the unprecedented dominance of humans over other species and the role of language and thought in this, it is extremely unlikely that there is no effect of conscious thought on our actions, for better or for worse.

An influential theory of how consciousness works is the *global workspace theory*.[68,69] This relates to Morsella's aforementioned idea that the primary function of consciousness is that of a common language, allowing different brain processes to influence each other. This allows for a flexible response and for a response to be tailored to the context. Language plays a crucial role here; research has shown that the meaning of a single word can have an unconscious effect on behavior, but when it comes to more than a single word, consciousness is required for an effect.[70]

The language we use to communicate with others is internalized in our thought language—an idea that dates back to Russian developmental psychologist Vygotsky.[71] The global workspace provides coherence and alignment of various brain processes and allows us to reason about issues beyond the here and now. This can relate to the possible consequences of one's own actions, but also to further questions, such as those concerning the origin of everything or about life after death. Without language there would be no myths, religions, philosophy or meaning of life. Nor education: we are the only species that directly instructs our offspring through education, which is part of "the secret of our success".[27,56,61]

Contemporary psychologist Roy Baumeister and colleagues have summarized all the psychological research examining the added value of conscious thought.[27] First, it is important to define what is meant by consciousness. At least two levels should be distinguished: a basic level of being awake and aware of your surroundings, which we share with many animals and is distinct from when we are asleep or in a coma. The second level is about conscious reasoning, which is especially developed in humans and has a lot to do with free will: it involves control over our actions based on reasons. Like: I take an umbrella with me because I heard it might rain this afternoon and I don't want to get wet.

The studies summarized by Baumeister and his team focus on how the second form of consciousness (including reasoning) influences behavior. In a typical experiment in this line of research, participants are randomly divided into two groups, where participants have to solve a decision task, while in one group conscious reasoning is interfered with, for example by having to count down from 1000 in multiples of 3, a task that severely hinders other conscious thought (try it!). The results are then compared with the group that performed the same task without this interfering countback task. Over many studies, a better result was found in the group that was not hindered in reasoning about a decision to be made. In other studies, imagination of a possible future was explicitly called upon. For example, participants in one group had to imagine that they continued going to therapy for four weeks, while the other group did not. People in the first group stayed in therapy longer on average.[72]

The bottom line is that the evidence that we can intentionally influence our behavior is empirically strong: it is supported by a wealth of studies, and the effects are strongest for the indirect effects, on later behavior rather than on the choice at the moment. When you make people think about what they could have done better in a given situation, they typically indeed do better the next time. This is especially true of the influence of emotions on behavior: if we have regrets, we are more likely not to do the thing we regret again.[73] Research has shown that playing an alternative scenario plays a crucial role in this.[27]

We can conclude that thinking about what we could have done differently is useful, while recognizing that it can also lead to psychological problems. If thoughts about what you could or should have done differently keep recurring (so called ruminations), it may result in depressive symptoms. Hence, from the present perspective, that is an unfortunate consequence of a psychological function that normally has a positive effect: you get stuck thinking about what you could have done differently. This is in line with the functional view of emotions by scientists like Nico Frijda[74] and with evolutionary theories about the relationship between emotions and psychological problems.[75] The general idea is that emotions are useful, in the sense that they have evolutionary value. Being afraid is useful in general, and even negative feelings can be useful because they can signal to you that you need to change course. But this useful mechanism can also lead to problems, when, for example, you keep fretting about something you can no longer change.

The conclusion of Baumeister and colleagues in their systematic review was that there is a lot of convincing research indicating that consciously thinking about a problem has an effect, albeit mostly on optimizing future decisions. But didn't the Dutch psychologist Ap Dijksterhuis and colleagues show that people make better decisions when they cannot think, in an influential Science paper?[76] They had participants make decisions in complex situations—for example, about whether or not to buy a house or car—and reported that the decisions turned out better in a condition in which thinking was hindered because the participants had to simultaneous perform another task designed to hinder conscious thought (again counting backwards in threes).[76,77] The first question with such counterintuitive research findings is how replicable the effect actually is: is it really the case that people make better decisions when they cannot think? The conclusion in a recent publication that summarized all previous research (a meta-analysis) is that the effect likely does not exist, which was supported by a large-scale study to replicate the effect in different labs that yielded no support.[78]

This doubt about the reality of spectacular counterintuitive findings is not isolated. In the aftermath of the Stapel affair,[vii] much psychological research was critically tested for replicability and, shamefully, often not replicated.[79] This is not to say that the results of such research were fabricated (à la Stapel), but rather that the findings proved to be unreliable, for example, because they were found in a small study, while other larger studies that did not confirm the effect were not published. This is not only a problem in psychology, but plays at least as strongly in medical research (where the stakes are often even higher),[80] and even the aforementioned meta-analyses are not immune from this problem.[81]

Thus, the counterintuitive conclusion that conscious thought only affects decisions negatively is in all likelihood incorrect, which is not to say that conscious thought always has only positive effects. For example, there is research that shows that consciously thinking about an action has a positive effect in novice athletes, but can actually have a negative effect in more experienced athletes.[27] When you have too much time to think about your next great stroke, as a tennis player, it can lead to an incomprehensible miss (*been there, done that*). This points to the functional role of conscious thought in learning *new* behavior. Once the behavior has been automated (e.g., driving a car), unconscious processes drive the behavior and your awareness can focus on something else, such as a conversation with a fellow passenger or strategy in the match. But when unexpected circumstances cause problems (the road is blocked off), consciousness is necessary to come up with a solution and you break off a conversation with a fellow passenger for a while. Conveniently, a passenger also sees what is going on and therefore typically stops talking for a moment, when routine driving is interrupted by something unexpected, which is not the case when the other person is on the phone, which is therefore more dangerous.[82]

All in all, then, there is every reason to believe that the "naive assumption" that we can use our conscious thinking and reasoning to influence our behavior,[83] is actually true: our consciousness allows us to imagine things and learn based on experiences of others, with our culture influencing our thinking and actions. We can also use this ability in choices relevant to addiction: is Martin going to accept that cigarette because of the pleasant feeling he thinks he will get from it at that moment (*bonding* with his old friends), fueled by the smell of burning tobacco, or is he going to turn down the cigarette because he has sworn

vii Diederik Stapel was a professor of social psychology at Tilburg University and a successful researcher until he was accused of fraud, which he confessed after a while. The case rocked international psychology and helped lead to the *open science* and replication movement in psychology.

off smoking for all sorts of good reasons, and wants to maintain his new self-image as an ex-smoker?

Therapy that helps people overcome addictions will emphasize the long-term positive effects of quitting. In doing so, it can help to paint that alternative picture as clearly and in as much detail as possible, as we will see in Chapter 7. Once this alternative goal is clear enough, you can devise ways (or help someone do so) to achieve that goal. That's why it makes sense to treat addiction. And that is why it makes sense to talk about a conscious influence on our behavior, sometimes perhaps a bit too loosely called "free" will. In doing so, I acknowledge on the one hand that the influence of the will on our behavior is limited—as research has shown, and mostly indirect affecting future choice—but on the other hand, I therefore do not go along with the claim that free will is just an illusion.

Following authors of a chapter in an edited book on free will,[84] I prefer to compare positions on free will to different forms of boating. We subjectively *experience* free will as if we were driving a motorboat: we feel that we can turn the rudder completely without much effort to control our behavior. This is consistent with the "naive" idea of free will that we always fully consciously direct our choices—but this view turns out to be false, as research has shown (e.g., decision making in the supermarket). At the other extreme, if the hard determinists are right, we are on a raft with a mast on which only a wind vane flutters. Floating along on the current of unconscious processes, we think the vane sets the course and make up all sorts of reasons why we are going in a certain direction. This picture doesn't seem to fit reality either: much research shows that we can indeed influence our choices with our conscious thinking and reasoning. The compatibility view can instead be compared to sailing: we can set sail for something (a goal in mind), but we cannot always steer straight to it. However, we can learn to sail better in order to reach our goals, even when they are located against the wind. In this metaphor, parenting is helping your children better master sailing techniques, and we all do that, as Protagoras said: just as children learn Greek from everyone. We teach children to pursue long-term goals and control impulses that go against them, for example, with everyday games.[85]

By now, the conclusion of this chapter will come as no surprise: a form of free will does exist, even if we cannot always influence our behavior with it as directly as we sometimes think. This indicates that indeed, there is something to lose in terms of steering power, for example, due to brain trauma or a progressive chronic brain disease such as Alzheimer's. Therefore, the thesis that addiction is a chronic brain disease that affects the will is a meaningful one. For this reason, this book does not end after this chapter. In the next chapter, we will look at the substantiation of this thesis.

References

1. Heather N, Segal G. Understanding addiction: Donald Davidson and the problem of akrasia. Addict Res Theory. 2013;21:445–52.
2. Babb S, Malarcher A, Schauer G, Asman K, Jamal A. Quitting smoking among adults—United States, 2000–2015. Morb Mortal Wkly Rep. 2017; 65:1457–64.
3. Nisbett RE, Fong GT, Lehman DR, Cheng PW. Teaching reasoning. Science (80–). 1987;238:625–31.
4. Steele CM, Josephs RA. Alcohol myopia: its prized and dangerous effects. Am Psychol. 1990;45:921–33.
5. Kahneman D. A perspective on judgment and choice: mapping bounded rationality. Am Psychol. 2003;58:697–720.
6. Kahneman D. Thinking, fast and slow. NY: Macmillan; 2011.
7. Wiers RW, Stacy AW. Handbook of implicit cognition and addiction. In RW Wiers, AW Stacy (Eds.). Handbook of implicit cognition and addiction. Thousand Oaks: SAGE; 2006.
8. Wiers RW, Stacy AW. Implicit cognition and addiction. Curr Dir Psychol Sci [Internet]. 2006;15:292–6. Available from: http://cdp.sagepub.com/lookup/doi/10.1111/j.1467-8721.2006.00455.x
9. Bechara A. Decision making, impulse control and loss of willpower to resist drugs: a neurocognitive perspective. Nat Neurosci. 2005;8:1458–63.
10. Wiers RW, Bartholow BD, van den Wildenberg E, Thush C, Engels RCME, Sher KJ, et al. Automatic and controlled processes and the development of addictive behaviors in adolescents: a review and a model. Pharmacol Biochem Behav [Internet]. 2007 [cited 2013 Feb 28];86:263–83. Available from: www.ncbi.nlm.nih.gov/pubmed/17116324
11. Stacy AW, Wiers RW. Implicit cognition and addiction: a tool for explaining paradoxical behavior. Annu Rev Clin Psychol [Internet]. 2010 [cited 2013 Mar 13];6:551–75. Available from: www.pubmedcentral.nih.gov/articlerender.fcgi?artid=3423976&tool=pmcentrez&rendertype=abstract
12. Volkow ND, Fowler JS, Wang GJ. The addicted human brain viewed in the light of imaging studies: Brain circuits and treatment strategies. Neuropharmacology. 2004;47:3–13.
13. Heatherton TF, Wagner DD. Cognitive neuroscience of self-regulation failure. Trends Cogn Sci [Internet]. 2011;15:132–9. Available from: http://dx.doi.org/10.1016/j.tics.2010.12.005
14. Goldstein RZ, Volkow ND. Drug addiction and its underlying neurobiological basis: Neuroimaging evidence for the involvement of the frontal cortex. Am J Psychiatry. 2002;159:1642–52.
15. Goldstein RZ, Volkow ND. Dysfunction of the prefrontal cortex in addiction: neuroimaging findings and clinical implications. Nat Rev Neurosci. 2011;12:652–69.
16. Cesario J, Johnson DJ, Eisthen HL. Your brain is not an onion with a tiny reptile inside. Curr Dir Psychol Sci. 2020;29:255–60.
17. Cobb M. The idea of the brain: a history. London: Profile Books; 2020.
18. Zilverstand A, Huang AS, Alia-Klein N, Goldstein RZ. Neuroimaging impaired response inhibition and salience attribution in human drug addiction: a systematic review. Neuron [Internet]. 2018;98:886–903. Available from: https://doi.org/10.1016/j.neuron.2018.03.048
19. Gladwin TE, Figner B, Crone EA, Wiers RW. Addiction, adolescence, and the integration of control and motivation. Dev Cogn Neurosci [Internet]. 2011 [cited 2013 Feb 28];1:364–76. Available from: www.ncbi.nlm.nih.gov/pubmed/22436562

20. Wiers RW. Slaaf van het onbewuste. Over emotie, bewustzijn en verslaving. Amsterdam: Bert Bakker; 2007.
21. Hofmann W, Friese M, Strack F. Impulse and self-control from a dual-systems perspective. Perspect Psychol Sci [Internet]. 2009;4:1–15. Available from: http://research.chicagobooth.edu/cdr/docs/DualSystemsPerspective-Hofmann.pdf%5Cnpapers3://publication/uuid/9F1AABF1-D1F1-4022-80CC-177184AC822F
22. Friese M, Hofmann W, Wiers RW. On taming horses and strengthening riders: recent developments in research on interventions to improve self-control in health behaviors. Self and Identity 2011;10:336–51.
23. Wiers RW, Gladwin TE. Reflective and impulsive processes in addiction and the role of motivation. In: R Deutsch, B Gawronski, W Hofmann (Eds.). Reflective and impulsive determinants of human behavior. Abingdon, UK: Routledge; 2016. pp. 173–88.
24. Volkow ND. Addiction is a disease of free will [Internet]. National Institute on Drug Abuse Blog. 2015. Available from: www.drugabuse.gov/about-nida/noras-blog/2015/06/addiction-disease-free-will
25. Asma L. Mijn intenties en ik. Filosofie van de vrije wil. Amsterdam: Boom; 2021.
26. Levy N. Consciousness and moral responsibility. Oxford: Oxford University Press; 2014.
27. Baumeister RF, Masicampo EJ, Vohs KD. Do conscious thoughts cause behavior? Annu Rev Psychol. 2011;62:331–61.
28. Harris S. Free will. Simon and Schuster; 2012.
29. Wegner DM. The illusion of conscious will. Cambridge, MA: MIT Press; 2003.
30. Swaab D. We are our brains: from the womb to Alzheimer's. London: Penguin Random House; 2015.
31. Libet B. Unconscious cerebral initiative and the role of conscious will in the initiation of action. Behav Brain Sci. 1985;8:529–66.
32. Gazzaniga MS. Forty-five years of split-brain research and still going strong. Nat Rev Neurosci. 2005;6:653–9.
33. Swaab D. Wij zijn ons brein: van baarmoeder tot Alzheimer. Amsterdam: Atlas Contact; 2010.
34. Lamme V. De vrije wil bestaat niet. Amsterdam: Prometheus; 2011.
35. Mele AR. Effective intentions: the power of conscious will. Oxford University Press; 2009.
36. Nachev P, Hacker P. The neural antecedents to voluntary action: a conceptual analysis. Cogn Neurosci [Internet]. 2014;5:193–208. Available from: http://dx.doi.org/10.1080/17588928.2014.934215
37. Khalighinejad N, Schurger A, Desantis A, Zmigrod L, Haggard P. Precursor processes of human self-initiated action. Neuroimage [Internet]. 2018;165:35–47. Available from: https://doi.org/10.1016/j.neuroimage.2017.09.057
38. Asma L. There is no "Free won't". J Conscious Stud. 2017;24:8–23.
39. Schurger A, Sitt JD, Dehaene S. An accumulator model for spontaneous neural activity prior to self-initiated movement. Proc Natl Acad Sci U S A. 2012;109:2904–13.
40. Travers E, Khalighinejad N, Schurger A, Haggard P. Do readiness potentials happen all the time? Neuroimage [Internet]. 2020;206:116286. Available from: https://doi.org/10.1016/j.neuroimage.2019.116286
41. Gholipour B. A famous argument against free will has been debunked. The Atlantic. 2019. Available from: www.theatlantic.com/health/archive/2019/09/free-will-bereitschaftspotential/597736/

42. Gazzaniga MS. Cerebral specialization and interhemispheric communication. Does the corpus callosum enable the human condition? Brain. 2000;123:1293–326.
43. Roser M, Gazzaniga MS. Automatic brains—interpretive minds. Curr Dir Psychol Sci. 2004;13:56–9.
44. Nisbett RE, Ross L. Human inference: strategies and shortcomings of social judgment. Englewood Cliffs (NJ): Prentice-Hall; 1980.
45. Baumeister RF. Free will in scientific psychology. Perspect Psychol Sci. 2008;3:14–9.
46. Clark A. Whatever next? Predictive brains, situated agents, and the future of cognitive science. Behav Brain Sci. 2013;36:181–204.
47. Butterfly effect. Wikipedia. Available from: https://en.wikipedia.org/wiki/Butterfly_effect
48. Dennett DC. From bacteria to Bach and back: the evolution of minds. WW Norton & Company; 2017.
49. Dennett DC. Consciousness explained. New York: Little Brown; 1991.
50. Oomen P. vrije wil en determinisme Een verkenning met een open einde. In: Vrije wil—een hersenkronkel? zoetermeer, NL: Klement; 2013. pp. 117–40.
51. Seth A. Being you. The new science of unconsciousness. London: Penguin; 2020.
52. Pennartz C. De code van het bewustzijn. Amsterdam: Prometheus; 2021.
53. Hume D, Millican PF. An enquiry concerning human understanding. Oxford: Oxford University Press, 2007. Oxford: Oxford University Press.
54. Spencer JP. The development of working memory. Curr Dir Psychol Sci. 2020;29:545–53.
55. MacDonald KB. Effortful control, explicit processing, and the regulation of human evolved predispositions. Psychol Rev. 2008;115:1012–31.
56. Baumeister RF, Masicampo EJ. Conscious thought is for facilitating social and cultural interactions: how mental simulations serve the animal—culture interface. Psychol Rev. 2010;117:945–71.
57. Burgoyne AP, Engle RW. Attention control: a cornerstone of higher-order cognition. Curr Dir Psychol Sci. 2020. Available from: www.animalsandsociety.org/wp-content/uploads/2015/10/beirnes.pdf
58. Beirnes P. The law is an ass: reading E.P. Evans' The Medieval Prosecution and Capital Punishment of Animals. Soc Anim. 1994;2:27–46.
59. Harari YN. Sapiens: a brief history of humankind. Random House; 2014.
60. Harari YN. Homo deus: a brief history of tomorrow. Random House; 2016.
61. Henrich J. The secret of our success: how culture is driving human evolution, domesticating our species, and making us smarter. Princeton, NJ.: Princeton University Press; 2016.
62. Gardner H. The mind's new science: A history of the cognitive revolution. NY: Basic books; 1987.
63. Johnson A, Redish AD. Neural ensembles in CA3 transiently encode paths forward of the animal at a decision point. J Neurosci. 2007;27:12176–89.
64. Dennett D. De vrije wil, natuurlijk bestaat die! De Psycholoog. 2016;2.
65. Jackson F, Pettit P. In defence of folk psychology. Philos Stud. 1990; 59:31–54.
66. Morsella E. The function of phenomenal states: supramodular interaction theory. Psychol Rev [Internet]. 2005;112:1000–21.
67. Pörtner HO, Roberts DC, Adams H, Adler C, Aldunce P, Ali E, et al. Climate change 2022: impacts, adaptation and vulnerability [Internet]. IPCC; 2022. Available from: www.ipcc.ch/report/ar6/wg2/
68. Baars BJ, Ramsoy TZ, Laureys S. Brain, conscious experience and the observing self. Trends Neurosci. 2003;26:671–5.

69. Dehaene S, Naccache L. Towards a cognitive neuroscience of consciousness: basic evidence and a workspace framework. Cognition. 2001;79:1–37.
70. Baars BJ. The conscious access hypothesis. Trends Cogn Sci. 2002;6:47–52.
71. Wertsch J V. Vygotsky and the social formation of mind. Boston, MA: Harvard University Press; 1985.
72. Sherman RT, Anderson CA. Decreasing premature termination from psychotherapy. J Soc Clin Psychol. 1987;5:298–312.
73. DeWall CN, Baumeister RF, Chester DS, Bushman BJ. How often does currently felt emotion predict social behavior and judgment? A meta-analytic test of two theories. Emot Rev. 2014;8:136–43.
74. Frijda NH. The emotions. Cambridge University Press; 1986.
75. Nesse RM. Good reasons for bad feelings insights from the frontier of evolutionary psychiatry. NY: Dutton; 2019.
76. Dijksterhuis A, Bos MW, Nordgren LF, Van Baaren RB. On making the right choice: 'the deliberation-without-attention effect. Science (80–). 2006;311:1005–7.
77. Dijksterhuis A. Think different: the merits of unconscious thought in preference development and decision making. J Pers Soc Psychol. 2004;87:586–98.
78. Nieuwenstein MR, Wierenga T, Morey RD, Wicherts JM, Blom TN, Wagenmakers EJ, et al. On making the right choice: a meta-analysis and large-scale replication attempt of the unconscious thought advantage. Judgm Decis Mak. 2015;10:1–17.
79. Aarts AA, Anderson JE, Anderson CJ, Attridge PR, Attwood A, Axt J, et al. Estimating the reproducibility of psychological science. Science (80–). 2015;349.
80. Ioannidis JPA. Why most published research findings are false. Get to Good Res Integr Biomed Sci. 2018;2:2–8.
81. Ioannidis JPA. The mass production of redundant, misleading, and conflicted Systematic reviews and meta-analyses. Milbank Q. 2016;94:485–514.
82. Drews FA, Pasupathi M, Strayer DL. Passenger and cell phone conversations in simulated driving. J Exp Psychol Appl. 2008;14:392–400.
83. Churchland PM. Folk psychology and the explanation of human behavior. Philos Perspect. 1989;3:225–41.
84. Shariff AF, Schooler J, Vohs KD. The hazards of claiming to have solved the hard problem of free will. In: Are we free?: Psychology and free will. Oxford University Press; 2008. pp. 181–204.
85. Diamond A, Lee K. Interventions shown to aid executive function development in children 4 to 12 years old. Science (80–) [Internet]. 2011;333:959–64. Available from: www.pubmedcentral.nih.gov/articlerender.fcgi?artid=3159917&tool=pmcentrez&rendertype=abstract
86. Elfeddali I, de Vries H, Bolman C, Pronk T, Wiers RW. A randomized controlled trial of web-based attentional bias modification to help smokers quit. Health Psychol. 2016;35.
87. Smith ER, DeCoster J. Dual-process models in social and cognitive psychology: conceptual integration and links to underlying memory systems. Personal Soc Psychol Rev. 2000;4:108–31.
88. Strack F, Deutsch R. Reflective and impulsive determinants of social behavior. Pers Soc Psychol Rev. 2004;8:220–47.
89. Liu Y, Van Den Wildenberg WPM, González GF, Rigoni D, Brass M, Wiers RW, et al. "Free won't" after a beer or two: chronic and acute effects of alcohol on neural and behavioral indices of intentional inhibition. BMC Psychol. 2020;8.

3 A chronic brain disease?

Since the 1990s, addiction has been described as a chronic brain disease, particularly in the biomedical and neuroscience literature. In the words of the aforementioned Alan Leshner, then director of the US National Institute on Drug Abuse (NIDA):

> The more common view is that drug addicted people are weak or bad people, unwilling to lead moral lives and to control their behavior and gratifications. To the contrary, addiction is actually a chronic, relapsing illness, characterized by compulsive drug seeking and use.[1]

Here, two views of addiction are contrasted: the everyday view that addicted people are characterized by a weak or flawed character (the moral view) and the scientific view that addiction is a chronic brain disease. Note that Leshner did state: "Addiction is not just a brain disease. It is a brain disease for which the social contexts in which it has both developed and is expressed are critically important." Hence, addiction is a chronic brain disease, but the social environment plays a critical role in its development. Before diving into the world of biomedical research on the chronic brain disease of addiction, it is worth briefly describing the interesting background of one of its protagonists: Nora Volkow, the successor of Alan Leshner and since 2004 the director of the US National Institute on Drug Abuse (NIDA), the world's largest sponsor of addiction research.

Nora Volkow was one of the top researchers on brain changes in addiction before she became director of NIDA. She has an interesting family history: she is a great-grandchild of Leon or Lev (he was born in the Ukraine) Trotsky, the Russian revolutionary who, after the revolution, opposed some of Lenin's plans and was therefore exiled from Russia, a lenient punishment; most opponents were killed right away. He defected to Mexico, where he found refuge with the help of the painter

DOI: 10.4324/9781032634548-3

Diego Rivera and his wife Frida Kahlo. From Mexico he opposed the non-aggression treaty that Lenin's successor Stalin made with Hitler, leading to his assassination in his heavily guarded home—the same house in Mexico-city where Nora grew up with her parents and two sisters. Nora studied medicine and became fascinated by the newly developed imaging techniques in the 1990s (PET and fMRI)[i]. This was the decade of the brain, where there was growing enthusiasm and optimism that these techniques would finally make us understand the machinery of the human mind and its vulnerabilities. The link to addiction was also personal for Nora: her maternal grandfather was addicted to alcohol and committed suicide, after many unsuccessful attempts to recover. She talked about this in a lecture to the American Psychiatric Association in Toronto.[2] In this personal account she explained her motivation to study the brain science of addiction: she wanted to understand how it is possible for people to lose their free will and become addicted. She called on psychiatrists to treat addiction just like other chronic brain diseases, rather than condemning those affected and thus contribute to their stigmatization. Volkow is a passionate researcher and advocate in the area of addiction, and I had the pleasure of meeting her a couple of times, due to a personal link: my second cousin Corinde Wiers (a researcher who will return in Chapter 8), worked with her as postdoc at NIDA for several years. In addition to being the director of NIDA, Nora Volkow is well known for her own contributions, including her work on the effects of different addictive substances on dopamine in the brain[3] and the influential iRISA model[4,5] that she developed with Rita Goldstein, discussed below.

What is meant by scientists who declared addiction a chronic brain disease? Over the past 30 years, much research has been done on the brain mechanisms underlying addiction. Some of this research is done with laboratory animals and some with humans. The great advantage of animal research is that real experimental designs can be used: individuals can be randomly assigned to different groups ("conditions"), for example, a group that is exposed to a drug and another group that is not given the same drug, after which the effect of that drug on the brain can be studied. This is not possible with humans for ethical and practical reasons; they determine for themselves whether they start using a drug or not (or at least that's what they believe, but let's not go there now). Random assignment to conditions is the "gold standard methodology"

i PET stands for positron emission tomography, a functional imaging technique using radioactive tracers to visualize brain activity in relation to a specific task; fMRI stands for functional magnetic resonance imaging, which does not need radioactive tracers but assesses and visualizes changes in blood flow in relation to a task.

to study causal relations, although it should be noted that recently other methods have been developed.[ii]

In animal studies, you can also vary other aspects in a controlled way, such as whether substance use begins during adolescence or during adulthood (in rats only a few weeks later). Then differences in behavior and related brain changes can be systematically studied. If you then find, for example, that negative effects are greater when the animals are given the drug during adolescence than when they are given the exact same amount during adulthood, you can convincingly demonstrate that the effect of substances during adolescence on brain development is greater (and indeed this has been found across many animal studies).[6–8]

As noted, random assignment to drug initiation conditions is not possible with humans for ethical reasons. However, we can examine the extent to which the brains of adolescents who drink or use other addictive substances at an early age differ from those of adolescents who start to take them at a later age, but then we cannot distinguish between the effects of the substances and differences that were already there before they started to use the substance. This is not some theoretical issue only, because indeed individuals who start using substances at an early age differ in many other aspects; the group that starts early has a different genetic profile, a different character, different friends, they come from different families, from different neighborhoods and more often experienced more misery in childhood, etc. (discussed further in Chapter 6). Therefore, by definition, it remains comparing apples and oranges, if you have not been able to randomly distribute people among the research groups.[9] For this reason, the strongest evidence regarding changes in the brain caused by (excessive) substance use comes from animal studies, but these have their own limitations (discussed in Chapter 4).

It is clear—from both animal and human research (each with its own limitations)—that the brain changes as a consequence of substance use. There is currently much debate about the extent to which such changes

ii The past decades the "causal revolution" was announced, where statistical methods have been developed to infer causality from patterns of correlations, by systematically testing what may or may not have caused the other factor. A lot of this work was developed to establish the causal link between tobacco smoking and lung cancer, which was clearly important to demonstrate (and has since led to legislation to reduce smoking), without the possibility of a true experimental design in humans (forcing some kids to smoke and others not). Famous statisticians held it possible that there were genes that influenced both the likelihood that someone would smoke and the risk of developing lung cancer (a third variable explaining a correlation). Using causal analysis (and supporting biomedical research on tissue and animals), the case could finally be made that indeed there was a causal link between smoking and lung cancer. For a nice introduction to this line of work, see the work of Judea Pearl.[80]

also occur in behavioral addictions such as excessive gambling, gaming or porn viewing, and perhaps also in excessive eating resulting in obesity (a topic that I will return in Chapter 9). Changes that have often been studied can be broadly divided into three groups, as summarized in an influential review by Nora Volkow and George Koob:[iii]

> Drug addiction is a chronically relapsing disorder that has been characterized by (1) compulsion to seek and take the drug, (2) loss of control in limiting intake, and (3) emergence of a negative emotional state (e.g., dysphoria, anxiety, irritability) reflecting a motivational withdrawal syndrome when access to the drug is prevented. Drug addiction has been conceptualized as a disorder that involves elements of both impulsivity and compulsivity that yield a composite addiction cycle composed of three stages: "binge/intoxication", "withdrawal/negative affect", and "preoccupation/anticipation" (craving).[10]

Given their prominent positions (directors of NIDA and the alcohol equivalent NIAAA), this model of addiction can be considered the standard biomedical model for the development of addiction, although it should be noted that the details vary by drug.[11] For example, positive reinforcement, the siren's call to experience a euphoric kick (predicted reward), is especially important with stimulants (cocaine, amphetamine) and to some extent with alcohol, while countering the negative consequences of use (withdrawal symptoms) plays an important role in the case of opiates and alcohol.[11]

People generally start substance use because of the expected positive effect. These may be expectations about pharmacology (the kick) or about associated social enhancement effect, such as helping to fit in with a peer group and easing social interactions.[12,13] This typically takes place in adolescence or young adulthood, when most addictive behaviors originate, and establishing friendships and partner relations constitutes an important developmental task, as described by influential developmental psychologists like Erik Erikson.[14] The early phase of the addiction cycle is the binge/intoxication phase, in which expected positive effects are usually reinforced; using substances together can be an experience that creates a bond, caused to some extent by the substance, but largely by the social setting surrounding early use, as highlighted by psychologist Mark Goldman and colleagues.[15,16] Essentially, the basic problem with

iii George Koob is director of NIAAA, the US National Institute for Research on Alcohol Addiction and Alcohol Problems. For historical reasons, alcohol research is organized separately from the rest of drug research, which is not because alcohol is less harmful as a drug compared to most other drugs (see an analysis by David Nutt and colleagues).[53]

addiction is that the negative effects occur later than the positive ones; should negative effects occur immediately, there is little or no risk of addiction. A famous example concerns Asian people who, because of a genetic variation, do not break down alcohol efficiently and therefore feel sick directly after ingesting alcohol.[17] While chances are these individuals do not develop alcoholism, this does not imply that alcoholism is rare in Asia.[18] Back to the bigger picture: most young people experience positive effects immediately after intake and negative effects only later, and the longer it takes until an effect occurs, the less likely it is that this predictive relationship is recognized. Hence, most people initially develop mostly positive expectations when they start using addictive substances.[15]

Over time, negative effects also occur, for example, the user experiences negative moods and feels lethargic. When someone starts using substances to counteract negative feelings, we speak of "negative reinforcement". Consider, for example, someone who drinks or smokes to counteract gloom or physical pain. It is easy to see that this reason to use quickly leads to escalation, because the after-effect of substance use exacerbates the malaise. This mechanism is particularly important in the development of addiction to opiates and alcohol, but plays a role in excessive use of other substances as well. For example, weekend use of stimulants and MDMA (ecstasy) can lead users to experience a *midweek low*, which can spur renewed use heading into the next weekend to overcome the low.

Finally, there is an influential theory that states that addictive behavior becomes compulsive over time (like compulsive cleaning or hand washing), proposed by Cambridge neuroscientists Barry Everitt and Trevor Robbins. From this perspective, the most important change in the brain when someone develops an addiction is the loss of control: once the opportunity to use the drug (or to gamble, play video games etc.) is present, there is no way back and the behavior has to be performed, especially when there is stress or a negative mood.[10,19,20] These are strong claims, and if they are true, it seems right to characterize addiction as a brain disease in which free will is at least compromised, and maybe in extreme cases lost. And when these brain changes do not recover after prolonged abstinence, one could legitimately speak of a *chronic* brain disease. Let us consider each of these changes in some more detail.

Positive reinforcement: sensitivity to the Siren's call

Addiction develops through normal neuropsychological systems that had evolutionarily useful functions.[21] A key brain system in recognizing signals that predict rewards is the mesolimbic dopamine system located centrally in the brain. Think of Pavlov's famous dog: a bell announcing that food was coming caused anticipatory physiological responses, such as the production of saliva, after the dog had experienced only a few pairings of the bell with food. Although dopamine is often equated with a reward response in the brain, it has been more accurately identified as an important learning signal in the brain, signifying something like: *pay attention: something important!*[iv] When reward is unexpected, a strong dopamine peak occurs in the midbrain (mesolimbic) dopamine system, which does not happen if the same reward was already predicted, as famously demonstrated by Wolfram Schultz from the University of Cambridge.[22] As a consequence, signals that preceded the reward subsequently attracts attention. This could be anything: Pavlov's bell, the smell of a cigarette, the five in the clock, or the singing of the Sirens in ancient Greece.

Contemporary American researchers Terry Robinson and Kent Berridge from the University of Michigan have shown in a famous series of studies that dopamine is crucial in developing *incentive salience*. This concerns the ability of signals of upcoming reward to attract attention and motivate efforts to approach and consume. They labelled this process *neural "wanting"*, which they distinguished from subjective wanting.[23–25] They showed that, neurobiologically, this is a different process from the neural process evoked when we find something pleasant or enjoyable ("liking")—that is, the hedonic response to a drug, in which endorphins play an important role. These two neurobiological systems—"wanting" and "liking"—normally work closely together: we generally want what we like or enjoy. Importantly, drugs directly activate the dopamine system, which is normally activated when something of strong relevance occurs, such as finding an unexpected source of good food or access to an attractive mate. Whereas such a strong learning signal would normally only occur in response to evolutionarily relevant rewards, such a spike now occurs after ingestion of a drug, or after an unexpected reward in gambling or gaming. As a consequence, predictors of that reaction (the smell of beer, the colorful lights of the slot machine), develop incentive salience, which mean that they become attractive—like the rewarding experience itself. This can be clearly observed in animal research, when rats start licking a light that indicates that a food reward is coming up, as though the light itself has taken on some of the attractive, tasty properties of the food that it signals. Pavlov's dog doubtlessly loved the sound of that bell, just like some of us love the sound of beer pouring down the glass of a fresh draft.

iv That dopamine should not be equated with a reward has been demonstrated in research in which a dopamine spike was found in the same system for a signal announcing a painful shock, that can be actively avoided.[81]

Addictive drugs (stimulants, opioids, alcohol, nicotine) cause dopamine neural mechanisms of the "*wanting-reaction*" to become stronger and stronger in vulnerable individuals, which is called "incentive sensitization". Somebody developing an addiction at some point typically begins to recognize negative outcomes associated with it, such as a complaining spouse or facing the results of an accident that happened while being intoxicated, which may decrease the liking of the drug. However, this will *not* decrease the (neural) "wanting", which can still easily be evoked with cues that predict the opportunity to take the drug again. Hence, according to this theory, addicted people are strongly drawn to continue their addictive behavior, even when they do not like it anymore. This can explain the phenomenon that is difficult to grasp for outsiders, that despite all the misery involved, the addicted person continues the addiction and approaches drug cues like iron to a magnet. According to the authors, the sensitized lure of drug signals is long-lasting and perhaps permanent,[25] though this is difficult to establish definitively since it is hard to generalize from laboratory animals to humans (in rats, an effect after a year is already very long). The impact of sensitization also seems to vary between substances: hypersensitivity to signals of reward is most prominent in excessive use of stimulants and alcohol, and less so in opiate addiction,[26] although Robinson and Berridge point to evidence that while opioids do not directly act on mesolimbic dopamine neurons, they do so indirectly and also produce a sensitized dopamine reaction in rats.[27] Hence, opioid cues also become motivational magnets, which plays an important role in addition to the strong withdrawal effects.

During my time as a researcher in Maastricht, Kent Berridge—at the time already a world-renowned addiction researcher—gave a lecture at Maastricht University, and I invited him to visit us in the old picturesque village of Eijsden, where we lived at the time, near the Belgian border. Coincidentally, this visit took place during the so-called "Bronk" festivities, a historic festival that lasts three days. It begins with a procession, for which the habitants (including me) lay sacred patterns of flower beds at sunrise (very early, as it takes place in early summer). Even though we came "from above" (the north of the Netherlands) and didn't speak Limburgish (the strong local dialect), we were invited to participate from the first year and joyfully did so. I checked with the neighbor if you had to be Catholic to participate, which was not the case, so I was literally drummed out of my bed every Bronk Sunday at 4 a.m. to participate in creating the flower beds in front of the altar, where soon the pastor would pronounce his blessing. The nice thing was that the celebration brought a lot of cohesion in the neighborhood: first you make the flower beds with neighbors, after the procession you clean everything up again, followed by traditional line dancing in the street and a tour of the local bars with everyone living there (all ages included).

On the second day of the festivities, Kent Berridge stepped out of the local train on the famous small platform of Eijsden (famous because the last German emperor Wilhelm arrived there during the First World War to ask for exile). Kent is a very polite and modest academic, resembling more the stereotypical English than American academic.[v] Yet the surprise could be read off his face when we left the station, where the festivities were already under way that early afternoon. It was like stepping into an old Breughel painting: tipsy, dancing people everywhere, children walking around with large trays of beer. We quickly agreed that excessive drinking by humans involves more than just the neurobiological adaptations (which we share with laboratory animals) and that culture clearly plays an important role too.

Recently we met again, some 20 years later, after he had presented his latest work on wanting and liking at the annual conference of the Association for Psychological Science (APS). He had presented some of the latest research from his lab, using optogenetics, a recently developed technique used to control the activity of specific neurons through light. This technique has made it possible to map functional connectivity in the brain in great detail. In the studies he presented, the researchers had introduced to the central nucleus of the amygdala[vi] in one randomly selected group of rats a substance that allowed for optogenetic stimulation, while rats in a control group received the same operation and received an optically inactive version (a placebo control condition).[28] In a first study, rats could choose which of two holes to poke their nose into: nose-poking into one hole earned sugar, and the other cocaine. Control-rats nose-poked into both holes about equally often. The optogenetic rats that were selectively stimulated after one of the choices (randomly picked), soon only wanted that outcome (either sugar or cocaine), arguably creating the equivalent of narrowly focused sugar or cocaine addiction. In a next experiment Berridge and colleagues selectively paired to stimulation the voluntarily touching of a protruding rod which gave the rats a shock. Normal rats (without operation) and control rats alike, would avoid this rod with fearful motivation, covering it with sand and staying away from it. With optogenetic stimulation in their central amygdala when touching the rod that gave them a shock, the rats behaved very differently: they kept on approaching and touching the rod. This was

v Read David Lodge's brilliantly funny book "changing places", for the full stereotypes.

vi The fact that the amygdala was targeted may come as a surprise to some, as this structure deep in the brain is often equated with negative emotions, specifically fear.[82] However, it plays a central role in determining what is important, both in relation to positive and negative events.[83]

not because they enjoyed touching the rod and receiving a shock: on a day when the activation was switched off, they would not do it. The same could also be tentatively concluded from the behavior on days that the optogenetic activation was turned on: "they sometimes appeared to hold back their paw from the rod for a moment as though avoiding shock, yet within a few moments their fascination would bring paw or nose too close, and so receive another shock" (remember Tolman's rats!). This is arguably the clearest demonstration that "wanting" and "liking" are different processes.

One feature of incentive salience is that both people and laboratory rats put much effort into approaching the desired object. Would this also be the case with the rod that produced a shock, or would it be out of sight, out of mind? To test this, the experimenters blocked the view of the rod with a big obstacle, and sure enough, the optogenetically stimulated rats would climb over the obstacle to touch the rod and get more shocks. Another feature is that incentive salience can spread to associated cues—that's why the heavy drinker's local bar may appealing to him, even though this is hard to understand for an outsider, who sees a shabby place with an unpleasant smell. This is also why rats start licking the rod if it earlier produced sugar, cocaine or even shock (after optogenetic stimulation). In Pavlov's spirit, Berridge and colleagues tested whether a specific tone that sounded when the rat touched the rod (and got a shock), would also be preferred above a neutral sound, which indeed was the case. Clearly, when this brain structure in the amygdala was activated, the result was that the rat wanted whatever was associated with it. And this activation turned out to activate associated structures related to "wanting", including the ventral tegmentum, where dopamine neurons begin, and the nucleus accumbens (a structure in the ventral—or front part—of the striatum), where dopamine neurons end.

So the brain structure that was stimulated in the study—the central nucleus of the amygdala—is clearly important in the attribution of incentive salience (i.e., in establishing what we *want*). But (as noted in footnote vi above) this same structure is also widely known for its role in a brain circuitry that controls what we *fear*. In line with this idea, Berridge and colleagues demonstrated that indeed the same area was involved in fear conditioning: when this was done with optogenetic stimulation in the same area, fear-related defensive responses became stronger; anything that predicted an unavoidable shock became fear-inducing.[29] Could this structure therefore function as a switch, where activation under the right circumstances could change "wanted" stimuli into something to be avoided? And could that hint at new treatments? This is related to counterconditioning that has been tried in the treatment of addiction, which will return in Chapter 8. We continued our conversation over coffee after his recent talk about the extent to which incentive salience could also play a role in adolescent development in humans, when strong passions often arise: for a lover, an activity, or a type of music, or maybe under less optimal circumstances for drug use or other self-harming behaviors. Kent has become convinced over the years that these modern passions activate the same basic motivational mechanisms as those involved in substance use.

Individual differences in sensitivity to the Siren's call

While Kent Berridge and his colleagues further explored neural mechanisms underlying "wanting" versus "liking", his early collaborator Terry Robinson and colleagues began to study individual differences in sensitivity to reward signals.[30,31] This distinguishes between individuals who are highly attracted to learned reward signals and others who are less so and instead keep an eye on their ultimate goal, called "sign-trackers" and "goal-trackers", respectively. The experimental design developed to reveal these individual differences is essentially as follows: on one side of a cage a reward signal is given (a lever pops out of a wall announcing a reward, e.g., sugar or cocaine), while on the other side the actual reward is provided for a brief period. As we saw, one of the characteristics of incentive salience is that the cues announcing the reward become attractive as well. Sign-trackers strongly show this behavior: they will approach and lick the lever that signals the reward as if it is the reward itself, even if doing so causes them to miss the actual reward! Goal-trackers, in contrast, upon seeing the same lever signaling the availability of the reward, turn to where the actual reward is available and don't waste precious time at the lever, thus using the signal to reach their goal, even when that implies that they have to move away from the signal. Noteworthy here is that the aforementioned dopamine spike in response to signals of reward is most strongly found in sign-trackers, apparently indicating the attraction to the cue itself.[32]

Our dog often gives great examples of sign-tracking. When Tarzan (as the kids baptized our cute little white dog), at a walk, picks up signals that a female dog has been around, he is so mesmerized by interesting smells, that he does not notice an actual female present. Exemplary sign-tracking behavior. After this example, it may come as no surprise that there are gender differences in the percentage of sign-trackers versus goal-trackers, and probably even less that males are relatively frequently sign-trackers[33] (although this is not universally found).[34] This could well be related to the greater likelihood of developing addiction in males, which is common across addictions (with again some exceptions, such as addiction to tranquilizers).[vii] We ourselves concluded in a recent brain imaging study that responses to alcohol cues in the brain's classic reward and attention areas were much stronger in male than in female students with an alcohol problem.[35] It should be noted, however, that by no means all addicted people respond strongly to reward cues. As we will see, there are other pathways leading to addiction, where substance use (or other addictive behavior) is used as a means to an end (e.g., getting calm after stress, falling asleep, etc.), and this is common in both males and females. But the strong sensitivity to reward signals still seems to be primarily a vulnerability factor for addiction in males, probably for good evolutionary reasons.

A creative researcher at the University of New South Wales (Sydney, Australia), Mike Le Pelley (who also received a prize for growing the universities fiercest beard, easy to find online), has developed a task to distinguish sign-trackers and goal-trackers in people.[36] The basic task for the participant is simple: in an array of gray shapes, the participant must repeatedly find an odd-one-out (for example, a diamond among circles).[viii] Occasionally one of the nontarget circles is a brightly colored distractor, and the color of this distractor signals the size of the reward that participants will earn for quickly finding the target diamond. For example, a blue distractor might indicate that a high reward is available, whereas an orange distractor might signal a low reward. Importantly, participants only receive this reward if they find the target *without looking at the colored distractor*. The task for the participant should be simple: they should always ignore the colored distractor and respond as fast as possible to the diamond. Yet participants are sometimes distracted by the colored circle and look at it even though doing so means they lose the reward—and, interestingly, *especially when the color indicates a high reward*. This is crucial, because the different distractors are matched for their distracting properties (hue) and counterbalanced (for some participants blue indicates high reward, for others orange), and still the effect emerges. Like sign-tracking laboratory rats, some participants in this setup do exactly what should *not* be done: precisely

vii There is some evidence that females more readily escalate from moderate substance use into addiction,[84] which could be related to stronger bodily reactions to alcohol, that on the one hand may protect against developing addiction: if you strongly experience negative effects (similar to the genetic variety in Asians that is protective against developing an alcohol problem), this will keep most people from escalating. However, a more sensitive reaction could also to more rapid escalation of problems, in case these warning signals are ignored and heavy use is continued.

viii A different version of the task was developed by Texas A&M University's Brian Anderson.[40]

when you can obtain a big reward for ignoring the distractor, they get most distracted by it. This is why this effect (and the corresponding task) have been labeled value-modulated attentional capture (VMAC). The effect occurs when people first learn the value of the different distractors in a separate task (big rewards after one color, small after the other), after which they occur as distractors in the VMAC task, but the effect can also be obtained when you simply explain that one color signals high reward while the other signals low reward. Notably, people differ in the extent to which they get distracted by the signal of high reward, and this has been related to addiction (where addiction is associated with a particularly strong VMAC effect) and more tentatively to depression (small or no VMAC effect).[37,38]

One of Le Pelley's former PhD students, Lucy Albertella, has developed a variety of the task that also works without measuring eye movements, which allows for assessment over the Internet. With that

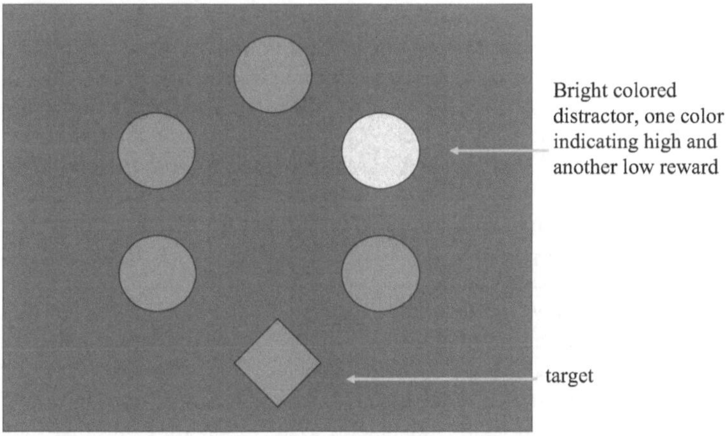

Figure 3.1 A computer screen of a variety of the Value-Modulated Attentional Capture (VMAC) task that measures distraction by a reward signal. Participants task is to look as quickly as possible to the odd one out of the dark grey figures (here the target in the bottom), without being distracted by a brightly colored distractor (here light grey). The distractor can come in one of two colors, one indicating the opportunity to win a small reward (say orange) and the other the opportunity to win a big reward (say purple). In both cases, the reward can only be won, when the participant does *not* look at the distractor. The VMAC effect is a measure of the extent to which the participant is more distracted by the distractor signaling high versus low reward opportunity (indicated by errors and slower reaction times to target).

task she found a relationship between the degree of sign-tracking and illicit substance use, in students with relatively weak executive control functions (another risk-factor for addiction, discussed later).[39] And in another recent collaborative study with volunteers participating in the Dutch equivalent of Dry January, we found that the degree of *sign-tracking* predicted who would or would not persevere through the end of January: the more participants were distracted by the reward signals, the more likely they were back to drinking before the end of the month.[40] A colleague unintentionally illustrated how this works. A solid social drinker and at the time also a therapist of addicted people, he participated in the Dry January challenge to experience what it was like not to drink for a month, as he often asked his patients to do. He even wore the colored bracelet provided by the campaign saying "No Thanks". After work, he joined colleagues in the local pub and ordered a sparkling water. Later the same evening, as he was walking back from the bar with a tray full of beer in his hands, his eye fell on that bracelet ... Oh yes, Dry January! He had forgotten his temporary abstinence goal in this context full of attractive signs ...

The initial brain adaptations ("neuroadaptation" in technical jargon) can thus be summarized as an enhanced sensitivity to signals of upcoming reward, or the siren's lure. Dopamine plays an important role in this, but it is now clear that this is in concert with other neurotransmitters.[25] Sign-tracking is also related to reward sensitivity, which is one of the risk factors for addiction, related to the personality traits impulsivity and sensation seeking, discussed in Chapter 6 on risk factors and development.[41] Finally, it is important to note that the differences are relative; that is, it is not the case that a sign tracker in the computer game is *always* distracted by the signal of high reward, or that they can *never* stick to a goal when there are distracting reward signals. However, sign trackers do have a little more trouble with ignoring reward cues compared to goal trackers. Also, the sex difference should not be exaggerated. It is just like height: usually men are a bit taller than women, but of course there are small men and tall women. Similarly, men are on average a bit more sensitive to reward signals than women, but there are also women who are very sensitive to reward signals and men who are not. So, the first neuroadaptation is enhanced sensitivity to reward signals, especially in those who were relatively sensitive to them anyway.

Impaired response inhibition and salience attribution

While Robinson and Berridge focused on increased salience attribution ("wanting") to drug-related cues as the driving mechanism in developing addiction, Goldstein and Volkow, in their iRISA model emphasized the combination of abnormal salience attribution and impaired response inhibition, two neuroadaptations that reinforce each other's effects. The first concerns the salience attribution, similar to the sensitized "wanting" response discussed above, while they also emphasize the reduced salience attribution to "normal" reinforcers. This is in line with the clinical wisdom that addiction really becomes problematic once the addictive behavior has become more attractive than sex, which was exactly what was suggested by an influential early brain imaging study in cocaine users and controls.[42] In addition to these midbrain dopamine-mediated changes, they emphasized changes in the prefrontal cortex (PFC), in particular those related to impaired response inhibition. Together with the increased salience of addiction-related cues and the reduced salience of other reinforcers, the impaired ability to inhibit an undesirable response-tendency makes it especially difficult to resist the cue-induced temptation to engage in the addictive behavior, even when one has resolved to refrain from it that night. Note that this model is conceptually close to the dual process models in psychology described briefly in the previous chapter. When exposed to cues that signal the possibility of use, the model predicts not only enhanced activity in midbrain dopamine ("wanting"), but also in PFC areas, mimicking the effects of actual use, related to anticipated positive effects (positive expectancies), attention allocation to the drug cues, and if necessary strategy selection (how to produce the high). These changes have been related to craving and to the high after actual drug use, although here also differences between drugs were noted (e.g., increase of frontal activity after cocaine and a decrease after heroin), which may correspond to a further increase in craving after cocaine and a decrease after heroin intake.[5] At the same time frontal activity related to the alternative to drug use, decreases: showing a blunted response to other rewards such as money. According to the model, executive or frontal functions become impaired as a consequence of long-term drug use, leading to problems in inhibition and working memory, while noting that relatively weak executive functions are also a vulnerability factor that increases the risk to develop addiction. For some drugs (cocaine, cigarettes), there is also some evidence for temporary normalization of these functions after drug use. As similar effects have been described for mood after smoking, this may be a specific maintaining mechanism in stimulant drugs: you feel worse and can't concentrate, which is remediated on a temporary basis by taking another "hit" (see below).

Negative reinforcement: "the dark side of addiction"

The second set of neuroadaptations that plays a major role in addiction is related to negative reinforcement and the negative moods that arise in addictions over the somewhat longer term. These neuroadaptations have poetically been called the "dark side of addiction" by the aforementioned George Koob (from the Scripps Research Institute, and director of NIAAA) and the French neuroscientist Michel LeMoal.[43] These changes have everything to do with two of the most classic characteristics of addiction: withdrawal and tolerance. At the heart of this mechanism is *homeostasis*, which refers to mechanisms that act to maintain the body in a desired state. For example, think of our body temperature: if we get too hot, we sweat to get our body temperature down and if we are too cold, we shiver.

Psychoactive substances have all kinds of effects on physiological systems, for example, your heart rate goes up when you drink coffee or smoke a cigarette. The first time you drink a cup of coffee, within minutes your heart rate shoots up. In reaction, regulatory systems are put to work that make your heart rate go down again. But more happens: the brain is learning in order to better predict the future.[44,45] In this case, we learn that the smell of coffee and the sound of the coffee machine predict the effects that follow, the taste of coffee and an imminent heart rate acceleration. In anticipation of this effect, a second process is initiated, which already slows down the heart rate, to counteract the upcoming stimulant effect of the drug. The net effect is that over time the coffee causes less heart rate acceleration, or in other words, you need more coffee for the same heart rate acceleration, and that is what is called tolerance.

Tolerance is thus not only about a physiological mechanism, but also about a learned (conditioned) response to signals announcing the drug. This was published back in the 1980s in a famous report in *Science* by Canadian psychologist Shep Siegel and colleagues.[46] Rats were given increasing doses of heroin in a particular cage. Some of them (randomly assigned) were subsequently given a high dose in an entirely different cage, while those remaining were given an equally high dose in the cage in which they had previously been administered heroin. Of the first group, a much higher proportion (two-thirds) died than of the second group (one-third). This experiment dramatically demonstrates the importance of that conditioned counter-reaction: when it occurs—provoked by the familiar cage in which the drug was previously used—the net effect of the drug is smaller. However, when the counter-reaction fails to occur, because the drug is taken in an unfamiliar environment, then the full dose takes effect without a counter-reaction, which proved fatal for the laboratory rats in many cases.

The same mechanism also seems to play a crucial role in cases of fatal ODs in humans. Often these do not involve an abnormally high dose of the drug, but a normal amount used in a different place than usual. As an example, a Spanish couple was described, who were addicted to heroin and decided to quit together. The first few days went well, but the boyfriend didn't keep it up and without telling her after a few days decided to buy his normal amount from his regular dealer. But he couldn't use it the normal way, at home, because his girlfriend was there, so he went to a public restroom, where he was later found dead.[47] The cause of death was diagnosed as "drug overdose". Hence, this tragic example illustrates that an overdose is often a normal dose used under abnormal circumstances, so the context cannot initiate the preparatory physical counter-reaction.

This preparatory counter-reaction, according to Koob and LeMoal, also has an effect on motivation and mood: the euphoria would diminish over time and an increasingly strong negative mood would remain, which would then encourage renewed use. This easily leads to escalation of use and addiction: the drug to counteract the negative feelings actually reinforces those same negative feelings in the long run. This neuroadaptation has a lot to do with stress. Indeed, the hormones that are amplified when stress is present also play a role in withdrawal symptoms, and stress can also trigger relapse, even when a person has been in rehab for some time.[48–50]

An additional neuroadaptation mentioned by these authors is the brain's diminished reward response to life's normal rewards. In a depressed state (whether caused by substance use or not), the brain sees only one clear way out of its misery: substance use. Depression is indeed very common in addiction, and fortunately in most cases the depression disappears after successful withdrawal, without further treatment for depression. In clinical practice, this is a good reason to first try to treat the addiction, in case of an depressed patient with addiction problems.[51] The second set of neuroadaptations in the chronic brain disease model of addiction revolve around tolerance and withdrawal, in relation to substance use as a means to (temporarily) alleviate negative feelings, which may resemble the *anti-reward state* caused by the drug use (e.g., stress and negative feelings). This makes a person more susceptible to relapse precisely when feeling low or stressed.[43]

Compulsion: from impulsive to compulsive use

The third mechanism involved in the view of addiction as a chronic brain disease is that it develops from impulsive to compulsive habits. Barry Everitt and Trevor Robbins, two Cambridge neuroscientists, developed this model.[19,20] The idea is that while addiction begins as voluntary goal-directed behavior, over time control shifts to brain circuits in which an eliciting signal invariably leads to an action, making that action involuntary and compulsive. This is associated with a shift in control of behavior from one circuit to another in the (mid)brain. Initially, control of rewarded and goal-directed behavior relies on a circuit in which the aforementioned *nucleus accumbens* in the anterior (*ventral*) part of the *striatum*, plays a significant role. After prolonged use, the addictive behavior becomes compulsive, which has been related to control moving to a circuit in the posterior (*dorsal*) part of the *striatum* that is important in automated actions. Addictive behavior thus develops from voluntary and purposeful to automated and compulsive; when a signal indicates that the drug is available, there is no more choice, it simply has to be taken.

In testing this mechanism, it is essential to study the effects of extinction or punishment on the automated response, because a compulsive habit should not diminish after extinction or punishment. This is done in a setup where a test animal decides for itself whether it will consume a drug (e.g., water with cocaine) or choose an alternative (e.g., sugar water), by pressing one of two pedals. If the animal prefers a high dose of the drug, the critical test is whether it will continue to press the pedal that previously provided the drug, even if it no longer does so, or even if pressing it results in an electric shock. Some of the experimental animals continued to press the drug-associated pedal regardless, which is seen as a model of a central symptom of human addiction: continued use despite expected negative consequences. For example, in one of their studies, rats that had previously had little experience of receiving cocaine for lever-pressing stopped pressing the lever—which had previously provided the cocaine—as soon as the task was changed so that they received a shock after pressing it. By contrast, rats that had had greater experience of cocaine reward actually continued pressing the lever, even though doing so now led to shocks instead of cocaine.[52] This result was not found when given a natural reward (sugar water), underscoring that concentrated drugs, such as cocaine (and artificial opiates and distilled spirits), provide stronger effects than natural rewards.

A strong point in this model is that not all animals started using compulsively, which is consistent with the behavior of humans—it is not the case that everyone who has ever tried an addictive drug becomes addicted: depending on the drug, it is about 10–20% of people.[53,54] In the animal experiment, the shock was set so that about 15–20% of the test animals continued to search for the drug (by pressing the lever), without getting it, while risking shock in the process.[20,55] Follow-up research has shown that these were not random animals, but rather those that had been previously labeled as above-average impulsive (on animal translations of human tasks to assess impulsivity).[55] On this finding (and much related animal research) the authors described the development of addiction as a shift from impulsive to compulsive behavior.

The transition of control over substance use from the anterior part to the more posterior part of the *striatum* has now been confirmed experimentally in several animal studies.[20] For example, researchers found that blocking activity in the anterior part of the *striatum* affected incipient use of a psychoactive drug but not compulsive continuation after frequent use, while the reverse was found after blocking the posterior part: that affected compulsive behavior but not incipient use.[56] In humans, there is also some evidence suggesting such a shift,[57] but the evidence is necessarily weaker, as people cannot be experimentally assigned to a group that becomes addicted and a group in which they do not.

The shift from purposeful controlled to compulsive use may also be partly due to the weakening of cognitive control abilities due to substance use, for which there is also some evidence,[20,58] but again, the evidence is stronger in animal studies than in humans.[59,60] In part, this has to do with the aforementioned lack of experimental studies in humans.[6] A key problem here is that relatively weak cognitive control functions are a predictor of early initiation of substance use,[61] making it difficult to determine to what extent relatively weak cognitive control functions are a consequence of addiction or a cause of it (or a combination of both), i.e., a variant of the age-old chicken-and-egg problem.[62,63]

An interesting research strategy is to examine family members of people with the problem under study for neurocognitive functions associated with addiction. In my dissertation some 25 years ago, I examined such functions in children of alcoholics compared to those of control children. We found relatively weak cognitive control (also known as executive functioning) in the children of alcoholics, and especially in those who themselves already exhibited behavioral problems.[64] This is consistent with other findings in children of addicted parents: they have a slightly higher risk of becoming addicted themselves, in which relatively weak control functions seem to play a role.[65–67] Recent research has also shown subtle brain abnormalities in siblings of addicted people who were not themselves addicted people. These were abnormalities of brain regions that play an important role in self-control functions, suggesting that this is a mechanism related to the hereditary side of addiction (about which more in Chapter 6).[68]

The hidden island of addiction

Neuroscientist Antoine Bechara, from the University of Southern California, has done a lot of research on the role of hunches in decision making, and their neural substrate, involving the insula deep in the brain. He developed a card game in which participants take cards from one of four stacks, often done on a computer. Some stacks occasionally provide large rewards, but also many losses, while other stacks mostly provide small gains but turn out to be more profitable in the end. Most participants draw some cards from all stacks until they realize that some stacks are more profitable in the long run, after which they draw mostly from the more profitable stack of cards. Bechara and colleagues argued in an influential article that physical cues indicate this change even before the participant is aware of it.[69] Note that the conclusion unconscious markers can be detected before the person becomes subjectively aware of which stacks are profitable, has later been challenged on methodological grounds.[70] Bechara also showed that addicted people in general persisted for longer in drawing cards from stacks that occasionally caused large gains but overall resulted in long-term losses compared with non-addicted people.[71] The insula plays an important role in developing the hunch that a particular stack is "not OK", and lack of becoming aware of such a signal is likely to play a role in the development of addiction,[72] as has recently also been underscored with a different task in animals and humans.[73] If the insula does not give a "not fluff signal" or does so too late, it may prevent people from adjusting their (addictive) behavior in time.

The insula plays an important role in becoming aware of feelings evoked in the body. Bechara's collaborator Antonio Damasio described "somatic markers", that indicate that we become aware of a bodily state.[74] In addiction, these signals can manifest themselves in an extreme craving of a substance or activity, in which the insula plays a central role. This can be seen as the subjective counterpart of the neural "wanting" response described earlier. This idea received a lot of attention after an inveterate smoker suffered brain damage in the insula, after which he was suddenly able to quit smoking, which he had tried many times in vain before. This was attributed to the disappearance of the strong desire for a cigarette after the brain damage.[75] The great influence of the insula in craving has also been confirmed in later research, after which these structures, hidden deep inside the skull, received their nickname "the hidden island of addiction" ("insula" is Latin for island).[72] In craving, anticipated feelings play a strong role. The insula causes you to anticipate, as it were, the relaxation or euphoria that the drug will bring about, which brings the decision to take it closer.

The insula, together with other frontal areas, also play a role in self-insight, which is often impaired in addiction. For one thing, the large majority of people meeting criteria show little awareness of the problem and do not seek treatment. In clinical encounters, addicted people often minimize their problems, if not plainly denying them, which was traditionally attributed to their immoral character. The aforementioned Rita Goldstein, Bechara, Volkow and colleagues wrote an intriguing paper on the neural basis of impaired insight in addiction.[76] The suggestion, in line with the original claims of the chronic brain disease model, is that these characteristics may be part of the neurological problems associated with addiction. One of the symptoms of addiction is that drug use is continued despite knowledge of negative consequences. Perhaps part of the problem is not so much intentional denial, but a lack of awareness of a relation between the addictive behavior and negative experiences, which "just happen" a lot. And this could also affect decision-making in addiction[77] (discussed further in Chapter 5).

What is the current status of the brain disease model?

A recent systematic review from Goldstein's team described differences in brain function between addicted people and controls in over 100 neuroimaging studies. Current neuroscience relates functions to large scale brain networks rather than to specific areas,[78] and they found impairments related to addictions in six of these brain networks, with similar effects for alcohol, cannabis and stimulants. First, not surprising, a reward network, including both the subcortical regions involved in incentive salience attribution ("wanting"), as well as frontal areas, important in determining expected subjective value (what is this action going to yield?). Activation in this network in reaction to drug cues not only differed between addicted and non-addicted people, it also predicted relapse after treatment in some studies. Second, a habit network, involved in automatizing of behavior, with different parts of the *striatum* playing a role, which was related to changes in the addictive behavior (initiation or quitting). The third network found to differ was the salience network, involving part of the insula and related structures. This gets activated when something is important, independent of valence (both for relevant good and bad things). Reactions by this network to drug cues were also related to the prediction of relapse. The fourth large-scale network was the executive control network, involving different frontal areas and executive control functions, such as inhibition and working memory. Its (lack of) activation in tasks with neutral cues (no alcohol or drugs) was also predictive of relapse. All of these networks can be related to the different neurobiological accounts described earlier in this chapter. In addition, the researchers found differences in the *default mode network*, which is important in self-directed processes, including self-awareness, where we also saw abnormalities in addiction. Finally, a memory network was found, including the hippocampus and related structures, which also appeared to be related to change, but, like the habit network, not to current use and problems. So … can we conclude that all accounts are partly right and that addiction should be considered as a multi-faceted chronic brain disease?

Perhaps, but, as we will see in the next chapter, the model has also come under increasing criticism during the past decade. Where there is no disagreement is that the neuroadaptations described in this chapter play a role in the development and maintenance of addictions, that is: previous use causes changes in the brain that facilitates the decision to use again. Where there is much debate is, on the one hand, about the relative importance of different neuroadaptations in the development of addiction—a debate among neuroscientists. For example, some believe that the *dark side of addiction is* especially crucial, while others believe that the same is true of sensitization, negative reinforcement or the development of compulsive use.[79] On the other hand, there is much debate between supporters of (variants of) the model of addiction as a chronic brain disease and opponents of that idea, who often come from the social sciences. I address their arguments in the next chapter.

References

1. Leshner AI. Addiction is a brain disease, and it matters. Sci New Ser. 1997;278:45–7.
2. Volkow ND. Addiction is a disease of free will [Internet]. 2015. Available from: www.youtube.com/watch?v=X1AEvkWxbLE
3. Volkow ND, Fowler JS, Wang GJ, Swanson JM Dopamine in drug abuse and addiction: results from imaging studies and treatment implications. Mol Psychiatry. 2004;9:557–69.
4. Goldstein RZ, Volkow ND. Drug addiction and its underlying neurobiological basis: Neuroimaging evidence for the involvement of the frontal cortex. Am J Psychiatry. 2002;159:1642–52.
5. Goldstein RZ, Volkow ND. Dysfunction of the prefrontal cortex in addiction: neuroimaging findings and clinical implications. Nat Rev Neurosci. 2011;12:652–69.
6. Spear LP Consequences of adolescent use of alcohol and other drugs: studies using rodent models. Neurosci Biobehav Rev [Internet]. 2016;70:228–43. Available from: 10.1016/j.neubiorev.2016.07.026
7. Crews FT, Robinson DL, Chandler LJ, Ehlers CL, Mulholland PJ, Pandey SC, et al. Mechanisms of persistent neurobiological changes following adolescent alcohol exposure: NADIA consortium findings. Alcohol Clin Exp Res. 2019;43:1806–22.
8. Spear LP. Effects of adolescent alcohol consumption on the brain and behaviour. Nat Rev Neurosci. 2018;19:197–214.
9. Meehl PE. Nuisance variables and the ex post facto design. In: M Radner, S Winokur (Eds.), Minnesota Studies in the philosophy of science: Vol. IV. Analyses of theories and methods of physics and psychology. Minneapolis: University of Minnesota Press. pp. 373–402. Available from: https://meehl.umn.edu/sites/meehl.umn.edu/files/files/084nuisancevariables.pdf
10. Koob GF, Volkow ND. Neurocircuitry of addiction. Neuropsychopharmacology [Internet]. 2010;35:217–38. Available from: www.ncbi.nlm.nih.gov/pubmed/19710631%5Cnwww.pubmedcentral.nih.gov/articlerender.fcgi?artid=PMC2805560
11. Badiani A, Belin D, Epstein D, Calu D, Shaham Y. Opiate versus psychostimulant addiction: the differences do matter. Nat Rev Neurosci

[Internet]. 2011;12:685–700. Available from: www.ncbi.nlm.nih.gov/pubmed/21971065%5Cnwww.nature.com/nrn/journal/v12/n11/pdf/nrn3104.pdf
12. Wiers RW, Hoogeveen KJ, Sergeant JA, Gunning WB. High- and low-dose alcohol-related expectancies and the differential associations with drinking in male and female adolescents and young adults. Addiction [Internet]. 1997 [cited 2013 Apr 5];92:871–88. Available from: http://doi.wiley.com/10.1111/j.1360-0443.1997.tb02956.x
13. Cooper ML, Frone MR, Russell M, Mudar P. Drinking to regulate positive and negative emotions: a motivational model of alcohol use. J Pers Soc Psychol [Internet]. 1995;69:990–1005. Available from: www.ncbi.nlm.nih.gov/pubmed/7473043
14. Erikson EH. Identity and the life cycle. NY: WW Norton & Company; 1980.
15. Goldman MS, Brown SA, Christiansen BA. Expectancy theory-thinking about drinking. In: H Blane & KE Leonard (Eds.), editor. Psychological theories of drinking and alcoholism. NY: Guilford; 1987. pp. 181–226.
16. Goldman MS. Risk for substance abuse: memory as a common etiological pathway. Psychol Sci. 1999;10:196–8.
17. Luczak SE, Glatt SJ, Wall TJ. Meta-analyses of ALDH2 and ADH1B with alcohol dependence in Asians. Psychol Bull. 2006;132:607.
18. Belay GM, Lam KKW, Liu Q, Wu CST, Mak YW, Ho KY. Magnitude and determinants of alcohol use disorder among adult population in East Asian countries: a systematic review and meta-analysis. Front Public Heal. 2023;11.
19. Everitt BJ, Robbins TW. Neural systems of reinforcement for drug addiction: from actions to habits to compulsion. Nat Neurosci. 2005;8:1481–9.
20. Everitt BJ, Robbins TW. Drug addiction: updating actions to habits to compulsions ten years on. Annu Rev Psychol [Internet]. 2016; 67:150807174122003. Available from: www.annualreviews.org/doi/abs/10.1146/annurev-psych-122414-033457
21. Nesse RM, Berridge KC. Psychoactive drug use in evolutionary perspective. Science (80–). 1997;278:63–6.
22. Schultz W, Dayan P, Montague PR. A neural substrate of prediction and reward. Science (80–). 1997;275:1593–9.
23. Robinson TE, Berridge KC. The neural basis of drug craving: an incentive-sensitization theory of addiction. Brain Res Rev. 1993;18:247–91.
24. Berridge KC, Robinson TE. Parsing reward. Trends Neurosci. 2003; 26:507–13.
25. Berridge KC, Robinson TE. Liking, wanting, and the incentive-sensitization theory of addiction. Am Psychol. 2016;71:670–9.
26. Nutt DJ, Lingford-Hughes A, Erritzoe D, Stokes PRA. The dopamine theory of addiction: 40 years of highs and lows. Nat Rev Neurosci. 2015;16:305–12.
27. Robinson TE, Berridge KC. The incentive-sensitization theory of addiction 30 years on. Annu Rev Psychol. 2024;in press.
28. Warlow SM, Naffziger EE, Berridge KC. The central amygdala recruits mesocorticolimbic circuitry for pursuit of reward or pain. Nat Commun [Internet]. 2020;11:1–15. Available from: 10.1038/s41467-020-16407-1
29. Berridge KC. Separating desire from prediction of outcome value. Trends Cogn Sci [Internet]. 2023;27:932–46. Available from: 10.1016/j.tics.2023.07.007
30. Flagel SB, Watson SJ, Akil H, Robinson TE. Individual differences in the attribution of incentive salience to a reward-related cue: influence on cocaine sensitization. Behav Brain Res. 2008;186:48–56.

31. Robinson TE, Yager LM, Cogan ES, Saunders BT. On the motivational properties of reward cues: individual differences. Neuropharmacology [Internet]. 2014;76:450–9. Available from: 10.1016/j.neuropharm.2013.05.040
32. Flagel SB, Robinson TE. Neurobiological basis of individual variation in stimulus-reward learning. Curr Opin Behav Sci [Internet]. 2017;13:178–85. Available from: 10.1016/j.cobeha.2016.12.004
33. Barker JM, Taylor JR. Sex differences in incentive motivation and the relationship to the development and maintenance of alcohol use disorders. Physiol Behav [Internet]. 2017;online fir. Available from: 10.1016/j.physbeh.2017.09.027
34. Bien E, Smith K. The role of sex on sign-tracking acquisition and outcome devaluation sensitivity in Long Evans rats. Behav Brain Res [Internet]. 2023;455:114656. Available from: 10.1016/j.bbr.2023.114656
35. Kaag AM, Wiers RW, de Vries TJ, Pattij T, Goudriaan AE. Striatal alcohol cue-reactivity is stronger in male than female problem drinkers. Eur J Neurosci. 2019;50:2264–73.
36. Le Pelley ME, Pearson D, Griffiths O, Beesley T. When goals conflict with values: counterproductive attentional and oculomotor capture by reward-related stimuli. J Exp Psychol Gen. 2015;144:158–71.
37. Anderson BA. Relating value-driven attention to psychopathology. Curr Opin Psychol [Internet]. 2021;39:48–54. Available from: 10.1016/j.copsyc.2020.07.010
38. Pearson D, Watson P, Albertella L, Le Pelley ME. Attentional economics links value-modulated attentional capture and decision-making. Nat Rev Psychol. 2022;1:320–33.
39. Albertella L, Copeland J, Pearson D, Watson P, Wiers RW, Le Pelley ME. Selective attention moderates the relationship between attentional capture by signals of nondrug reward and illicit drug use. Drug Alcohol Depend [Internet]. 2017;175:99–105. Available from: 10.1016/j.drugalcdep.2017.01.041
40. Albertella L, Van den Hooven J, Bovens R, Wiers RW. Reward-related attentional capture predicts non-abstinence during a one-month abstinence challenge. Addict Behav. 2021;114:106745.
41. Flagel SB, Waselus M, Clinton SM, Watson SJ, Akil H. Antecedents and consequences of drug abuse in rats selectively bred for high and low response to novelty. Neuropharmacology [Internet]. 2014;76:425–36. Available from: 10.1016/j.neuropharm.2013.04.033
42. Garavan H, Pankiewicz J, Bloom A, Cho JK, Sperry L, Ross TJ, et al. Cue-induced cocaine craving: neuroanatomical specificity for drug users and drug stimuli. Am J Psychiatry. 2000;157:1789–98.
43. Koob GF, Le Moal M. Addiction and the brain antireward system. Annu Rev Psychol [Internet]. 2008;59:29–53. Available from: www.annualreviews.org/doi/abs/10.1146/annurev.psych.59.103006.093548
44. Friston K. The free-energy principle: a rough guide to the brain? Trends Cogn Sci. 2009;13:293–301.
45. Clark A. Whatever next? Predictive brains, situated agents, and the future of cognitive science. Behav Brain Sci. 2013;36:181–204.
46. Siegel S, Hinson RE, Krank MD, Mccully J, Mauk D, Warren JT, et al. Heroin "overdose" death: contribution of drug-associated environmental cues. Science (80–). 1982;216:436–7.
47. Gerevich J, Bácskai E, Farkas L, Danics Z. A case report: Pavlovian conditioning as a risk factor of heroin "overdose" death. Harm Reduct J. 2005;2:1–4.

48. Koob GF, Le Moal M. Plasticity of reward neurocircuitry and the "dark side" of drug addiction. Nat Neurosci. 2005;8:1442–4.
49. Haber SN, Rauch SL. Neurocircuitry: a window into the networks underlying neuropsychiatric disease. Neuropsychopharmacology. 2010;35:1–3.
50. Blaine SK, Sinha R. Alcohol, stress, and glucocorticoids: from risk to dependence and relapse in alcohol use disorders. Neuropharmacology [Internet]. 2017;122:136–47. Available from: 10.1016/j.neuropharm.2017.01.037
51. Brown SA, Schuckit MA. Changes in depression among abstinent alcoholics. J Stud Alcohol. 1988;49:412–7.
52. Vanderschuren LJMJ, Everitt BJ. Drug seeking becomes compulsive after prolonged cocaine self-administration. Science (80–). 2004;305:1017–9.
53. Nutt DJ, King LA, Phillips LD. Drug harms in the UK: a multicriteria decision analysis. Lancet. 2010;376:1558–65.
54. Van Amsterdam J, Opperhuizen A, Koeter M, Van Den Brink W. Ranking the harm of alcohol, tobacco and illicit drugs for the individual and the population. Eur Addict Res. 2010;16:202–7.
55. Belin D, Mar AC, Dalley JW, Robbins TW, Everitt BJ. High impulsivity predicts the switch to compulsive cocaine-taking. Science (80–). 2008; 320:1352–5.
56. Murray JE, Belin D, Everitt BJ. Double dissociation of the dorsomedial and dorsolateral striatal control over the acquisition and performance of cocaine seeking. Neuropsychopharmacology. 2012;37:2456–66.
57. Vollstädt-Klein S, Wichert S, Rabinstein J, Bühler M, Klein O, Ende G, et al. Initial, habitual and compulsive alcohol use is characterized by a shift of cue processing from ventral to dorsal striatum. Addiction. 2010; 105:1741–9.
58. Jentsch JD, Taylor JR. Impulsivity resulting from frontostriatal dysfunction in drug abuse: implications for the control of behavior by reward-related stimuli. Psychopharmacology (Berl). 1999;146:373–90.
59. Wiers RW, Boelema SR, Nikolaou K, Gladwin TE. On the development of implicit and control processes in relation to substance use in adolescence. Curr Addict Reports [Internet]. 2015;2:141–55. Available from: http://link.springer.com/10.1007/s40429-015-0053-z
60. Lees B, Mewton L, Stapinski LA, Squeglia LM, Rae CD, Teesson M. Neurobiological and cognitive profile of young binge drinkers: a systematic review and meta-analysis. Neuropsychol Rev. 2019;29:357–85.
61. Nigg JT. On inhibition/disinhibition in developmental psychopathology: views from cognitive and personality psychology and a working inhibition taxonomy. Psychol Bull. 2000;126:220.
62. Verdejo-García A, Lawrence AJ, Clark L. Impulsivity as a vulnerability marker for substance-use disorders: review of findings from high-risk research, problem gamblers and genetic association studies. Neurosci Biobehav Rev. 2008;32:777–810.
63. De Wit H. Impulsivity as a determinant and consequence of drug use: a review of underlying processes. Addict Biol. 2009;14:22–31.
64. Wiers RW, Gunning WBW, Sergeant JAJ. Is a mild deficit in executive functions in boys related to childhood ADHD or to parental multigenerational alcoholism? J Abnorm Child … [Internet]. 1998 [cited 2013 Apr 5];26:415–30. Available from: http://link.springer.com/article/10.1023/A:1022643617017
65. Sher KJ. Children of alcoholics: a critical appraisal of theory and research. University of Chicago Press; 1991.

66. Nigg JT. Temperament and developmental psychopathology. J Child Psychol Psychiatry Allied Discip. 2006;47:395–422.
67. Finn PR, Hall J. Cognitive ability and risk for alcoholism: short-term memory capacity and intelligence moderate personality risk for alcohol problems. J Abnorm Psychol. 2004;113:569–81.
68. Ersche KD, Jones PS, Williams GB, Turton AJ, Robbins TW, Bullmore ET. Abnormal brain structure implicated in stimulant drug addiction. Science (80–). 2012;335:601–4.
69. Bechara A, Damasio H, Tranel D, Damasio AR. Deciding advantageously before knowing the advantageous strategy. Science (80–). 1997;275:1293–5.
70. Maia TV, McClelland JL. A reexamination of the evidence for the somatic marker hypothesis: what participants really know in the Iowa gambling task. Proc Natl Acad Sci USA. 2004;101:16075–80.
71. Bechara A, Dolan S, Hindes A. Decision-making and addiction (part I): impaired activation of somatic states in substance dependent individuals when pondering decisions with negative future consequences. Neuropsychologia. 2002;40:1675–89.
72. Naqvi NH, Bechara A. The hidden island of addiction: the insula. Trends Neurosci. 2009;32:56–67.
73. Jean-Richard-dit-Bressel P, Lee JC, Liew SX, Weidemann G, Lovibond PF, McNally GP. Punishment insensitivity in humans is due to failures in instrumental contingency learning. Elife. 2021;10:e69594.
74. Damasio AR, Everitt BJ, Bishop D, Damasio AR. The somatic marker hypothesis and the possible functions of the prefrontal cortex. Philos Trans Biol Sci. 1996;351:1413–20.
75. Naqvi N, Rudrauf D, Damasio H, Bechara A. Damage to the insula disrupts addiction to cigarette smoking. Science (80–). 2007;315:531–5.
76. Goldstein RZ, Bechara A, Garavan H, Childress AR, Paulus MP, Volkow ND. The neurocircuitry of impaired insight in drug addiction. Trends Cogn Sci. 2009;13:372–80.
77. Schoenbaum G, Chang CY, Lucantonio F, Takahashi YK. Thinking outside the box: orbitofrontal cortex, imagination, and how we can treat addiction. Neuropsychopharmacology. 2016;41:2966–76.
78. Menon V. Large-scale brain networks and psychopathology: a unifying triple network model. Trends Cogn Sci [Internet]. 2011;15:483–506. Available from: 10.1016/j.tics.2011.08.003
79. Robinson TE, Berridge KC. Addiction. Annu Rev Psychol. 2003;54:25–53.
80. Pearl J, Mackenzie. D. The book of why: the new science of cause and effect. NY: Basic Books; 2018.
81. Oleson EB, Gentry RN, Chioma VC, Cheer JF. Subsecond dopamine release in the nucleus accumbens predicts conditioned punishment and its successful avoidance. J Neurosci. 2012;32:14804–8.
82. Nader K, Schafe GE, Le Doux JE. Fear memories require protein synthesis in the amygdala for reconsolidation after retrieval. Nature. 2000;406:722–6.
83. Cunningham WA, Raye CL, Johnson MK. Neural correlates of evaluation associated with promotion and prevention regulatory focus. Cogn Affect Behav Neurosci. 2005;5:202–11.
84. Becker JB, McClellan ML, Reed BG. Sex differences, gender and addiction. J Neurosci Res. 2017;95:136–47.

4 Why addiction is (usually) not a chronic brain disease

In the previous chapter, I discussed research showing that addiction is associated with various neuroadaptations or changes in the brain. These cause cues announcing the availability of the substance or activity to attract attention and become attractive themselves (incentive salience). Furthermore, substance use creates negative feelings, coupled with an easy recipe for making them disappear (i.e., taking the drug again). In some individuals, especially in impulsive ones, this subsequently develops into compulsive use where the signal always leads to use. Some develop an enormously strong desire for drug use, in which "hidden island of addiction" (insula) play an important role, and all of these neuroadaptations together "hijack" the addicted brain. Logically, given all these neuroadaptations and their effects, it becomes difficult, if not impossible, to quit addiction and as a result the brain disease becomes chronic. This is what proponents of the brain model of addiction believe we must recognize; we should help addicted people, rather than blaming them for their addiction or punishing them.

Over the past decade, there has been an increasingly strong dissenting voice arguing that addiction is *not* a chronic brain disease. What are the arguments? As we saw, the strongest evidence for changes in the brain due to addiction necessarily comes from animal research, because that's where true experiments can be done, in which laboratory animals are randomly distributed among different experimental groups, from which causal effects can be derived. A major line of criticisms of the chronic disease model of addiction is about the value of animal research for understanding addiction in humans. A related second is about the usefulness of the chronic disease model for understanding and dealing with addictions in humans, who are more than isolated brains. Finally, the claim that the brain disease model would reduce blame and stigma has been challenged.

DOI: 10.4324/9781032634548-4

Animal research does not say much about addiction in humans

Over forty years ago, Canadian psychologist Bruce Alexander believed that animal models of addiction had little relevance to understanding addiction in humans because experimental animals—usually rats—were kept in unnatural ways in solitary cages, whereas they are social animals by nature. Alexander therefore developed an alternative experimental setup, which would later be called "Rat Park", in which the animals were housed in a colony, with plenty of room to play. The researchers compared how much morphine water the rats from the Rat Park used compared with those confined in solitary cages according to then-standard procedures.

The results were clear: the rats in solitary cages drank much more morphine water than the animals in Rat Park, which often preferred plain water. Even caged animals that were first addicted in isolation generally preferred water when given the opportunity to play with the other rats in Rat Park.[1–3] These results went directly against the established view that animal models are a good model for addiction in humans, and emphasized the importance of social context in addiction. According to Alexander, addiction is primarily a social problem: when people are lonely and unhappy (in our lonely apartment-cages in modern society) and narcotics are available, addiction can easily develop.[4]

As is often the case with results that go against a dominant view, the Rat Park studies were initially ignored or dismissed by researchers studying brain mechanisms in addiction. As the model of addiction as a chronic brain disease became dominant, opponents of this perspective began to refer more to these pioneering experiments. Animal researchers have now also become more aware of the influence of social context on substance use. In addition, animal models have evolved further. For example, animals in current experiments are usually no longer raised in isolation and forced into addiction, but can choose whether or not to use a drug, and in some cases a choice is created between the drug and access to other rats.[5] To illustrate, a recent study (forty years after Rat Park, which was not referred to), in Yavin Shaham's lab[i] examined how rats chose between drugs and social interactions.[6] The results confirmed those of the Rat Park study: virtually all rats preferred playing with peers (social interaction) to substance use, even animals that had already been made addicted to two of the most addictive drugs: methamphetamine and heroin.[6] The researchers indicated that the minority of animals that

i Perhaps surprisingly, this study was conducted at NIDA, where the chronic brain disease model is still the official doctrine, see www.nida.com.

preferred to take drugs under these conditions may provide a better animal model of addiction than mainstream models.

A related interesting study, in terms of clinical implications, compared rats that had first been forced into addiction, and then were forced to rehab (alone again, in their cages), with rats that chose social interactions when possible and therefore stopped ("voluntarily") with using the same drug. The first group showed characteristic drug-seeking behavior in the form of endlessly pressing a pedal that had previously provided the drug, while this was not the case in the animals that had chosen social interactions above drugs. One could take this as support for the idea that in addiction therapy it is crucial to encourage a person's own motivation to change, which is also central to a widely used technique in addiction treatment: motivational interviewing. I discuss this in Chapter 7.

The aforementioned studies undermine the value of much of the previous animal research, in which the animals were mostly isolated and made addicted. Indeed, the research indicates that addiction traits would disappear like snow in the sun in most individuals, if given the opportunity to play with their peers.[6] This raises the question of what the findings on brain changes in these animals tell us about addiction in humans. The good news is that some animal researchers are now convinced of this and are making efforts to develop better models in which voluntary choice and social interactions do play a role.

Addictive behavior is habitual, but not compulsive

A second line of criticism targets the idea that in addiction, impulsive use turns into compulsive use.[7] The studies on which this theory is built investigates laboratory animals that first learn to press a pedal after which it is given a drug, followed by a period in which touching same pedal gives no more drug (extinction) or even a shock, as we saw in the previous chapter. The critical test was what happens after the change—does the drug seeking stop or continue? According to supporters of the theory that addiction develops from impulsive to compulsive behavior, the animals should then continue to press the pedals. English researcher Lee Hogarth recently performed a systematic review of all the studies on this phenomenon, including both animal and human studies. Across both lines of research, he found little support for the theory: most addicted animals and humans alike do change their behavior when they receive punishment instead of reward.[8] These findings go against the idea that the habit of taking the drug becomes compulsive in addiction. Of course, it is possible that this mechanism does play a role, but only in a small minority of individuals of which high impulsivity was a predictor.

This is also not to say that habits do not play a role in addiction: in human substance use, they are a factor of importance: the drink before dinner, the wine with dinner, the cognac afterward, etc. The question is to what extent in addiction, the usual habitual use turns into *compulsive* use. This is important because the difference is that we can correct habitual behavior if it does not lead to the desired result (a shock rather than a drink! or more likely, a headache the next morning after that cognac), which is very difficult with a compulsive act. Let's consider an everyday example: you finish work and walk to the office's front door to leave and ... oh yes, there was a renovation so you now have to leave the building through the backdoor. Much of our behavior is driven by habitual control mechanisms, you don't need to pay attention how you exit the building when your goal is to leave, but as soon as we notice that the habit no longer leads to the desired result, we focus our attention on finding a new solution.[9] If the behavior were compulsive, the person in this example would just keep pulling the front door, which always worked, even though it is locked because of the ongoing renovation works. Habitual behavior is originally purposeful (I go in and out through that door every day), and the frequent repetition eliminates the need for conscious control.[9,10] The same argument against the compulsive model of addiction has been used by researchers Robinson and Berridge,[11] whom we encountered earlier in describing the sensitized response to reward signals or the call of the Sirens.[ii]

Good arguments have now been made against the idea that addiction is compulsive behavior, although it could play a role in some cases. The alternative is that it resembles highly motivated but still flexible behavior. For example, when a smoker's lighter does not work, he looks for alternatives and does not compulsively keep trying the broken lighter to get a flame out of it (although perhaps longer than the non-smoker). That seems obvious, but that search for alternatives indicates that addictive behavior is not entirely automatic, that people want to achieve a goal (in this case to light the cigarette with the motive to temporarily relief tension, for example) and think creatively about how to succeed.

People have self-control and long-term goals that can influence their behavior

A third line of criticism concerns the important role that language and conscious intentions play in human behavior. People can direct their behavior in view of a goal they have in mind, and that goal may be far in the future. Although there is much overlap between the brains of

ii Note that this was done in the context of discussions about which neuroadaptations are most important in addiction, a discussion between neuroscientists adhering to variants of the brain disease model of addiction.

experimental animals like the rat and humans, especially where primary reward systems are concerned, there are also major differences. We are constantly weighing our behavior against different goals, which enables us to make our behavior serve a long-term goal, even if that means foregoing short-term gratification—one of the virtues already discussed by Socrates and Protagoras in their discussion of *akrasia*: sometimes you have to do something unpleasant or forego something pleasant in order to achieve an important goal later. This virtue has been labelled self-control.

In psychology, research on the development of self-control was made famous by the marshmallow experiment by Columbia psychologist Walter Mischel and his team. That experiment found that children who managed to not eat a marshmallow at a young age, in order to receive a larger reward (two marshmallows) after waiting, did better years later as adolescents than the children who ate the marshmallow—both in terms of their health and school performance.[12] The famous Dunedin study (named after a city in New Zealand where some 2000 newborns were assessed from birth, discussed in more detail in Chapter 6), individual differences in self-control also predicted a more positive development in the future, including a lower likelihood of addiction and other mental health problems later in life, and they included many more measures of self-control than a single marshmallow test. This indicates that self-control is an important trait for humans. And that is exactly something other animal species are notoriously bad at. Another illustration by our late dog Tarzan, from the previous chapter. When we had dinner, we put him in his cage, where he would get his dog cookie, allowing the people in the house to eat without a begging dog around the table. When Tarzan picked up signals that we are about to eat (time of day, handling of cutlery), he ran to his bench wagging his tail—in fact, he was typically the only one to respond when the day's chef announced dinner. After being allowed into the cage to receive his cookie, the door closed behind him and he would soon realize that he was locked in again and turned his back to these mean people (yes, dogs can turn their backs to you). However, none of this leads to him running towards the cage less enthusiastically at the next meal announcement: the foresight of the close reward clearly overpowered any other thought.

In comparative psychology, cognitive functions that play an important role in human behavior, like working memory and other executive functions have been compared between different species, often between great apes and children.[13] Working memory has been related to self-regulation abilities in humans,[14] and consists of different functions, including a system temporarily keeping decaying information active, in humans supported by language (called the phonological buffer by Baddeley[15]), a strategic sub-system to support goal-directed behavior and an attentional control subsystem, to focus on relevant aspects in the environment, in light of currently active goals.[13,16] In human children, working memory gradually increases, to plateau in puberty at the famous "magical number" of 7±2 (i.e., the number of items an average person can hold in their short-term memory). In non-human great apes, there is a parallel increase, but the capacity in great apes is surpassed from toddlerhood in human children, as a recent systematic review concluded.[13] Cognitive functions that are distinctively human or only nascent in other species include causal understanding and prospective memory, or thinking about how the future could be, rather than how it is now.[13] These functions are important in the development of addiction, including recovery, which limits the relevance of theories based on animal models to understanding addiction in humans.

People can flip a switch

It is clear that it is difficult for many people to change ingrained patterns of behavior, especially in addiction, given the neuroadaptations described in the previous chapter, but at the same time it is possible. Some addicted people manage to "flip a switch: and stop smoking and sometimes even the use of alcohol or other drugs overnight.[17] This often happens after something profound has happened that puts everything in a different light, such as the death of a family member or close friend from smoking related illness.[18] Others, like Bill Wilson, one of the founders of AA, describe having suddenly beholding the divine light and radically quit excessive use. There are also people who suddenly see themselves through someone else's eyes, so to speak, which gives a new perspective. University of Mexico psychologist Bill Miller, a famous clinical researcher who developed the treatment method of motivational interviewing (discussed further in Chapter 7), provides an example:

> A father went to pick up his children from school because it was raining hard. He was waiting in the car and noticed that he was out of cigarettes and thought he could get some quickly before the children arrived. He drove off to the tobacco store and in his rearview mirror saw the children running outside, and realized that they saw their father driving away, standing in the rain. It had apparently gotten to the point where he considered his addiction more important than his children, and that realization was a strong motivator to radically quit smoking.

The point is that an event like the one described above can change a person's perspective on the world, resulting in a radical change in behavior. It seems difficult if not impossible to capture such a change in an animal models. You can gain insight into changes in brain networks that have to do with learning and reward, but you miss the factors of human behavior that have to do with longer-term goals and values, and those are precisely what have been shown to be of great importance in overcoming addiction.[19,20] This in turn has to do with "free will", as discussed in Chapter 2: people can adjust their behavior based on a representation of the outcomes of various choices. Not that it is easy, but at least there is the ability to do so.

Most people quit addictions without treatment

A related argument concerns the course of addiction in humans. The view that addiction is a chronic brain disease, where relapse is the norm, leans heavily on studies with patients most of whom indeed relapse after treatment.[21] But the vast majority of people who struggle with addiction at some point in their lives are not treated at all and overcome the problem without professional help. Estimates vary by substance, but for the common addictions of alcohol, tobacco and cannabis, less than 10% of people are treated for their addiction.[22]

American psychologist Gene Heyman wrote a groundbreaking book provocatively titled *Addiction: A Disorder of Choice*,[23] in which he argues that throughout history the vast majority of people who use a drug excessively for some time, eventually greatly reduce use or stop using it. This happens when the use gets too much in the way of other goals in life. According to Heyman, both immediate rewards and later disadvantages play a role in the onset of excessive use and in the cessation of use. It is a continuous balancing act that can change over time. Often in young people, the benefits are stronger—the substances play a role in building friendships and relationships—while later, the drawbacks become stronger: not showing up fresh to work the next day. Hence, the peak in human addictions is in young adulthood and most people mature out after that.[24–26] In terms of *akrasia*, according to Heyman, there is no *akrasia* in most people who use substances excessively for some time: the trade-off between pros and cons at the time of use leads to the decision to use the substance and the later trade-off is precisely to reduce or stop. While this may be true for common substance addictions like alcoholism or cigarette smoking, is it also true for hard drugs like heroin?

The natural "Vietnam experiment" showed that this is indeed the case, at least when there is a change in context: many American soldiers were addicted to heroin during the Vietnam War, which was readily available there, along with the negative and often traumatizing events of war.[27] Before they were allowed to fly home, they had to kick their drug use habit and because the army was worried that many ex-soldiers would wander around as junkies after returning, they followed the soldiers up to see how they were doing. Perhaps surprisingly, the number of ex-soldiers who relapsed into heroin addiction was low: after three years, only 12% had relapsed into heroin addiction. The explanation is often sought in the changed context: the soldiers had become addicted during the war in Vietnam, in order to stay afloat under the extreme conditions of that war, but back in the US, the environment was completely different; heroin was less readily available, and the new context did not provide cues that would reawaken the *craving*. But it also shows that the model of a brain chronically addicted to hard drugs that no longer has a choice ("once addicted always addicted") was wrong, at least for the vast majority of these young adults.[28] Note that the helpful effect of a change in context can be used when you wish to change a maladaptive habit (or someone else's): take advantage of a natural change in context (e.g., move of house, new job). For example, if you are used to smoking in the car and want to quit, make it easy on yourself and quit when you buy a new car, in which you will never smoke. In this way you make sure your new car does not become a new smoking context and chances are that you will not develop a strong urge to smoke in the new car.

While these changes have been related to the dramatic change in context between war in Vietnam and the very different situation back home in the US, the question may arise what the natural course of addiction is without such a dramatic change in context. Large population studies in the US have shown a similar pattern: most people who were addicted in young adulthood were no longer so by later measurements (over a decade later, three-quarters were no longer addicted). The minority who was still addicted often suffered from other mental health problems, often using substances to cope with these problems—as we saw, a strategy that typically exacerbates problems in the long term. Indeed, many people in addiction treatment suffer from additional mental health problems, which makes this group not representative of all people who face addiction sometime in their lives.[23,28]

The question, then, is whether the descriptions of heavily addicted people who successfully kick their habit and move on with their lives should be considered the exception or rather as examples of the normal course and that those who *fail* to quit addiction are the exception and therefore seek professional help. I would argue that based on the epidemiological data, the people whose addiction is best described as a chronic brain disease are the proverbial black swans, not the people who successfully quit.[29]

The brain is constantly changing

A second line of criticism focuses on the argument that addiction is a chronic brain disease because it is characterized by persistent changes in the brain (the neuroadaptations summarized in the previous chapter). The Canadian neuroscientist Marc Lewis, a leading voice in this debate, put forward the counter-argument that yes, changes occur in the brain when someone becomes addicted, but that the same is always true when people learn something or fall in love and that the brain is plastic.[17,30,31] He wrote a book about his own addiction problems before making a career as a neuroscientist,[32] describing his life as an undergraduate in Berkeley in the 1970 s, where he experimented with all sorts of drugs to end up, as an increasingly addicted intern in a hospital, stealing morphine to satisfy his strong need for drugs. He details the effects of various substances on mind and brain together with his own experiences. After a broken marriage and career (the proverbial hitting *rock bottom*, in addiction recovery stories), he was able to build a new life and career as a neuroscientist. In a later book, he turned against the disease model of addiction and illustrates it with interviews of long-term addicted people after recovery.[17]

When we learn something, the brain changes, as illustrated by studies of the brains of London taxi drivers. Researchers found that parts of the hippocampus, a key brain area in memory processes, are larger in taxi drivers than in bus drivers with the same number of years of service. The difference between these groups is that taxi drivers determine their own routes, for which a mental map is crucial (this was before navigational devices), while bus drivers drive fixed routes.[33] When you learn something, your brain changes, whether it's riding a bike, learning a language or using a drug and what comes with it. Therefore, by analogy, the brain changes that occur in addiction are not necessarily evidence of a chronic brain disease; they could simply show that the addict has learned something and developed an affectionate relationship with some objects and a related activity. What is key, is that it is demonstrated that the brain changes are related to the addictive behavior and that they make a discontinuation of this behavior difficult if not impossible.[34]

Lewis discusses the various learning mechanisms involved in addiction and discussed in the previous chapter. Relatively weak control, according to Lewis, is normal when an immediate reward is available, whether sex, gambling, snacking, or an addictive drug, and thus not a unique characteristic of addicted brains either. The crucial question is whether the control over impulses also increases again after abstinence; perhaps surprisingly, little is known about that. Lewis cites some studies that show an improvement in brain connections related to self-control after total abstinence.[35,36] That's promising, but there are also studies that show poor recovery after abstinence.[37,38]

Above all, Lewis gives a different perspective: a perspective of development, including the possibility of growth in recovery, similar to growth after a crisis. This idea comes from positive psychology, which in recent years has paid much attention to psychological growth after trauma.[39,40] As the proverb says, "What does not kill you makes you stronger". This is a hopeful idea, but questions have been raised about the research methods used to demonstrate the phenomenon: it almost always involved retrospective data, that is, people report after the trauma that they are doing much better now than right after the trauma, and indeed even better than before the trauma. The problem with this is that research has shown that such retrospective data is only moderately correlated with objectively measured growth.[41] Note that the critical authors do not deny the existence of psychological growth after trauma, but they do believe that, when measured objectively, it is not the most common response after trauma.[41] This could also be the case after addiction (maybe Lewis did interview "black swans" or exceptional cases of recovery after long severe addiction).

The least we can conclude from Lewis' story and those of other people who managed to overcome their addiction is that addiction is not always a chronic brain disease.[29] At the same time, it is clear that there are also people who cannot get rid of their addiction.[42] For this small group of severely addicted people, programs have been set up in which the drug is provided (e.g., providing heroin to long-term heroin addicted people), with the primary goal of improving participants' quality of life, while at the same time reducing the nuisance. For these severe cases (participants were selected to have been long-term addicted and tried everything to quit in vain), it appears to make sense to speak of addiction as a chronic brain disease, as it leads to humane action.[42,43] However, this concerns only a small fraction of all people classifying with the diagnosis sometime in their lives, as the epidemiological data have shown.

How strong is the evidence for irreversible brain changes in addiction?

Over ten years ago I received a request from the Dutch governmental health care research organization (ZonMW, the small Dutch nephew of NIH), which requested me to do a literature review on what exactly we know about changes in the brain as a result of addiction. There was an interesting addition after this clear question: *so not from abuse or problematic use*. The addition caused some further questions: can someone be addicted *without* problematic use? Here a brief foray into definitions of addiction is relevant.

At the time of the assignment (2011), the fourth edition of the *Diagnostic and Statistical Manual of Mental Disorders* (DSM-IV) published by the American Psychiatric Association (APA) was still the leading classification scheme, distinguishing between abuse of and dependence on psychoactive substances. Abuse was the lighter diagnosis, where you only had to meet one of four criteria, and it mainly came down to putting yourself or others at risk through substance use, such as using under dangerous circumstances (e.g., drunk driving), neglecting social roles (you don't pick up your kids because you're drunk on the couch) or violations of the law. The more severe diagnosis of "substance dependence" required meeting at least three out of seven criteria, including the classic indications of physical dependence (tolerance and withdrawal), as well as characteristics of loss of control (continuing for longer than planned, intending to quit but failing, giving up other activities in order to use, etc.).

The more recent edition of the manual, the DSM-5, introduced in 2013, not only departed from the Roman numeration, but also combined the 11 criteria of abuse and dependence.[iii] Now a person had to meet at least two of those 11 criteria to be diagnosed as an addict. Furthermore, the criterion "problems with the law" varied too much between countries (in one country you can ask a police officer for a light for your joint, in another you go straight to jail) and was therefore replaced by craving. Increasing the minimum number of criteria for a diagnosis from one to two was generally welcomed. A "severity score" was also added, referring to the number of symptoms added up (2–11).

What is striking about all these criteria is that nowhere is there any mention of how much you have to drink, inhale or inject to meet criteria. This makes sense in a way, because people differ in how sensitive they are to the effects of substances. But ... they also differ in interpreting loss of control. Some think (wrongly) that they are still fully *in charge* after a night of drinking, and get in the car. Therefore, we have laws that are not about the extent to which people *thinks* they are in control, but about how much alcohol is found in the blood at the time of driving, which not only depends on how much was drunk, but also on gender, weight and factors influencing digestion rate. When we now turn to health damage by alcohol (or other addictive substances), it also increases with increased use. And that increase in many areas is non-linear but exponential, that is, the damage from drinking eight glasses of alcohol is not double of that of four, but more.[44]

I discussed these issues with a European group of researchers after which we wrote a "target article", in which we argued that we should define problematic substance use primarily based on how much a person uses and not on subjective assessments of control over use. Take that

iii Furthermore, problematic gambling was also added to the category, which previously dealt only with addictions to psychoactive substances (*substance use disorders*). Behavioral addictions return in Chapter 9.

nice daily glass of wine with dinner in Mediterranean countries like France and Italy. That leads to few social problems and loss of control and thus to relatively few diagnoses given the amount of alcohol consumed. But the number of alcohol consumption-related liver problems in a country does correlate strongly with the total amount of alcohol consumed in that country, regardless of the percentage of people who qualify their use as problematic or not. An additional advantage of a diagnosis based on excessive consumption is that the solution is obvious (i.e., drink less). Furthermore, there is less stigma with a diagnosis that you drink too much than with a diagnosis of addiction, especially if the latter refers to a chronic brain disease, about which more in a moment.

From this alternative definition, with its emphasis on how much a person consumes, reducing becomes an alternative goal, which for many people is more realistic than total abstinence. Take Joanna, a sociable young woman who drinks a few glasses of wine five times a week. Okay, usually half a bottle, because she typically shares one with a friend. She basically only does so on special occasions, catching up with friends, at a nice dinner, after a nice game of tennis and Monday night after singing. That's too much according to the current understanding of health effects of alcohol and the advice based on that: a maximum of one glass a day, and not every day.[45] If Johanna manages to cut her consumption in half on these "special" occasions (of which there are always many more than we think, such special lives we lead!), then she is still drinking too much according to current advice, but has *more than* halved her risk of health damage. And those risks are not imaginary. For example, excessive drinking is linked not only to liver damage—which most people know about—but also to many cancers, including breast cancer, one of the leading causes of death in young women.

Hence, we argued that long-term excessive use is actually a much more meaningful definition of substance problems, than "addiction". From this perspective, the question to me and my lab about the effects of addiction on the brain *separate from excessive use* was unanswerable. After all, were there any studies in which two groups drank or used exactly the same amount, but one group was "addicted" and the other was not? The answer is no, and that is for good reasons: long-term excessive use is a prerequisite for addiction.

After this brief aside about definitions, the question remains what we now know about the effects of excessive substance use (or addiction) on the brain and to what extent any adverse effects recover after (long-term) abstinence. Our systematic literature review about 10 years ago showed that many neurocognitive functions recovered at least partially after long-term abstinence (usually 6 to 12 months).[46] The tricky part in interpreting the data was that measurements of the same functions had almost never been done *before* the person had become addicted. This is understandable, because that process takes many years and then a person still needs to enter treatment. In the studies we included in the review, one measurement had been taken shortly after detoxification and then another one sometime later (often 3 months later). The general pattern was that addicted people did better on the test after several months of successful abstinence, but generally scored lower than their peers from similar backgrounds. "Partial recovery" was often the conclusion in the original papers.

As we argued, this conclusion is problematic, because the lower score immediately after detoxification could be due to many things, such as the effects of detoxification on brain functioning or years of excessive substance use. Another possibility is that the relatively weak functions in these people compared with non-addicted people may have been present before their addiction, and may have contributed to the onset of their addiction or to their failure to overcome it by themselves. The latter idea may seem far-fetched at first, but it is not, because many of the same functions play a role in the risk of developing addiction, as we will see in Chapter 6. These include brain functions related to self-control, planning, working memory and stopping undesired impulses, sometimes summarized as "executive" or "cognitive control" functions. So there is no good reason to assume that the suboptimal scores in people with addiction are caused by the addiction; they may have made the road to addiction more likely.[47,48] What's also possible is that both are true: brain functions related to relatively poor self-control and high impulsivity are a risk factor for an early onset of substance use, which in turn further compromises the further development of the same functions. The fact that scores in addicted people improve after abstinence is hopeful and is often interpreted as *partial* recovery, but so we don't actually know whether this is partial or *full* recovery (relative to a lower starting level), without measurement prior to addiction.

A more recent meta-analysis, combined data from nearly three thousand alcohol-dependent patients who had undergone neuropsychological testing. As standardized tests were used, the results could be compared with those of the general population.[49] The analysis showed that the patients scored lower on average in almost every domain compared to the general population, and that while many functions improved after long-term abstinence, they still scored relatively poorly a year later, especially on verbal and memory tests. Again, although we cannot say with certainty to what extent this was cause or effect, it is likely that at least some of the problems were caused by excessive alcohol consumption, given the breadth of the problem. It should also be noted that the damage may have been amplified by vitamin deficiency, which is often associated with alcohol dependence

(Korsakoff syndrome). So let there be no mistake: long-term excessive consumption of alcohol has negative effects on the brain in virtually all areas, and the same can be said for other drugs, as the meta-analysis of brain networks at the end of the previous chapter indicated.[50] But some of those functions seem to recover at least partially after long-term abstinence, and perhaps this can be enhanced with targeted cognitive training (discussed in Chapter 8).[51]

Brain problems caused by adolescent drinking and smoking

Given the difficulties in interpreting the neuropsychological problems of long-term addicted people due to the lack of measurement before they were addicted, a relatively large amount of research has been done on the effects of excessive use of alcohol and other substances in adolescence. Here, unfortunately, the same problem applies as with the studies comparing the brain functioning in addicted versus non-addicted adults: many studies do not have assessments prior to the addiction, which does not allow us to properly determine cause and effect. Based on animal research and scarce human data, it was decided at the time that there was sufficient evidence to assume that excessive alcohol consumption at an early age caused negative effects on brain development. Partly for this reason, the age limit for alcohol in the Netherlands was raised from 16 to 18 in 2013. This followed a hearing in the parliament of experts in the field a couple of years before, who all witnessed that the state of the science was that an earlier age of onset was related to an increased chance of developing problems later in life. I was one of them, and when the change of law took effect, my oldest son had just turned 16 and could no longer legally drink for another year and a half. He wanted to have a word with me, with his friends.

Shortly after, a comprehensive study by the Dutch Trails consortium cast doubts: the researchers had followed more than 2,000 adolescents in the northern provinces and had a premeasurement of neuropsychological functions at age 11 before drinking. With the data at later ages, they categorized participants into a number of groups according to their drinking habits during adolescence—from teetotalers to heavy drinkers—and compared the scores on the same neuropsychological tests at age 19. Perhaps surprisingly, they found no differences whatsoever.[52] Universities value publicity these days, so a press release was published by the communications department of Utrecht University, where the first author, Sarai Boelema, was to defend her PhD thesis on this research. It was picked up by one of the main national newspapers, *The Volkskrant*, which put it as headline on the next day's front page: "Alcohol and Teens: The Damage Doubted" (December 3, 2014). This was followed a day later by an analysis examining the policy implications: now that alcohol has been shown to have no effect on the adolescent brain, was the minimum drinking age rightly raised from 16 to 18? I was asked for a response, but I was in a quandary: I was on the promotion committee and had yet to pose my critical questions to the candidate, and it would be odd if she would be able to read these in the paper, the morning before the actual defense. We agreed that my response would appear a day later, after the PhD defense.[53]

I made a number of comments about the research. The main point was that previous research had shown that there are broadly two types of changes in brain functioning when young people start drinking (a lot): first, there are general executive control functions that we use to inhibit unwanted impulses, and these may become relatively weaker (or rather, excessive drinking frustrates further development). In addition, there are motivational responses, such as to what extent alcohol attracts your attention or tends to move you toward it, but these were not measured in this study. As for the weakening of control processes by alcohol consumption at a young age, this has emerged mainly from animal studies.[54] The evidence in humans is weaker, and as we saw, one can question to what extent findings on addiction from animal research can be translated well to humans.

There are indications that negative effects in humans after a period of excessive alcohol consumption can already be measured at the brain level, but not yet at the behavioral level. For example, the Belgian psychologist Pierre Maurage did a premeasurement of both neuropsychological behavioral tasks and brain measurements (EEG) freshmen, after which some of the students would start to drink a lot and some did not.[iv] He then indeed found effects on brain functioning that could be characterized as a weaker version of effects in long-term alcoholics, but found no differences (yet) on neuropsychological tasks.[55] The overall conclusion should probably be that brain damage in terms of these general control functions after excessive drinking during adolescence was not that bad yet, which a meta-analysis recently confirmed. It found generally small effects of drinking, except on tasks involving decision-making.[56] It should be noted that the ability to make wise decisions does constitute a crucial brain function when it comes to addiction, as we will see in the next chapter.

iv I asked him later how he had so beautifully selected those groups that would or would not start drinking heavily in the following year, while no difference between the groups had been observed beforehand. "That was simple," he replied: "I asked incoming students: are you here primarily to study or to party?" The higher the freshmen scored on "partying", the more they drank in the year to follow. This nicely indicates that excessive drinking during study time is goal-directed behavior, rather than something that happens to them due to a supposed immaturity of their brains.

As noted, our brain not only uses general control functions, but substance use at an early age also affects motivational processes (reward and salience networks in terms of contemporary neuroscience). However, those were not measured in the Trails study, so the conclusion that there are no effects on the brain when you start drinking at an early age could not be drawn. In fact, the researchers had cast their conclusions cautiously,[57] but before you know it, sweeping conclusions are drawn in news reports. The doubt was sown, and questions were raised in Parliament in response to the *Volkskrant* reports. Thereupon, the minister set up a committee at the Health Council to review all the evidence on effects of drinking during adolescence in various fields. Now, was there or was there not evidence of negative effects of alcohol consumption at an early age?

I was on that committee, and we examined effects of alcohol use in a number of areas: brain development (both structure and functioning), neuropsychological functioning, school and study, and later psychological problems.[58] The sub-reports and the final report can be found on the health council website, and the summary article was recently published.[59] Because of the aforementioned chicken-and-egg problems when comparing heavy drinkers with non-drinkers, we included only studies with pre-measurements, before the person in question drank (a lot). The general conclusion was that surprisingly little research had actually been done in which pre-measurements had been taken and in which you could demonstrate a difference in development between (heavy) drinkers and total abstainers.[v]

The development of gray brain matter (neurons) showed an abnormal and accelerated decrease in young people who drank excessively. As for the development of white brain matter (myelin, important for efficient connections between brain regions) and studies of brain responses to certain stimuli, this conclusion was not (yet) justified, although there were indications of negative effects of alcohol. We can therefore conclude that early drinking is in all likelihood not good for brain development, but in order to clarify this, larger studies are needed in which there is also a pre-measurement. There are now a number of such studies in Europe, including the Imagen study (with about two thousand European adolescents) and more recently an even larger study was initiated in America, the ABCD study, in which thousands of American adolescents are scanned and followed.[60]

One of the first publications of the Imagen study showed that personality is a much stronger predictor of early drinking onset than

v To draw reliable conclusions, we required at least three good independent studies with similar results.

all brain measures and genetics combined (while noting, of course, that personality is partly heritable): children who score high on impulsivity and sensation seeking are more likely to begin substance use at an early age.[61] Evidence was also found that excessive drinking affects personality development: the normal decline in impulsivity with age occurred less among excessive drinkers,[62] which had also been reported in an American study.[63] The negative effects of alcohol on cognitive functioning (the kind of neuropsychological tasks in the Trails study) were not clearly demonstrable. There were indications of negative effects on school performance, but these studies were generally not methodologically strong enough to draw clear conclusions (most studies had no pre-assessment).

The clearest link found between excessive drinking in adolescence and later outcomes was an increased risk of later alcohol problems: the likelihood of this increased greatly when someone had started drinking (a lot) at a young age.[59,64] All in all, there was enough evidence to report to the minister that drinking alcohol at a young age indeed still had negative effects according to our review of the science and that there was enough reason to maintain the 18-year age limit. In addition to the long-term negative effects of early drinking, there are of course the acute dangers of drunkenness, both to the person and to the environment (nightlife violence). When a young and healthy person dies or is seriously injured, chances are that alcohol or drugs were involved.

In summary, it is clear that starting to use alcohol and other substances at an early age creates an increased likelihood of various negative outcomes, which can be measured both at the brain level, and at the behavioral level (especially later addiction and longer persistence of impulsive behavior). In general, the changes are still relatively small during adolescence, although by then strong effects have been reported on decision processes that can influence further escalation of use. All the more reason, then, to curb use at an early age, and research, mostly from the US (from the time when States could determine their own legal drinking age), has shown that legislation can help.[65] In addition to an age limit, other effective policies include limiting advertising that encourages young people to drink,[66] making alcohol expensive and using minimum prices.[67] At this moment, in the Netherlands, weak versions of these measures are being introduced in the Netherlands based on the National Prevention Agreement, which is not surprising as the alcohol industry took part in the discussions (which was not the case for the tobacco industry, and indeed more effective measures have been taken to prevent smoking). In the US, attention has largely shifted to cannabis, after some states have legalized it, while others have not. There was an understandable fear that this would lead to an increase in youth marijuana use and use of other substances, but this was not found and there was evidence for a reduction in nondrug crimes.[68] However, one worrying aspect is marketing,[69] which some states allow, and which is likely to attract new young users, as has been convincingly demonstrated for alcohol.[66]

Although most of the research on effects of adolescent substance use has been on alcohol, there is also evidence of such negative effects with the use of other substances, such as tobacco smoking—something many people see as relatively harmless in terms of the effect it has on the brain (its often lethal effects on the lungs are well known). In a recent meta-analysis, we found the strongest negative effects on the ability to stop ("inhibition") for cigarette smoking, while looking at all possible substances and their combinations.[70] In another line of research, identical twins were studied, of whom one started smoking and the other did not. As they were genetically identical and were raised in the same family, differences in cognitive functions could be reasonably attributed to smoking. The researchers found that those who smoke show more attention problems than those who don't,[71] an interesting finding, as many smokers believe they can concentrate better when they smoke. In reality, smokers are on average *less* able to concentrate, something that may be temporarily alleviate by smoking. The same is true of their generally more negative mood, which is temporarily lifted somewhat by smoking (see Figure 4.1). But when they quit, their average mood and their ability to concentrate improves markedly after some time. Showing people this bigger picture may help them to quit smoking.

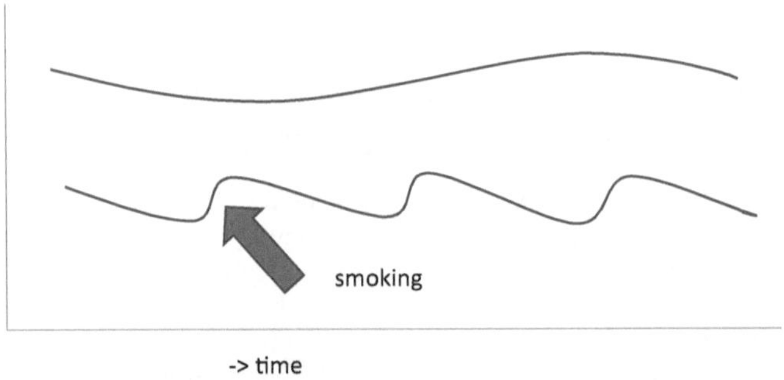

Figure 4.1 Sketch of differences in mood and ability to concentrate between smokers and non-smokers. For both mood and concentration, the average score is lower for the smoker, but it may temporarily improve after smoking. This creates the illusion that smoking helps against a negative mood or to improve concentration, while the non-smoker (and ex-smoker) in fact scores better.

So, all in all, there is strong evidence that alcohol has a negative effect on the development of various brain functions when started at a young age and quite some evidence that this is more generally the case with substance use. This does not imply that a substance-using adolescent has acquired a chronic brain disease, but it does lead to the conclusion that discouraging substance use before adulthood is a good recommendation, while leaving the question open what the most effective way is to do so, a question that will return in Chapter 6.

Excessive focus on the brain leads to ignoring social factors

A further criticism of the model of addiction as a chronic brain disease is that it ignores social factors, even though they are very influential in the development of addiction. Note that Leshner and later proponents of the chronic brain disease model of addiction, often mention social factors as contributing to addiction. However, the focus of the biomedical research has since been on unravelling mechanisms underlying the chronic brain disease.[72,73] For example, smoking is strongly related to socioeconomic status (a combination of education and income): people from poor neighborhoods smoke more than people from rich ones.[74] A child is much more likely to start smoking at a young age if many people around them smoke, so this is a problem that can be self-sustaining. How does this come about? One can look at changes in the brain that contribute to this. As we saw, it becomes harder to quit smoking later in life if you started at a young age. The argument here is that focusing on changes in brain processes ignores most important causes. One example is living in poverty without much prospect of improvement. In the case of minorities, who relatively often live in poor neighborhoods, negative experiences such as discrimination and exclusion add to the equation. This situation is even more dire in the US, where the image of addiction as a chronic brain disease prevails.

Carl Hart wrote a fascinating book on the subject, entitled *High Price*.[75] In it, he combined his own story, about an African-American boy growing up in a poor neighborhood in Miami, with a description of the development of his views on addiction. He is now a professor at Columbia University (NY), while some of his old friends have become dealers or ended up in prison. Hart described the difficult life in such a neighborhood and the easy way out by using alcohol and drugs. He himself managed to escape it by studying neuroscience, initially with the goal of contributing to solutions to the enormous problem of addiction. But over time, he came to the conclusion that research into addiction as a chronic brain disease was getting in the way of attention to its social and economic causes, and that the one-sided investment in this type of research was at the expense of research into effective prevention in the neighborhoods where the problems were most prevalent. He more recently criticized the aforementioned large American ABCD study, which spends billions to measure early changes in the brain, while there is virtually no money for research into socioeconomic causes of addiction[vi] and ways to counteract them.[76]

Related to this is the "war on drugs", which costs billions and has caused more African-Americans to be in prison now than there were slaves when slavery was abolished. A striking detail is that prisoners often work for a couple of dollars per day, which could be seen as a continuation of slavery, as a recent report from the University of Chicago Law School concluded.[77] Many young African-American men are incarcerated for drug use, and once they enter prison, they lose the right to refuse to work, otherwise they face additional punishments such as solitary confinement, lose opportunities to reduce their sentence and family visits. The link between poverty and (excessive) use of addictive substances undoubtedly contributes to the prejudice against young African-American men, in whom death from police brutality is one of the leading causes of death.[75] It is now widely acknowledged that the *war on drugs* has not worked. The question is what is the alternative: releasing all drugs? Given the intertwined nature of criminality and illegal drugs, there is certainly something to be said for that; the main issue is to protect the vulnerable, such as young people from using at an early age and developing addiction.[78] Carl Hart's more general point is that money should be allocated to doing research on ways to prevent addiction in vulnerable groups, rather than (almost) only to neuroscience research to unravel the supposed chronic brain disease.[34,73] And the answers won't always be easy.

Consider the following example; about ten years ago, a new medication (varenicline) was added to basic health insurance in the Netherlands, after a number of controlled studies showed that the drug could help people quit smoking. The idea behind this measure was that many poor people have difficulty quitting smoking and thus would not use this new medication if they had to pay for it themselves.[79] However, the main effect was that the new medication was used more by rich smokers wanting to quit. How could this be? The unexpected effect appeared to be related to so-called "social norms": people of low socioeconomic status were relatively more likely to find smoking normal and socially accepted (which is indeed the case in their neighborhoods). As people found it more normal to smoke, they became less likely to use a drug to quit smoking, whether that drug

vi You may wonder if this is not an exaggeration or solely a problem in the US. Consider this recent call from the British Wellcome trust, where 50 million dollars is spent solely on research into untangling the chronic brain disease addiction. https://wellcomeleap.org/ua/, especially the full program makes the priorities clear.

was reimbursed or not.[79] As long as that norm held, people saw little reason to stop smoking; neither the cost of the medication nor the high costs of smoking were perceived as an insurmountable problem. This would suggest that something would have to be done about that norm before this kind of help would be effective with this vulnerable group. The follow-up question is how to get that done, but that is not a question that can be answered in the sort of biomedical approaches that typically receive funding.

The brain disease model has done little for treatment or prevention

A related objection to the chronic brain disease model of addiction is that the huge investments have yielded little in terms of treatment or prevention. As someone remarked in an online network on the topic: "What did all these billions of dollars NIDA invested in brain research yield for treatment? NADA!" This problem, by the way, is not unique to addiction but applies to the treatment of many mental health problems, with the result that the pharmaceutical industry has reduced its investment in developing drugs for these supposed brain diseases.[80] Why is that the case?

One of the people who has written about this is Steve Hyman, a Harvard biomedical researcher and former provost. He blames the lack of progress on the use of animal models that do not cover the essence of mental health problems in humans. An animal model is useful for research on psychiatric problems only if the disease mechanism is conserved in evolution between the animal model and humans. Assuming that the mental life of the rat is more limited than that of humans, the value of animal models will be limited in diseases where thoughts about the future play an important role. This appears to be the case with many mental health problems, whether it is rumination in depression or obsessive desires in addiction. This supports the argument that animal models often miss the essence of psychological problems in humans.[28]

Another influential piece in *Lancet Psychiatry* also argued that the model of addiction as a chronic brain disease has yielded surprisingly little in the way of addiction treatment, despite large investments.[72] Instead, health gains have come from policies such as banning indoor smoking and limiting cigarette advertising. These authors did not conclude that research on neurobiological mechanisms in addiction should be abandoned or that no more new medications should be developed, but rather that the strong emphasis on this work has come at the expense of other research that has much more effect at the population level. Nora Volkow and George Koob wrote a rebuttal to this paper[81] claiming that the brain disease model did provide new molecular targets for medication and brain regions for neurostimulation, and updated the evidence restating the advances achieved in understanding addiction as a chronic brain disease.[82]

No underlying disease but an interplay of symptoms

The idea that mental health problems should best be conceived as brain diseases, chronic or not, is widespread. In a sense, it is almost trivial: if we assume that brains are indispensable to our mental life, then it makes sense study what has gone wrong in the brain when mental problems arise. As a result, the cause is sought in the underlying substrate: for example, in a misbalance of messenger substances ("neurotransmitters") in specific brain regions, such as serotonin in depression[83] or dopamine in addiction,[84] (which have both been criticized), or in overactive or underactive brain regions (e.g., in anxiety: your amygdala is oversensitive![85]). It is a variant of the medical model: you look for the cause of a problem in the underlying tissue, in the case of mental problems, it must be somewhere in the brain. As we saw in the previous critique, this has accomplished little when it comes to progress in treating these common mental health problems, perhaps because mental and social levels are crucial, and those are difficult to capture in animal models.[80]

In psychology, an alternative model for explaining the origins of psychological problems has been developed over the past decade, the "symptom network approach.[vii] The general idea is that symptoms are not caused by an underlying biological mechanism, as the medical model assumes, but that symptoms cause each other. Take Rosa, who worries a lot because of the many hassles she experiences at work. As a result, she does not sleep well and feels even more listless the next day. In order to still function at work, she drinks more coffee than she should, which leads to further turmoil in her head and the need to drink alcohol in the evening to relax and fall asleep. But the coffee and alcohol are not good for her sleep quality, which leads to awakenings almost every night, too often followed by ruminations about what she should do at work, where she finally arrives in a rather drowsy and irritable state, despite many morning coffees. What we see here is how symptoms cause each other, not only symptoms of one disorder, but symptoms affecting other symptoms regardless of borders by disorder. What began with worry

vii Researchers from the psychological methods group at the department of psychology at the University of Amsterdam, such as Denny Borsboom, Angelique Cramer and Han van der Maas, took the lead in this effort.

brings further problems, such as anxiety (whether influenced by the coffee or not) and excessive substance use.

For many medical problems, the reductionist disease model has worked well. For example, a person suffers increasing headaches, forgetfulness and impaired vision. To identify the cause, a brain scan is performed, which reveals that a brain tumor is at the root of these symptoms. If the tumor can be successfully operated on, the cause of the problems is removed and the symptoms are relieved. Importantly, one can also have headaches and suffer from forgetfulness without having a brain tumor. So in this example, the disease and the disease mechanism can be separated from the symptoms.[86] With psychological problems, this is different: it is hard to imagine a person feeling gloomy for a long time, losing appetite, thinking a lot about death and having sleep problems *without* having depression. The reverse is also difficult to imagine: could someone really be depressed when there are no symptoms of gloom and lethargy? That seems nonsensical. In short, in the case of mental disorders, the symptoms *are* the mental disorder, and the symptoms affect each other.[87–89]

The symptoms often take place at the psychological level, and the core of the mental disorder is an interplay of symptoms at this level, which cannot be reduced to a biological correlate in the brain or genes,[90] just like my mentor Nico Frijda explained to me, in my search for the right study. Which is not to say that biological factors don't play a role: for example, they can increase the likelihood that you will develop a symptom in the first place[91] or that you develop a related symptom if you already had an initial symptom.[viii]

Importantly, from the network perspective, it is misleading to refer to mental health problems as chronic brain diseases, or as Denny Borsboom, one of the pioneers of the network approach and colleagues provocatively called a "target paper": Brain disorders? Not really: Why network structures block reductionism in psychopathology research.[90]

This discussion is also relevant to the view of addiction and of former addicted people who, both from (biomedical) science and from the AA perspective, are likely to hear variations of the slogan "once addicted always addicted".[28] But to what extent does it make sense that someone who has not been drinking (or using) for years can still be called addicted? Like the partner of a fellow researcher who introduced herself to me at a reception: "Hi, I am Monica and I am an alcoholic". She drank only sodas and turned out to have been in recovery for 12 years.

viii The word "symptom" is historically related to the disease model and refers to an expression of an underlying problem. But to avoid confusion, this word is still widely used in the network approach.

Was she really still addicted? Or was being an (ex-)alcoholic an important identity for her? This recognition may have helped her quit drinking in the beginning, but now came across as a bit strange and appeared more of a hindrance for further development (would she announce this at job applications too?). And does it make sense that someone who has had depression before but is recovered also "really" is still depressed? In either case, this doesn't seem like a very useful idea, even though people who have dealt with the problem before do have an increased vulnerability to develop the disorder again, and it may be wise to avoid relapse, using relapse prevention techniques that have been developed in both disorders; in depression by my colleague Claudi Bockting and collaborators[92] and in addiction by ourselves, which will be discussed in Chapter 8.

In network models of mental problems, the causes of problems can be diverse, either external (e.g., loss of a loved one and one's reaction to it) or internal (e.g., a neurological problem that makes a person hear voices). The crux is that the symptoms subsequently activate other symptoms. This creates person-specific links of symptoms. Ideally, you would personalize treatment based on an individual's personal network of symptoms. Initial attempts are being made to do that, but the limiting factor is that this requires a lot of data, from a single participant, including multiple daily multiple assessments for weeks if not months.[93–97] Therefore one of the ways to optimize this approach that are currently studied is to combine individual data with those of a relevant group (e.g., people who became addicted to substance X at a late age). A major research program has recently started in the Netherlands to further develop and critically test this approach and its clinical applications: the *New Science of Mental Disorders*, led by Anita Jansen from Maastricht University.[98]

At the University of Amsterdam, another big interdisciplinary research program has been initiated, *Urban Mental Health.* It focuses on the interplay of factors that determine mental health in urban environments. These range from individual factors, including genetic and biological vulnerabilities, to all sorts of environmental factors ranging from noise, the feeling of insecurity or discrimination (minorities are overrepresented in urban areas) to the presence of greenspaces in the neighborhood. In doing so, mathematical models are used from complexity science, with the aim to arrive at new interventions for common mental problems (addiction, anxiety and depression), as described in a recent article in *Lancet Psychiatry.*[99] For addiction, this means that rather than focusing on the addicted brain only, as if living in a vacuum, environmental factors are assessed, in the family and social environment, in the neighborhood and at the city level. There are relatively many people in urban environments who develop mental health problems (above average), while there are also people who thrive in cities.[ix] Aim is to find out how this works and what we can learn from it to develop better interventions.

Relapse as a sign of chronic brain disease?

One of the grounds to call mental health disorders *chronic* brain diseases, is the high likelihood of relapse after treatment; for the most common mental health problems (anxiety, depression and addiction), about half of the treated patients relapse after treatment. The large American project Match study (described in more detail in Chapter 7) showed that 70% of people treated for alcoholism had relapsed three years after treatment.[21] However, we must keep in mind when interpreting this, that only a small group of all addicted people enter treatment and most people who struggle with addiction in their lives get over it without professional help.[23,100] All addiction therapies aim to prevent relapse, which is the hardest thing about addiction, harder than quitting. To quote Mark Twain: "Giving up smoking is the easiest thing in the world. I know because I've done it thousands of times."

An related question here is whether it is wise to advise people to never ever get close to the drug again, to prevent relapse (steered by their still addicted brain). There are people who take a cigarette after years of not smoking and then relapse, even though they know how bad it is for their health (the *akrasia* example in Chapter 2). At the same time, there are ex-smokers who have come to find the cigarette really disgusting after quitting and don't think about ever smoking again. With the already mentioned researcher Corinde Wiers (my second cousin who independently entered addiction research), we did a study of the automatically initiated approach responses to smoking-related pictures in smokers and non-smokers, with the result that we found a stronger tendency to approach these stimuli in smokers compared to non-smokers, as expected. She raised the interesting question whether this would still be found in ex-smokers: would they, having quit for years, still be sensitive to smoking pictures and show a tendency to approach them?[x] This would be expected based on the chronic brain disease model. Perhaps surprisingly, unlike the current smokers, the ex-smokers showed no tendency to approach smoking pictures, and were indistinguishable

ix See www.centreforurbanmentalhealth.com. I lead the center together with Claudi Bockting.

x This automatically initiated tendency to approach drug-cues has been related to sensitization and "sign-tracking", discussed in the previous chapter. This tendency can be influenced, which can help overcome alcohol addiction, which comes back in Chapter 8.

from the never-smokers.[101] So on this measure, there was no indication of ex-smokers to "really" still be addicted. It should be noted, however, that these were *successful* ex-smokers, to which one could counter that those in whom there was an automatic tendency to approach cigarettes would have relapsed after quitting. In another study, ex-smokers, like smokers, still showed an attentional bias for smoking cues, this is the degree to which smoking-cues attract and capture attention, which was not found in people who had never smoked.[102] So it is an interesting question to what extent different cognitive biases that influence decision processes in substance use normalize after successful cessation of use, or not; perhaps this differs between people, substances and cognitive biases (this will be further discussed in Chapter 8).

There is some evidence that for a subgroup of severely addicted people, it is indeed good advice to never use the substance again, because the risk of relapse is too high. At the same time, there are also many people who meet the criteria of alcohol addiction for a time and successfully reduce to lower levels of intake.[103] In (Dutch) clinical practice, counselor and client generally determine the goal together and some of the people want to reduce rather than stop, with that goal sometimes having to be adjusted in the long run because it does not seem to be working. In the US, likely under the stronger influence of AA and the chronic brain disease model, total abstinence is often the only possible treatment goal. A recent study modeling transitions from abstinence to recreational use and to problematic use and back, found that the intermediate state (recreational use) was less stable for cigarette smoking than for drinking alcohol and smoking marijuana,[104] confirming clinical wisdom that total abstinence is a wise goal for most who want to quit smoking.

Does the chronic brain disease model reduce or reinforce the stigma of addicted people?

In his aforementioned *Science* article Alan Leshner not only claimed that science had shown that addiction is a chronic brain disease, but also that accepting this stance, would reduce the stigma associated with it. Addicted people should no longer be blamed for their self-destructive behavior any more than you can blame someone with Alzheimer's for forgetting things. As we have seen in this chapter, the scientific support for the theory that addiction is a chronic brain disease is controversial, with some supporting evidence presented in the previous chapter and some caveats presented here. Relatively separate from the question of the scientific status of the chronic brain disease theory of addiction is the question of the *effect* of this view on the blame and stigma surrounding addiction: will it decrease, as Leshner argued, or not?

Previous research had shown that genetic explanations of mental health problems could indeed reduce associated feelings of guilt, but at the same time created more distance and reinforced idea that people with mental health problems are qualitatively different from normal people and therefore unpredictable and dangerous. It was also shown to create pessimism about the expected outcomes of treatment, both among the therapist and the patient. These conclusions are based on two meta-analyses, from University of Melbourne's Nick Haslam and colleagues, that systematically summarized the research on the topic. The first meta-analysis included correlational studies, examining the extent to which people who endorsed biological and genetic explanations of mental health problems blamed people with mental problems less.[105] That correlation was confirmed: don't blame me, it's my genes! At the same time, addicted people were considered more dangerous and unpredictable and people showed a somewhat stronger tendency to stay away from people with mental disorders if they believed the causes to be biological. People who believed more strongly in addiction than chronic brain disease also more strongly endorsed statement *once addicted is always addicted.*

These conclusions were supported by a second meta-analysis that examined experimental studies[106] from which, as we saw earlier, stronger conclusions about cause and effect can be drawn. In those studies, participants are randomly assigned to an experimental condition; for example, they first read either a paper on a genetic explanation of a mental health problem or, conversely, a paper on its social causes, after which their attitudes towards patients suffering from mental problems were examined. In line with the cross-sectional findings, after reading biological explanations for mental health problems, patients were blamed less. However, negative effects were also found here, related to the idea that people with mental health problems are fundamentally different from "normal" people. Statements that characterized mental problems as brain diseases produced an even more negative effect: people then had a greater tendency to keep distance from persons with mental problems, because they were considered dangerous.[107]

These studies summarized the literature on the effects of biogenetic explanations of mental health disorders in general, not specifically about addiction. Some recent studies did examine this more specifically. First, John Kelly, from Harvard Medical School, and colleagues tested the effects of different labels (from chronic brain disease to social problem) to describe a person addicted to opiates. Again, the brain disease label caused less blame, but also caused pessimism about the continuation of the addiction and increased the ascribed danger this person would pose to others.[108] A recent study compared stigma for addiction with depression and with diabetes. Public stigma was highest for addiction, followed by the combined diagnosis of addiction and depression.[109] A study that just came out, examined the influence of different factors in predicting stigma: the health condition (alcohol use disorder or diabetes), the label ("chronically relapsing brain disease" or "problem") and stability for treatment seeking and outcome (low or high). It was found again that addiction comes with a (much) greater public stigma than diabetes, but in line with earlier findings, the mixed pattern appeared with less blame but more perceived danger and social distance.[110]

In conclusion, from research in the 25 years after Leshner's claim that calling addiction a chronic brain disease would reduce stigma, a different picture emerges from the studies that actually studied the effect: the degree to which addicted people are blamed for their problems does indeed reduce, but it also leads people to see addicted people as a fundamentally different kind of people, who are dangerous and best kept away from. One may wonder how this comes about. The authors of the meta-analysis relate the findings to psychological essentialism. Essentialism is the view that there is an immutable essence that distinguishes a certain type of human from other types of people. It is an ancient way of thinking about species, dating back to Plato and Aristotle, that made it difficult to accept evolution, both in history[111] and in children[112] (which happened to be the topic of my master's thesis).[xi]

Psychological essentialism has been related to racism: the more we see people of another race as fundamentally different, the stronger the tendency to discriminate against them.[113,114] As we saw, psychological essentialism may also have negative consequences in relation to mental disorders, with some of the strongest effects in addiction. It is important to note that this doubtlessly has not been the intention of scientists propagating the chronic brain disease model of addiction; most will themselves adhere to a model in which there is much overlap between "normal" people and people with mental health problems. Given the dominance of essentialism among non-experts, however, news reports about the abnormal brains of children with ADHD, patients with depression or addicted people can easily be interpreted as evidence for the idea that those patients are simply categorically different, with all related negative consequences. They are fundamentally different, for which they are not to blame, but better stay away from them. According to current estimates, about half of all people experience serious mental

xi We had initially submitted the accompanying article with the title "*On the origin of species,*" which seemed a nice entry into the scientific world, but after a long review process it was finally published with the title "*Children's Thoughts on the Origin of Species: A Study of Explanatory Coherence.*

health problems at some point in their lives, and fortunately most of these disappear, with or without professional help, showing that mental disorders are in most cases a temporary condition that can affect all of us.

Conclusion

Although most scientists would agree that long-term addiction changes the brain and that the brain enables our mental life, the model of addiction as a chronic brain disease has met controversy, both regarding its scientific status and regarding its impact. The scientific debate is still open, on the one hand there is growing understanding of the changes in different brain networks related to the development of addictions and how these can make recovery more and more difficult. On the other hand, the strong claim that addiction is a chronic relapsing disease requires strong data, and the current state of affairs is far from that: one would have to show that these brain changes are caused by the developing addiction (and not due to risk-factors and other learning processes in the brain), then that these changes remain long after a person has successfully quit, and finally that they likely lead to relapse into addiction.[34] This has clearly not been done: often the first step is missing (no pre-assessment before the addiction), as are subsequent steps. The strong experimental evidence comes from animal studies, but questions have been raised on their validity or what they can teach us about addiction in humans, beyond a better understanding of (often fascinating) basic motivational mechanisms that play a role. As Harvard scientist Heyman concluded, there may be a deeper reason behind the lack of progress when it comes to translating promising new medications from animal models of mental disorders to treatment: some of the important mechanisms involving language and foresight may be missed. This has been a reason for the pharmacological industry to reduce investments in addiction and mental health research, and could be a reason to reconsider spending the large bulk of money on research into mechanisms underlying the chronic brain disease rather than on intervention development in humans.

The second claim was that the chronic brain disease model was not only the current scientific state of affairs, but that it would also reduce stigma. In line with Leshner's claim, blame is typically reduced when people believe the chronic brain disease model of addiction, but stigma increases, related to increased perceived danger and an associated tendency to stay away from dangerous people. In addition, the chronic brain disease perspective has been shown to diminish hope of recovery, both among people struggling with addiction themselves and those around them, including their treatment providers. Is it all nonsense, then, that addiction can be described as a chronic brain disease? In the words of two prominent voices in the debate, Yale psychiatrist Sally Satel and the late Emory professor of psychology Scott Lilienfeld: "Like many misleading metaphors, the brain disease model contains some truth."[28] Yes, there is a genetic factor in addiction, and yes, long-term substance use affects the brain, including brain processes that influence future use. But addiction is at the same time a problem involving multiple levels of description. Addiction is also a psychological problem; personality, motivation and goals play an important role, both in developing addiction and in overcoming it. And as we saw, the interplay between symptoms (and ideas how substance use can relieve some symptoms) also has an important role. At the same time addiction is also a social and cultural problem, with different addictions flourishing in different times and neighborhoods. There is no reason to assume that one level carries the most weight or that the psychological and sociocultural factors can be reduced to (neuro)biology.

A final statement in Leshner's paper was that addiction is either a chronic brain disease or the result of moral failure. I argue that (in the large majority of cases) it is neither, and that there is an alternative position: addiction as *biased choice*. That is the topic of the next chapter.

References

1. Alexander BK, Coambs RB, Hadaway PF. The effect of housing and gender on morphine self-administration in rats. Psychopharmacology (Berl). 1978; 58:175–9.
2. Hadaway PF, Alexander BK, Coambs RB, Beyerstein B. The effect of housing and gender on preference for morphine-sucrose solutions in rats. Psychopharmacology (Berl). 1979;66:87–91.
3. Alexander BK, Beyerstein BL, Hadaway PF, Coambs RB. Effect of early and later colony housing on oral ingestion of morphine in rats. Pharmacol Biochem Behav. 1981;15:571–6.
4. Alexander BK. The globalization of addiction. Addict Res Theory. 2000; 8:501–26.
5. Spanagel R. Animal models of addiction. Dialogues Clin Neurosci. 2017;19:247–59.
6. Venniro M, Zhang M, Caprioli D, Hoots JK, Golden SA, Heins C, et al. Addiction in rat models. Nat Neurosci [Internet]. 2018;21. Available from: 10.1038/s41593-018-0246-6
7. Everitt BJ, Robbins TW. Drug addiction: updating actions to habits to compulsions ten years on. Annu Rev Psychol [Internet]. 2016;67: 150807174122003. Available from: www.annualreviews.org/doi/abs/10.1146/annurev-psych-122414-033457
8. Hogarth L. Addiction is driven by excessive goal-directed drug choice under negative affect: translational critique of habit and compulsion theory. Neuropsychopharmacology [Internet]. 2020; Available from: 10.1038/s41386-020-0600-8

9. Kruglanski AW, Szumowska E. Habitual behavior is goal driven. Perspect Psychol Sci. 2020;15(5):1256–71.
10. De Houwer J. On how definitions of habits can complicate habit research. Front Psychol. 2019;10:1–9.
11. Robinson TE, Berridge KC. Addiction. Annu Rev Psychol. 2003;54:25–53.
12. Mischel W, Shoda Y, Rodriguez MI. Delay of gratification in children. Science (80–). 1989;244:933–8.
13. Read DW, Manrique HM, Walker MJ. On the working memory of humans and great apes: strikingly similar or remarkably different? Neurosci Biobehav Rev. 2022;134.
14. Hofmann W, Gschwendner T, Friese M, Wiers RW, Schmitt M. Working memory capacity and self-regulatory behavior: toward an individual differences perspective on behavior determination by automatic versus controlled processes. J Pers Soc Psychol [Internet]. 2008 [cited 2013 Mar 2];95:962–77. Available from: www.ncbi.nlm.nih.gov/pubmed/18808271
15. Baddeley AD. Working memory, thought, and action. Oxford University Press; 2007.
16. Munakata Y, Herd SA, Chatham CH, Depue BE, Banich MT, O'Reilly RC. A unified framework for inhibitory control. Trends Cogn Sci [Internet]. 2011;15:453–9. Available from: 10.1016/j.tics.2011.07.011
17. Lewis M. The biology of desire: why addiction is not a disease [Internet]. NY: Public Affairs; 2015. Available from: https://books.google.com/books?hl=en&lr=&id=CRtpCQAAQBAJ&pgis=1
18. Miller WR. Rediscovering fire: small interventions, large effects. Psychol Addict Behav. 2000;14:6.
19. de Wit H, Epstein DH, Preston KL. Does human language limit translatability of clinical and preclinical addiction research? Neuropsychopharmacology [Internet]. 2018;43:1985–8. Available from: 10.1038/s41386-018-0095-8
20. Field M, Kersbergen I. Are animal models of addiction useful? Addiction [Internet]. 2019;add.14764. Available from: https://onlinelibrary.wiley.com/doi/abs/10.1111/add.14764
21. Cutler RB, Fishbain D a. Are alcoholism treatments effective? The Project MATCH data. BMC Public Health [Internet]. 2005 [cited 2013 Jun 28];5:75. Available from: www.pubmedcentral.nih.gov/articlerender.fcgi?artid=1185549&tool=pmcentrez&rendertype=abstract
22. Kohn R, Saxena S, Levav I, Saraceno B. The treatment gap in mental health care. Bull World Health Organ. 2004;82:858–66.
23. Heyman GM. Addiction: a disorder of choice. Harvard University Press; 2010.
24. Jackson KM, Sher KJ. Alcohol use disorders and psychological distress: a prospective state-trait analysis. J Abnorm Psychol. 2003;112:599.
25. Littlefield AK, Sher KJ, Wood PK. Is "maturing out" of problematic alcohol involvement related to personality change? J Abnorm Psychol. 2009;118:360–74.
26. Vergés A, Haeny AM, Jackson KM, Bucholz KK, Grant JD, Trull TJ, et al. Refining the notion of maturing out: results from the national epidemiologic survey on alcohol and related conditions. Am J Public Health. 2013;103:67–73.
27. Robins LN, Helzer JE, Davis DH. Narcotic use in Southeast Asia and afterward: an interview study of 898 Vietnam returnees. Arch Gen Psychiatry. 1975;32:955–61.
28. Satel S, Lilienfeld SO. Addiction and the brain-disease fallacy. Front Psychiatry. 2014;4:1–11.

29. Fenton T, Wiers RW. Free will, black swans and addiction. Neuroethics. 2017;10.
30. Lewis M. Addiction and the brain: development, not disease. Neuroethics [Internet]. 2016;10:7–18. 10.1007/s12152-016-9293-4
31. Lewis M. Brain change in addiction as learning, not disease. N Engl J Med [Internet]. 2018;379:1551–60. Available from: www.nejm.org/doi/10.1056/NEJMra1602872
32. Lewis M. Memoirs of an addicted brain: a neuroscientist examines his former life on drugs. London: Scribe; 2012.
33. Maguire EA, Woollett K, Spiers HJ. London taxi drivers and bus drivers: a structural MRI and neuropsychological analysis. Hippocampus. 2006;16:1091–101.
34. Heather N, Best D, Kawalek A, Field M, Lewis M, Rotgers F, et al. Challenging the brain disease model of addiction: European launch of the addiction theory network. Addict Res Theory [Internet]. 2018;26:249–55. Available from: 10.1080/16066359.2017.1399659
35. Connolly CG, Bell RP, Foxe JJ, Garavan H. Dissociated grey matter changes with prolonged addiction and extended abstinence in cocaine users. PLoS One. 2013;8:4–11.
36. Bell RP, Garavan H, Foxe JJ. Neural correlates of craving and impulsivity in abstinent former cocaine users: towards biomarkers of relapse risk. Neuropharmacology [Internet]. 2014;85:461–70. Available from: 10.1016/j.neuropharm.2014.05.011
37. Schulte MHJMHJ, Cousijn J, den Uyl TETE, Goudriaan AEAE, van den Brink W, Veltman DJDJ, et al. Recovery of neurocognitive functions following sustained abstinence after substance dependence and implications for treatment. Clin Psychol Rev [Internet]. 2014;34:531–50. Available from: 10.1016/j.cpr.2014.08.002
38. Le Berre AP, Fama R, Sullivan E V. Executive functions, memory, and social cognitive deficits and recovery in chronic alcoholism: a critical review to inform future research. Alcohol Clin Exp Res. 2017;41:1432–43.
39. Bensimon M. Elaboration on the association between trauma, PTSD and posttraumatic growth: the role of trait resilience. Pers Individ Dif [Internet]. 2012;52:782–7. Available from: 10.1016/j.paid.2012.01.011
40. Blackie LER, Jayawickreme E, Tsukayama E, Forgeard MJC, Roepke AM, Fleeson W. Post-traumatic growth as positive personality change: developing a measure to assess within-person variability. J Res Pers [Internet]. 2017;69:22–32. Available from: 10.1016/j.jrp.2016.04.001
41. Infurna FJ, Jayawickreme E. Fixing the growth illusion: new directions for research in resilience and posttraumatic growth. Curr Dir Psychol Sci. 2019;28:152–8.
42. Fischer B, Oviedo-Joekes E, Blanken P, Haasen C, Rehm J, Schechter MT, et al. Heroin-assisted treatment (HAT) a decade later: a brief update on science and politics. J Urban Heal. 2007;84:552–62.
43. Blanken P, van den Brink W, Hendriks VM, Huijsman IA, Klous MG, Rook EJ, et al. Heroin-assisted treatment in the Netherlands: history, findings, and international context. Eur Neuropsychopharmacol [Internet]. 2010;20:S105–58. Available from: 10.1016/S0924-977X(10)70001-8
44. Rehm J, Marmet S, Anderson P, Gual A, Kraus L, Nutt DJJ, et al. Defining substance use disorders: do we really need more than heavy use? Alcohol Alcohol [Internet]. 2013 [cited 2014 Jul 13];48:633–40. Available from: www.ncbi.nlm.nih.gov/pubmed/23926213

45. Gezondheidsraad. Alcohol—Achtergronddocument bij Richtlijnen goede voeding. Den Haag; 2015.
46. Schulte MHJ, Cousijn J, den Uyl TE, Goudriaan AE, van den Brink W, Veltman DJ, et al. Recovery of neurocognitive functions following sustained abstinence after substance dependence and implications for treatment. Clin Psychol Rev. 2014;34.
47. Verdejo-García A, Lawrence AJ, Clark L. Impulsivity as a vulnerability marker for substance-use disorders: review of findings from high-risk research, problem gamblers and genetic association studies. Neurosci Biobehav Rev. 2008;32:777–810.
48. De Wit H. Impulsivity as a determinant and consequence of drug use: a review of underlying processes. Addict Biol. 2009;14:22–31.
49. Crowe SF, Cammisuli DM, Stranks EK. Widespread cognitive deficits in alcoholism persistent following prolonged abstinence: an updated meta-analysis of studies that used standardised neuropsychological assessment tools. Arch Clin Neuropsychol. 2019;35:31–45.
50. Zilverstand A, Huang AS, Alia-Klein N, Goldstein RZ. Neuroimaging impaired response inhibition and salience attribution in human drug addiction: a systematic review. Neuron [Internet]. 2018;98:886–903. Available from: 10.1016/j.neuron.2018.03.048
51. Wiers RW, Verschure PFMJ. Curing the broken brain model of addiction: neurorehabilitation from a systems perspective. Addict Behav [Internet]. 2021;112:106602. Available from: 10.1016/j.addbeh.2020.106602
52. Boelema SR, Harakeh Z, Van Zandvoort MJE, Reijneveld SA, Verhulst FC, Ormel J, et al. Adolescent heavy drinking does not affect maturation of basic executive functioning: longitudinal findings from the TRAILS study. PLoS One. 2015;10.
53. Wiers RW. Wel bewijs voor effecten alcohol op puberhersenen. Volkskrant. 2014;6 December, 30.
54. Spear LP. Effects of adolescent alcohol consumption on the brain and behaviour. Nat Rev Neurosci. 2018;19:197–214.
55. Maurage P, Pesenti M, Philippot P, Joassin F, Campanella S. Latent deleterious effects of binge drinking over a short period of time revealed only by electrophysiological measures. J Psychiatry Neurosci. 2009;34:111–8.
56. Lees B, Mewton L, Stapinski LA, Squeglia LM, Rae CD, Teesson M. Neurobiological and cognitive profile of young binge drinkers: a systematic review and meta-analysis. Neuropsychol Rev. 2019;29:357–85.
57. Wiers RW, Boelema SR, Nikolaou K, Gladwin TE. On the development of implicit and control processes in relation to substance use in adolescence. Curr Addict Reports [Internet]. 2015;2:141–55. Available from: http://link.springer.com/10.1007/s40429-015-0053-z
58. Oosterlaan J, Braun K, le Cessie S, Leiden Durston S, Engels RCME, et al. Alcohol en hersenontwikkeling [Alcohol and brain development] [Internet]. 2018. Available from: www.gezondheidsraad.nl/documenten/adviezen/2018/12/17/alcohol-en-hersenontwikkeling-bij-jongeren
59. de Goede J, van der Mark-Reeuwijk KG, Braun KP, le Cessie S, Durston S, Engels RCME, et al. Alcohol and brain development in adolescents and young adults: a systematic review of the literature and advisory report of the Health Council of the Netherlands. Adv Nutr. 2021;1–32.
60. Garavan H, Bartsch H, Conway K, Decastro A, Goldstein RZ, Heeringa S, et al. Recruiting the ABCD sample: design considerations and procedures. Dev Cogn Neurosci [Internet]. 2018;32:16–22. Available from: 10.1016/j.dcn.2018.04.004

61. Nees F, Tzschoppe J, Patrick CJ, Vollstädt-Klein S, Steiner S, Poustka L, et al. Determinants of early alcohol use in healthy adolescents: the differential contribution of neuroimaging and psychological factors. Neuropsychopharmacology. 2012;37:986–95.
62. Ruan H, Zhou Y, Luo Q, Robert GH, Desrivières S, Quinlan EB, et al. Adolescent binge drinking disrupts normal trajectories of brain functional organization and personality maturation. NeuroImage Clin [Internet]. 2019;22:101804. Available from: 10.1016/j.nicl.2019.101804
63. White HR, Marmorstein NR, Crews FT, Bates ME, Mun EY, Loeber R. Associations between heavy drinking and changes in impulsive behavior among adolescent boys. Alcohol Clin Exp Res. 2011;35:295–303.
64. Kuntsche E, Rossow I, Engels R, Kuntsche S. Is "age at first drink" a useful concept in alcohol research and prevention? We doubt that. Addiction. 2016;111:957–65.
65. Wagenaar AC Ph D, Toomey TL Ph D, Able T. Effects of minimum drinking age laws: review and analyses of the literature from 1960 to 2000. 2002;206–25.
66. Anderson P, De Bruijn A, Angus K, Gordon R, Hastings G. Impact of alcohol advertising and media exposure on adolescent alcohol use: a systematic review of longitudinal studies. Alcohol Alcohol. 2009;44:229–43.
67. Room R, Babor T, Rehm J. Review: alcohol and public health. Lancet. 2005;365:519–30.
68. Anderson DM, Rees DI. The public health effects of legalizing marijuana. SSRN Electron J. 2021;61:86–143.
69. Ayers JW, Caputi TL, Leas EC. The need for federal regulation of marijuana marketing. Jama. 2019;321:2163–4.
70. Liu Y, van den Wildenberg WPM, de Graaf Y, Ames SL, Baldacchino A, Ragnhild B, et al. Is (poly-) substance use associated with impaired inhibitory control? A mega-analysis controlling for confounders. Neurosci Biobehav Rev [Internet]. 2019;1–17. Available from: 10.1016/j.neubiorev.2019.07.006
71. Treur JL, Willemsen G, Bartels M, Geels LM, van Beek JHDA, Huppertz C, et al. Smoking during adolescence as a risk factor for attention problems. Biol Psychiatry. 2015;78:656–63.
72. Hall W, Carter A, Forlini C. The brain disease model of addiction: is it supported by the evidence and has it delivered on its promises? The Lancet Psychiatry [Internet]. 2015;2:105–10. Available from: 10.1016/S2215-0366(14)00126-6
73. Grifell M, Hart CL. Is drug addiction a brain disease? This popular claim lacks evidence and leads to poor policy. Am Sci [Internet]. 2018;106:160+. Available from: http://link.galegroup.com.ezproxy.endeavour.edu.au/apps/doc/A537718669/AONE?u=61ench&sid=AONE&xid=d5874f8b
74. Hiscock R, Bauld L, Amos A, Fidler JA, Munafò M. Socioeconomic status and smoking: a review. Ann N Y Acad Sci. 2012;1248:107–23.
75. Hart CL. High price: drugs, neuroscience and discovering myself. London: Penguin; 2013.
76. Hart CL. Viewing addiction as a brain disease promotes social injustice. Nat Hum Behav [Internet]. 2017;1:1. Available from: 10.1038/s41562-017-0055
77. Report A and GR. Captive labor: exploitation of incarcerated workers. [Internet]. Chicago; 2022. Available from: www.aclu.org/wp-content/uploads/legal-documents/2022-06-15-captivelaborresearchreport.pdf
78. Crews FT, Robinson DL, Chandler LJ, Ehlers CL, Mulholland PJ, Pandey SC, et al. Mechanisms of persistent neurobiological changes following

adolescent alcohol exposure: NADIA Consortium findings. Alcohol Clin Exp Res. 2019;43:1806–22.
79. Benson FE, Nagelhout GE, Nierkens V, Willemsen MC, Stronks K. Inequalities in the impact of national reimbursement of smoking cessation pharmacotherapy and the influence of injunctive norms: an explorative study. Subst Abus Res Treat. 2016;10:45–53.
80. Hyman SE. Psychiatric drug development: diagnosing a crisis. Cerebrum [Internet]. 2013;5:5. Available from: www.ncbi.nlm.nih.gov/pubmed/23720708%0Awww.pubmedcentral.nih.gov/articlerender.fcgi?artid=PMC3662213
81. Volkow ND, Koob G, Mental D, Parity H, Act AE. Brain disease model of addiction: why is it so controversial? Lancet Psychiatry. 2015;2:677–9.
82. Volkow ND, Koob GF, McLellan AT. Neurobiologic advances from the brain disease model of addiction. N Engl J Med [Internet]. 2016;374:363–71. Available from: www.nejm.org/doi/10.1056/NEJMra1511480
83. Vashadze S V. Serotonin and depression. Klin Lab Diagn [Internet]. 2006;1771:19–21. Available from: 10.1136/bmj.h1771
84. Nutt DJ, Lingford-Hughes A, Erritzoe D, Stokes PRA. The dopamine theory of addiction: 40 years of highs and lows. Nat Rev Neurosci. 2015;16:305–12.
85. Bishop SJ, Duncan J, Lawrence AD. State anxiety modulation of the amygdala response to unattended threat-related stimuli. J Neurosci. 2004; 24:10364–8.
86. Borsboom D, Cramer AOJ. Network analysis: an integrative approach to the structure of psychopathology. Annu Rev Clin Psychol. 2013;9:91–121.
87. Cramer AOJ, Waldorp LJ, Van Der Maas HLJ, Borsboom D. Comorbidity: a network perspective. Behav Brain Sci. 2010;33:137–50.
88. Borsboom D. A network theory of mental disorders. World Psychiatry. 2017;16:5–13.
89. Fried EI, Robinaugh DJ. Systems all the way down: embracing complexity in mental health research. BMC Med. 2020;18:4–7.
90. Borsboom D, Cramer AOJ, Kalis A. Brain disorders? Not really: why network structures block reductionism in psychopathology research. Behav Brain Sci. 2019;42.
91. Borsboom D. A network theory of mental disorders. World Psychiatry [Internet]. 2016;16:5–13. Available from: www.ncbi.nlm.nih.gov/pubmed/28127906%5Cnwww.pubmedcentral.nih.gov/articlerender.fcgi?artid=PMC5269502
92. Bockting CL, Hollon SD, Jarrett RB, Kuyken W, Dobson K. A lifetime approach to major depressive disorder: the contributions of psychological interventions in preventing relapse and recurrence. Clin Psychol Rev [Internet]. 2015;41:16–26. Available from: 10.1016/j.cpr.2015.02.003
93. Bringmann LF, Vissers N, Wichers M, Geschwind N, Kuppens P, Peeters F, et al. A network approach to psychopathology: new insights into clinical longitudinal data. PLoS One. 2013;8:e60188.
94. van de Leemput IA, Wichers M, Cramer AOJ, Borsboom D, Tuerlinckx F, Kuppens P, et al. Critical slowing down as early warning for the onset and termination of depression. Proc Natl Acad Sci. 2014;111:87–92.
95. Epskamp S, van Borkulo CD, van der Veen DC, Servaas MN, Isvoranu AM, Riese H, et al. Personalized network modeling in psychopathology: the importance of contemporaneous and temporal connections. Clin Psychol Sci. 2018;6:416–27.

96. Burger J, Van Der Veen DC, Robinaugh DJ, Quax R, Riese H, Schoevers RA, et al. Bridging the gap between complexity science and clinical practice by formalizing idiographic theories: a computational model of functional analysis. BMC Med. 2020;18:1–18.
97. Mansueto AC, Wiers RW, van Weert J, Schouten BC, Epskamp S. Investigating the feasibility of idiographic network models. Psychol Methods. Advance online publication. 10.1037/met0000466
98. Roefs A, Fried EI, Kindt M, Martijn C, Elzinga B, Evers AWM, et al. A new science of mental disorders: using personalised, transdiagnostic, dynamical systems to understand, model, diagnose and treat psychopathology. Behav Res Ther [Internet]. 2022;153:104096. Available from: 10.1016/j.brat.2022.104096
99. van der Wal JM, van Borkulo CD, Deserno MK, Breedvelt JJF, Lees M, Lokman JC, et al. Advancing urban mental health research: from complexity science to actionable targets for intervention. The Lancet Psychiatry [Internet]. 2021;8:991–1000. Available from: 10.1016/S2215-0366(21)00047-X
100. Heyman GM. Addiction and choice: theory and new data. Front Psychiatry. 2013;4:1–5.
101. Wiers CE, Kühn S, Javadi AH, Korucuoglu O, Wiers RW, Walter H, et al. Automatic approach bias towards smoking cues is present in smokers but not in ex-smokers. Psychopharmacology (Berl). 2013;229.
102. Masiero M, Lucchiari C, Maisonneuve P, Pravettoni G, Veronesi G, Mazzocco K. The attentional bias in current and former smokers. Front Behav Neurosci. 2019;13:1–11.
103. Witkiewitz K, Tucker JA. Abstinence not required: expanding the definition of recovery from alcohol use disorder. Alcohol Clin Exp Res. 2020;44:36–40.
104. Epskamp S, van der Maas HLJ, Peterson RE, van Loo HM, Aggen SH, Kendler KS. Intermediate stable states in substance use. Addict Behav. 2022;107252.
105. Kvaale EP, Gottdiener WH, Haslam N. Biogenetic explanations and stigma: a meta-analytic review of associations among laypeople. Soc Sci Med. 2013;96:95–103.
106. Kvaale EP, Haslam N, Gottdiener WH. The “side effects” of medicalization: a meta-analytic review of how biogenetic explanations affect stigma. Clin Psychol Rev. 2013;33:782–94.
107. Loughman A, Haslam N. Neuroscientific explanations and the stigma of mental disorder: a meta-analytic study. Cogn Res Princ Implic. 2018;3:1–12.
108. Kelly JF, Greene MC, Abry A. A US national randomized study to guide how best to reduce stigma when describing drug-related impairment in practice and policy. Addiction. 2021;116(7):17757–67.
109. Rundle SM, Cunningham JA, Hendershot CS. Implications of addiction diagnosis and addiction beliefs for public stigma: a cross-national experimental study. Drug Alcohol Rev. 2021;40:842–6.
110. Pennington CR, Monk RL, Heim D, Rose AK, Gough T, Clarke R, et al. The labels and models used to describe problematic substance use impact discrete elements of stigma: a registered report. Psychol Addict Behav. In press.
111. Mayr E. The growth of biological thought: diversity, evolution, and inheritance. Cambridge, MA: Harvard University Press; 1982.
112. Samarapungavan A, Wiers RW. Children’s thoughts on the origin of species: a study of explanatory coherence. Cogn Sci. 1997;21:147–77.

113. Haslam N, Whelan J. Human natures: psychological essentialism in thinking about differences between people. Soc Personal Psychol Compass. 2008; 2:1297–312.
114. Chen JM, Ratliff KA. Psychological essentialism predicts intergroup bias. Soc Cogn. 2018;36:301–23.

5 Addiction as biased choice

Let's go back some 30 years in time. With a group of students I am searching for an empty classroom, in an almost deserted building of the University of Amsterdam. We find one and make ourselves comfortable with our coffees and teas and get our books out. There is no teacher: we are a self-organized group of graduate students from different disciplines, some from philosophy, some from psychology and some from biology and neuroscience, and we talk about self-organization in relation to brain and mind. What unites us is that we do not like what we get taught about the brain as information processing input–output machine. Where is the body in this account and what can we conclude about research solely focusing on the "ghost in the machine" to quote the American philosopher Gilbert Ryle? Our reading and discussion group, organized by Paul Verschure, met in the late 1980s and early 1990s.[i] One of the first books we read was on self-organizing biological systems, written by two Chilean biologists and philosophers, Maturana and Varela,[1] on autopoiesis and cognition.

Autopoiesis refers to self-organization and self-creation processes in living beings, and is a concept that brought us back to a fundamental question: how does an organism self-organize in an environment? According to the second law of thermodynamics, the entropy of a system will tend to increase; that is, the system will tend to become increasingly *dis*ordered. A living system has to actively counter this tendency, and create a stable state of low entropy (when the organism

i Looking back, it was a talented group of graduate students indeed. Apart from Paul Verschure and myself, there was philosophy student Fred Keijzer, who later wrote his PhD thesis on representation in embodied cognition, and is now an associate professor in philosophy in Groningen; Cyril Pennartz, now professor of neuroscience at UvA, where he is an expert on brain processes in consciousness; and Serge Wich, expert on the behavior of great apes, and now a professor in primate biology at Liverpool John Moores University. There were also some others, but I am afraid that their names did not survive the filter of time.

DOI: 10.4324/9781032634548-5

dies, the battle is lost, and its constituent elements will decay into a state of disorder). Living cells fight this battle against entropy by closing themselves off from their environment with a membrane, but the closure is necessarily incomplete, as energy and information have to come in. When there are nutrients around, the single-celled organism will move toward them as it will move away from toxic gradients. This simple cell is in itself already a self-organizing complex system. We now know that it incorporated another originally self-organized system, the mitochondria. In the further course of evolution, more complex ensembles of cells evolved, later evolving to complex systems made out of different organs. And somewhere down the line, this self-organized biological machine apparently produced a ghost in the form of our mental processes, but its bodily underpinnings should not be ignored, we strongly believed.

Edelman coined the term "neural Darwinism": an important mechanism in the self-organizing brain.[2] The idea behind neural Darwinism is that the brain, with all its connections, is far too complex to be genetically predetermined: the amount of information needed to encode all connections in the brain could never fit into the human genome. The same is true for the immune system, Edelman's previous topic of research, for which he was awarded the Nobel Prize. The immune system works by learning from the environment which pathogens the body must defend itself against and which invaders must be eliminated early on. This is not hard-wired in the genome, which would take up too much space and make the system inflexible, but the result of learning from interactions with the environment. The same mechanism underlies vaccination: the immune system learns to recognize pathogens without having to go through the disease. Back to the brain: there is competition among neurons that grow and make contact with other neurons, with connections that are not active dropping away like unfit animals ("use it or lose it"). This makes the brain adaptive, but also vulnerable to negative experiences, especially when these occur early in life. The same mechanism is the reason why the brains of identical twins differ in detail.

The idea of self-organizing brains interacting with the environment is also crucial for robots: they must learn for themselves what the environment looks like by interacting with it. This avoids the problem of classic AI (artificial intelligence), where the programmer had to program all the potentially relevant features of the world that a robot might encounter. As a student I had taken a minor in AI in the late 1980s, and spent whole afternoons entering all kinds of features to explain to the computer how the world works. A tree stands in the ground. Unless it stands in water. Unless it has fallen over. A tree has branches, unless they have been cut off. And more difficult: the tree still has branches, even though they are out of sight, because something else blocks the view, and so on ... This boring exercise was a useful way to get clear that this is *not* the way to learn to understand the world. After all, how do you explain to a computer that a car behind a tree is still a car (or the other way around)? It reminds me now of the test we have to do online, to prove we are human: recognizing fire hydrants on American streets. Dissatisfaction with classical AI was one of the driving forces for our reading group, and more generally, for exploring self-learning neural networks and even embodied little machines that learn by themselves to move in their environment (a topic Paul Verschure worked on as a postdoc with Edelman after his PhD).

Self-learning neural networks (nowadays in *deep learning* consisting of several interacting, self-learning layers) can learn these things, without explicit explanation. Paul and I wrote a paper on this 30 years ago, discussing the relevance of the neural network approach to understanding human development.[3] More recently, we have begun to think about how the current understanding of the power of self-learning systems might be applied to the case of the brain disease model of addiction.[4,5] In the years in between, we remained friends and shared ideas about the question that intrigued us both from our student years: how can the brain produce the machinery underlying the human mind? How can conscious thought result from such a biological machine? Anil Seth, another ex-postdoc of Edelman's lab, now based at the University of Sussex, recently wrote a nice and accessible book about this issue: how a self-learning and embodied system can develop a conscious mind.[6] The brain is viewed as a Bayesian prediction machine that continuously makes best guesses of what caused the current pattern of sensory input, and it can simulate the expected effects of actions. Seth calls our conscious experience a controlled hallucination; likewise, Paul Verschure talks about biological virtual reality (VR). This current perspective states that, unlike our intuitions, we do *not* have direct access to the world outside, in line with Plato's famous metaphor of the cave. Instead our brain, hidden in our skull-cave, creates a dynamic model of the world around us, based on all available input. That is the world we consciously experience, this creation of what our brain makes out of the available sensory input, based on previous experience and anticipated effects of our actions.

The brain is structured as a hierarchical control system. At the lowest level there are sensors that produce reflexes, for example in response to excessive stimulation. As a result we immediately withdraw our hand when it comes into contact with a red-hot stove, without losing precious time thinking about what is happening or what we should do. One level above is the reactive control system in which at an elementary level about the world around us. It is at this level that self-learning robot cars operate in the lab. With only this basic level of control they can learn to move around an environment—even in unfamiliar terrain, such as on the surface of Mars—while avoiding obstacles. The next level is the adaptive learning system, in which, for example, classical conditioning takes place. This involves making simple predictions about the world and the effect of our own actions on it, a mechanism we encountered in the context of the conditioned tolerance reaction, triggered by the smell of coffee or the context where a drug is typically taken. The highest level is the contextual layer, which creates more elaborate models of the world, that are continuously updated when new information indicates this is necessary.

Based on this idea "prediction error" is a crucial learning signal. Prediction error is the discrepancy between what our current model of the world predicted and what we experience as actually happening. It plays an important role in classical conditioning,[7] concerning simple predictions and also at a higher level concerning more elaborate belief systems. This higher level of mental representations also includes representations of other individuals and their predicted actions.[8,9] This highest level is what brought the cognitive revolution to the agenda; like Tolman's rats, we continuously make models of the world in order to better predict what is going to happen and how we can best act given the (changing) circumstances. And this is the level that is important in humans, because it is where expected outcomes of our different possible actions are continuously simulated, allowing for choice between alternatives, in light of the expected consequences. The more elaborate the belief system is, the less likely it is that a single prediction error will lead to changing the whole mental model. It has been shown that both lay people and scientists rather ignore evidence that is not in accordance with their belief system or discard or reinterpret it, and only start thinking about changing their belief system if counterevidence mounts.[10]

In Verschure's DAC (distributed adaptive control) theory,[8,9] these levels of control are linked to three interacting systems that represent the world around, someone's self and someone's actions. The latter system assumes that the other agencies also want things and we ought to anticipate what those are to act in a social environment, crucial for our survival. We almost can't help ourselves from attributing a will to other agents that we encounter—indeed, the Belgian psychologist Michotte showed that people even attribute willed agency to abstract circles and squares moving around on a computer screen.[11] This tendency is what philosopher Daniel Dennett has called the *intentional stance:*[12] our mental system has developed to attribute intentionality to apparently autonomously moving other objects.

Hence, according to Verschure's DAC theory (and similar ones, like the one from Anil Seth), we all move around in our internally created VR-world, without the need for special glasses. This internal VR is constructed by our brains, through interactions between memory and prediction systems, through which we constantly predict what will happen and how our actions may influence ongoing events.[9,13] The general idea of the predictive brain has become popular in neuroscience during the past decade. An important developer of the idea has been the University College London neuroscientist Karl Friston. He developed the mathematically formulated free energy principle, which holds that living systems act in the world in order to minimize surprise (discrepancies between predictions from their internal model and the incoming evidence about what is happening out there). The mechanism behind these predictions is active inference, the basis of the brain's model construction to deal with the environment.[14]

Hierarchical control works in such a way that a higher level is called in when the lower level can't figure out how to control the situation on its own. In principle, a higher level can suppress a lower level's call, for example, in the case of holding our breath underwater. In humans, language has enriched the contextual level by which we can influence behavior based on rules of the group (norms and values), by means of which we can detach ourselves from the immediate environment and the need to learn everything ourselves through direct experience. This "cultural revolution"[ii] has given the development of our species an enormous boost, as described eloquently in Harari's book *Sapiens*,[15] and Henrich's *The Secret of Our Success*.[16] Our linguistic and cultural abilities provide unique opportunities to continue where our predecessors left off, and allow us to stand on the proverbial shoulders of previous giants. However, this ability also involves dangers: ideas can influence our thinking in ways that can dehumanize people, with dire consequences, as witnessed by our past in the case of slavery and the Nazis' industrial killing. Precisely because we view the world through our brain's VR system, our experience of the world is always open to outside influence and propaganda can have terrifying effects. For example, flooding citizens with the message that certain groups of people are inferior and should be considered a plague (as in Nazi propaganda films) can eventually lead those citizens to perceive reality that way and act accordingly, resulting in pogroms and concentration camps. Perhaps surprisingly, neuroscientist Verschure also developed an actual VR model with his research team at the site of the Bergen-Belsen Nazi concentration camp, to enable people to experience what the camp looked like at its liberation, based on original film material and recent excavations. With a VR setup you can move around, just like the soldiers who liberated the camp, and get a more real sense of

ii Of man, not the disastrous cultural revolution of China's former leader Mao that killed millions of people.

the horrors of the past than would be possible by walking around the actual site in its current beautiful, peaceful and natural state. Why would a brain researcher engage in a VR model of a concentration camp during liberation? Beyond personal interest, Paul does so from his perspective on the brain as a dynamic self-learning system, from which the importance of education and prevention follow (elaborated upon in the next chapter).

The addicted situated brain

Now why is all this relevant to addiction, and more specifically to the model of addiction as a chronic brain disease? The same internal VR-tools, that are sensitive to propaganda, provides us with an ability to imagine effects about ourselves if we change in a positive direction. We can imagine a different reality, set goals, and adjust our behavior so that we work toward those goals. And this ability can be employed by heavily addicted people who successfully recover, as witnessed by the cases Marc Lewis described about long-term addicted people who managed to quit their addiction, described in the previous chapter.[17] As long as we can imagine ourselves in a better future and a path toward it, we can adjust our behavior, which does not mean it this easy. This fact is important not only for overcoming addiction, but also for the changes needed by all of us to preserve human life on Earth, discussed in Chapter 9.

The main point is that the brain does not stand alone: decisions are made by a situated agent in a body that can simulate the outcomes of its behaviors. As an alternative to the brain disease model, Paul and I proposed to view addiction from a systems-level perspective in order to more effectively capture the embodied and situated human mind and brain in relation to the development of addictions.[4,5] Our systems-theoretical framework includes high-level concepts related to the physical and social environment, motivation, self-image, and the meaning of alternative activities, which in turn dynamically influence subsequent brain adaptations. The human brain makes predictions about future states as well as expected (or counterfactual) errors, in the context of its goals. In line with motivational models of addiction,[18] we propose that human behavior—including addictive behaviors—is deeply goal-driven, but that the neuroadaptations in addiction may exert an effect on the machinery of our goal-driven behaviors. The good news is that some of this may be reversed through targeted cognitive training, as we will see in Chapter 8.

Decision-making is also influenced by one's learning history, which will be influenced by the environment in which that learning occurred. This is a crucial aspect that is neglected if one views addiction purely as an isolated "brain problem". Previous learning experiences have shaped the brain to make decisions the way it does. These decisions often involve trade-offs between short term positive effects and longer-term negative effects, in case of the choice for the addictive behavior and the reverse for an alternative choice (for example, Martin's cigarette versus a carrot with hummus, from Chapter 2). When people experience stress from poverty, this negatively shifts this balance to short-term fixes, as an influential paper in *Science* demonstrated.[19] And as we saw in the previous chapter, living in a poor neighborhood is an established predictor of later addiction. The effect of poverty and stress on self-control or the ability to forego the short-term fix and choose for an alternative with better expected long-term outcomes, could be one of the underlying mechanisms. We can conclude that both earlier experiences and environmental influences sculpt the brain processes that lead to later choice. Why is smoking prevalent in neighborhoods with many people of low socioeconomic status? Because their brains are different? But based on brain images alone, you can't distinguish smokers from non-smokers. Instead of merely considering the anatomy of their brains, you would get further by asking them about their ideas about smoking, about the sociability associated with it, and a reluctance to go with "state control", even when these aim at health improvement. Ironically, tobacco advertising has associated smoking with freedom, while in fact, it reduces people's freedom and health. But as a result, many poor people resist to be curtailed by the state, in their freedom to smoke. As we will see in the next chapter, bringing this mechanism to the surface can be useful to prevent smoking in adolescents.[20]

As we saw earlier when we talked about the concept of *homeostasis*, our nervous system constantly registers the state of our bodies and the environment in an effort to maintain a constant state; for example, if we are too hot or too cold autonomous mechanisms kick in, such as sweating or shivering. Many responses to small disturbances in our systems are triggered unconsciously so that we don't notice them until there is an (upcoming) issue.[21] The brain is made up of several interacting modules, each pursuing its own goals. The system responsible for ensuring a stable temperature has a clear purpose: if we are in danger of cooling down too much, it should take care of warming us up, and if it gets too hot, it should take care of cooling us down. Note that even in this simple example, it is important to predict: it would be better to take measures *before* you became too hot or too cold, because once the change has occurred, it might be too late to act appropriately. This implies that even basic self-regulatory mechanisms benefit from prediction by our predictive brain, which implies the mechanism of *allostasis* (regulation based on prediction) rather than *homeostasis* (like the simple mechanism of the thermometer in most houses: switch on when a threshold is reached and off when another threshold is reached).[iii] This can be done in part with automatically initiated physiological mechanisms, like sweating or shivering, but also with behavior. This is where conflicts can arise: when two different modules suggest opposing trends of action.

Let's look at such an inner struggle. Suppose I have the idea that it's good for my health to swim in open water during the winter, which is currently popular, in part due to the influence of Dutch "iceman" Wim Hof. Research has indicated that his method, which combines breathing techniques, meditation and exposure to cold, can have positive effects on the immune system, opening up possibilities for an alternative approach for some chronic diseases: swim in cold open water instead of taking pills.[22,23] At the same time, the method is not without risks, and a number of deaths have been attributed to it, especially when the breathing exercises are done in cold water—a combination that the iceman himself now advises against after fatalities.[24] The point here is that this is an almost prototypical case of willpower: when you enter the cold water, you have to counteract an enormously strong tendency *not to* enter the cold water, and, once entered, to climb straight back out. So, while the system that is supposed to take care of your constant body temperature is sending urgent messages in an effort to do something to prevent you from cooling down (internally screaming that you need to get out of that water), you can overcome this tendency and stay in it for a while—and with some practice for a little longer. Similarly, we can teach ourselves to swim underwater by holding our breath while getting an increasingly strong urge to breathe.[25] And as a teenager we can teach ourselves to smoke a cigarette, while we know how bad it is for future health, have to cough at the first puff and start to feel dizzy and nauseous at the next. Why would we do this? In all cases, we must have a strong motivation, for example, the idea that our action will increase our social status among peers (very important in puberty as we will see in the next chapter). In essence, the end justifies the means, and in some cases that implies suppressing strong urges to do otherwise: we can often ignore even a strong physical urge at least temporarily with conscious control. As we saw in Chapter 2, according to current neuroscientist Morsella, this is the function of consciousness: it provides a common language to coordinate the desires of various semi-autonomous control systems in the brain, echoing an early idea of AI pioneer Marvin Minsky, who described communication between

iii Recent books by Peter Sterling[76] and Anil Seth[6] provide excellent introductions to these ideas.

different brain modules the "society of mind".[26] So is there an internal language of thought where we can weigh the expected outcomes of our acts in a single currency?

Biased decision making as alternative to chronic brain disease or immoral character

Is there an alternative to the view that addiction is either a chronic brain disease or a manifestation of an immoral character? As we saw in the first chapter, until the nineteenth century, excessive drinking was judged as a "common sin": someone who got drunk often, apparently had an immoderate character and liked to drink a lot. Thus, there was no *akrasia*; a person simply drank a lot because they voluntarily chose to do so. This was interpreted as a sign of an intemperate character, and one could argue that this applies to most heavy drinkers who don't face problems yet.[27] As we saw in Chapter 1, Benjamin Rush in the late eighteenth century introduced the disease model: by drinking a lot, people could lose control over their drinking, which in turn could lead to compulsive use, even in face of immediate negative consequences ("the cannon to be passed", from Rush's first description of addiction as a disease of the will). Is there an alternative between the two evils, the Scylla and Charybdis, between addiction as an immoral choice and no longer having a choice?

The alternative perspective proposed here, is to view addiction as a manifestation of biased choice in a situated agent. Neuroadaptations as a consequence of previous (addictive) behavior limit the freedom in choice, but do not erase it in the large majority of cases. The choices our predictive brain makes are influenced by previous choices and their outcomes: learned reward signals are hard to ignore, especially for sign-trackers (as we saw in Chapter 3). This biases the choice toward learned reward signals. We have a general tendency to automatize behaviors so that limited conscious capacity remains available for new problems, in case there are signals that our autopilot is in trouble and we need our attention to solve an unexpected problem, such as the barred normal entrance of our office building or the empty lighter of a smoker. Addictive behaviors are strongly habitual, therefore a strong signal is needed that "something is wrong" in order to prevent the repetition of the habitual behavior. If the strong signal cannot change the course of action anymore, the action can be regarded as compulsive, which could perhaps be the case in some severe cases of addiction, although the evidence is meagre at best as we saw in the previous chapter. Of course, our choices are also influenced by our social environment, and in the case of a developing addiction, the neural mechanisms underlying choice (and the intimately related processes of attention),[28] will influence our decision making, but it still is decision making.

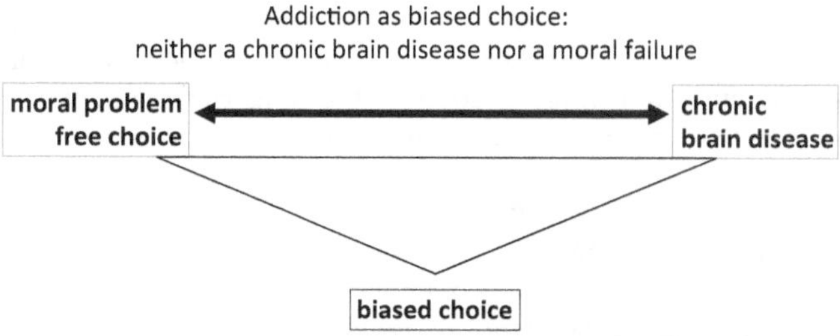

Figure 5.1 The dichotomy introduced by Leshner that addiction is either a moral failure or a chronic brain disease is false, according to the present perspective. The alternative is that addiction concerns biased choice. How we make choices is influenced by our character and early experience (which we could relate to the moral model) and after the addictive behaviors have commenced, by neuroadaptations that bias future choice—due to learning—in line with the chronic brain disease model. Crucially, these neuroadaptations bias decision making, but the decision-making process can still be influenced via changes in value of the addictive behavior and increasing attractiveness of alternatives.[iv]

A common neural currency?

When it comes to making choices by our single body that is composed of modules with their own suggested courses of action, there must be a common "currency" in which the expected effects of different choices can be expressed. University of Zurich-based neuroscientist Todd Hare and colleagues have mapped the brain-circuit responsible for this internal trading process, in which the ventromedial prefrontal cortex (vmPFC), and the nearby orbitofrontal PFC—both central, frontal brain regions—are important, as well as evolutionarily older areas traditionally associated with reward, such as the nucleus accumbens in the anterior striatum.[29–31] In this circuit the value of the expected outcomes of different possible actions is calculated, integrating the expected outcomes of different systems. Recent research has demonstrated that this system can be measured also in the context of decision making in drinking and other health-relevant behaviors. It can predict responses to alcohol-related messages: pro-alcohol from peers versus anti-drinking media messages.[32,33] Hence, maybe Plato was right and there is a single neural value-attribution mechanism, that makes us choose the option with the highest estimated value.

In neuroscientific versions of dual process models, the dorsolateral prefrontal cortex has often been proposed to act as a censor, inhibiting the tendency to choose attractive short-term options in the light of better long-term goals (e.g., Martin choosing to resume smoking to celebrate the now with old friends, disregarding the negative effects on his long-term health).[34] This led to the homunculus problem: how does this supervisory system know what is good in the long run? That would require that this brain region also determines value and makes decisions, which would lead to an infinite regression.[35,36] Many neuroscientists now agree that the dlPFC does *not* determine value, but that this system can influence (modulate) the general value system, based on our active goals. This is still based on values in the common value system. In doing so, choices that are seen as more favorable to longer-term goals start to weigh in more heavily,[v] as Hare and colleagues have shown in a landmark paper in *Science*.[30] In this process, attention plays a crucial role: by steering attention on positive features of the choice that better fits our long-term goal, the chance increases that this alternative indeed wins.[37]

Let's take this to our everyday lives. Suppose you are in a canteen for lunch and have to choose between salad and pizza. You realize the salad is healthier, but you're hungry and the tempting smell of the pizza's melted cheese is tingling your nose. One thing you can do is to focus on the attractive aspects of the salad (the fresh cherry tomatoes on top) and the positive health effects (I'll feel good when I'm on the weighing scale and not sleepy after lunch), which influences value assignment at the moment, based on modulation by the dlPFC.[37] Note that this explanation is different from that offered by dual process models, which would suggest that the impulsive system goes for the pizza, a behavioral tendency that must subsequently be censored by the reflective system because of the negative health effects.[38] Perhaps it feels as if there is some inner struggle going on, between passion for pizza and reason supporting salad, but that does not mean it is organized that way in the brain. As Elliot Berkman, professor of psychology at the University of Oregon stated it: the fact that self-control *feels* like an internal struggle between

iv Note that I am not alone in pointing to the importance of biased decision making in addiction. During the past decade, many scholars from different fields have done so, including Gene Heyman, who we encountered in the previous chapter (addiction a disorder of choice),[77] Nick Heather,[78] Matt Field and colleagues,[59] and Warren Bickel,[79] both of whom applied behavioral economic and neuroeconomic principles to choice in addiction, and who will return in Chapter 8. In addition, Geoffrey Schoenbaum and colleagues at NIDA, pointed to the importance of imagining future effects of our behaviors.[65]

v One can, of course, ask how the dlPFC then knows which choice is better for the long term, or whether there is no homunculus at play there. The answer is that the value of long-term goals and the corresponding tuning of choice based on longer-term goals is learned during development, which can also be modeled.[36] The issue here is that there is no separate value determination in the dlPFC, which leads to infinite regression (homunculus).

good and bad forces (heart and head) does not mean that it is neurologically organized that way.[39] Current evidence suggests that there is dynamic integration in one system, and that the values of our actions within it are determined by our goals and by our learning-history.[28,38,40] This has implications for interventions, in which it is important not only to discuss long-term goals, but also to try to maximize their influence at the moment when a relevant choice needs to be made, for example by teaching people to focus on the attractive aspects of the healthier choice and to imagine the positive long-term consequences, as in the pizza and salad example.

Basic models of attention and choice indicate that a continuously updated map of priorities is made of the environment, based on sensory input from different modalities, and that map determines where you allocate your attention.[28,41] How this map looks at a given moment, is influenced by different inputs: your physiological state and related input from modules that have to keep your body in good condition (if you are thirsty, anything that may signal an opportunity to drink grabs your attention), bottom-up external signals (e.g., a sudden loud noise), top-down goal-related signals (e.g., you want to stay in the cold water because you believe this will be good for your health), and learned signals of reward and threat. The latter we encountered before in the test of sign-tracking in humans, the value-modulated attentional capture (VMAC) task, developed by Mike Le Pelley from UNSW in Sydney.[42] The trick of the task (see Figure 3.1), is that the large reward signals are perfectly matched to the low reward signals in terms of bottom-up attention-grabbing potential, the goal is the same (ignore colored distractors) and still, the distractor that signals the availability of high reward distracts more, which has been related to a vulnerability for addiction.[28,43] Reactions to learned signals of reward are the reason why the decision making of a person is not only about rationally weighing of pros and cons of expected outcomes of possible choices: instead these signals of reward can act to bias attention and decision making toward the easy fix. Note again that these findings are not absolute: while addicted people are generally a bit more distracted by reward cues, it is not the case that they cannot find targets anymore when there is a distractor.

An important aspect of the integrated value model is that it has a decision criterion. You cannot go on collecting information endlessly; at some point, a decision must be made. People differ in the speed at which they make decisions (related to the personality trait impulsivity),[44] and this is something that is influenced by genes and early development and can be trained to some extent, as we will see in the next chapter. The upshot is not that making decisions quickly is necessarily bad and taking a long time to decide is always good. In all likelihood, it was evolutionarily beneficial to the group that people vary in this regard: where impulsiveness in today's society often has negative effects, it is quite conceivable it was beneficial to early groups of people to have some individuals with a tendency to immediately head for danger, while other, less impulsive individuals stayed at home.[45] And an individual has to find an optimum between a quick, reasonably good choice and the amount of effort and time it takes to weigh all the options.

Let us consider a real-world example: suppose you need to move to a new city and you start looking at apartments. It is unlikely that the first apartment you view will be the best you can get. But the only way to find out if you really have the best deal would be to view all apartments on the market. That is impractical if not impossible in a larger city, adding to the fact that an even better deal could come on the market sometime later (but when?). In short, based on a number of viewings in the new city and your ideas about the market, based on previous experience,[vi] you should try to get an idea of the market at that time, and then choose the best option of the set that you have viewed. Impulsive individuals will settle more easily with an option, and an adverse byproduct of this mechanism is that non-impulsive individuals may sometimes miss out on the best deal, as illustrated by a friend, a professor who was looking for a house in Utrecht with his partner. They had determined what they could spend and began viewing houses. Guess what? The very first viewing was the perfect house at an affordable price: a beautiful old mansion in a good state, close to the city center and the main train station. Too good to be true … They were excited, but didn't want to decide right away until they had seen some other houses to compare with. That's how sensible adults behave, we don't take important decisions on the fly. Sure enough, by the time they figured out that the first house was indeed by far the best deal, the house was long gone, and now they are living in a house in the suburbs (by their own admission with no regrets).[vii] Accordingly, it appears that even in modern society, there are situations in which making quick decisions is advantageous, although usually this is not the case, and impulsivity and lack of self-control is a strong predictor of later problems (including an increased risk of addiction), as we will see in the next chapter.

Thus, the integrated value system must eventually reach a decision, which happens when a threshold value is exceeded (see Figure 5.2). The

vi Research has indeed shown that expectations based on prices in your previous city influence the choice: if you come from a city where rents are high, you will on average settle on a more expensive apartment in your new city than if you come from a city with relatively low rents.[80]

vii This seems a typical case of cognitive dissonance reduction: a well-known psychological mechanism that causes you to better appreciate your choices after the fact.[81]

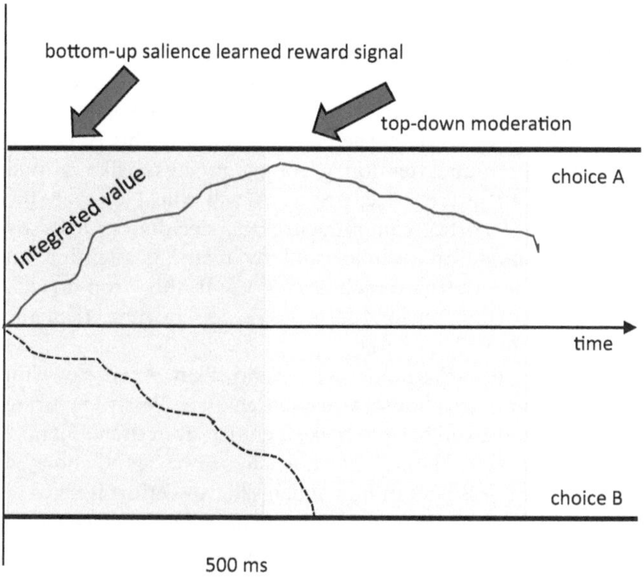

Figure 5.2 In the integrated valuation system, all influences on a choice are integrated dynamically over time (horizontal axis). When the integrated information exceeds a threshold (A or B), the choice is made, for example, pizza (A) or salad (B) in the lunch example, or a cigarette (A) or a carrot with hummus (B) in the case of the ex-smoker. The dorsolateral prefrontal cortex (dlPFC) can influence this process, for example, by focusing attention on the attractive aspects of the alternative choice (B, the cherry tomatoes on the salad, the fresh carrot with the fresh hummus). In the example, the moderation came just in time (response criterion A was almost reached), and in some cases the moderation may come too late and the decision has already been made even though there is a long-term goal that would argue for B. Impulsive people have lower decision thresholds in this model, so integrated value will tend to reach these thresholds sooner, resulting in more rapid choices (which will therefore tend to be more strongly influenced by "early" processes relating to learned reward signals). Neuroadaptations in addiction make the curve steeper, indicating a faster decision to take the drug or to engage in the addictive behavior again.

figure depicts the choice process based on dynamic value integration. There are two choices: choice A represents a choice that is attractive in the short term (e.g., the pizza from the example above or the cigarette for our ex-smoker Martin from the first chapter), and choice B represents a choice that the actor considers better in view of long-term goals (i.e., the salad or the carrot with hummus). There is a decision threshold for both choices, A and B. Furthermore, the lines are made squiggly on purpose because this is a probabilistic model, in which chance plays a role. As a consequence of previous learning, the simulation of the consequence of action A would more quickly reach its threshold, as a result of the attention-grabbing properties of learned cues of reward. This is a quick process, akin to bottom-up attention grabbing processes like a loud noise.[28] Hence, without interference, option A will win. However, the dorsolateral prefrontal cortex can influence the decision process by influencing the threshold for a choice and by focusing attention on positive aspects of the alternative choice.[30,38,46] If this "top-down", moderating influence based on long-term goals acts in time, then the result may be that option B is chosen.

What also plays a role in this model is time and effort. As we saw with the example of searching for a house, you can't go on endlessly exploring the market; at some point you have to make a choice, even though it may not turn out to be the optimal one. The choice has to be "good enough" for the situation. The assessment of how much time and effort it takes to choose is also factored into the value, with the *dorsal anterior cingulate cortex* (dACC) playing an important role.[38] Furthermore, it is important that the representations between which you choose (e.g., I eat pizza or salad, with different consequences) contain the representations of the corresponding actions: the moment the threshold is exceeded, you grab the pizza or the bowl of salad.[47] Thus, once the decision criterion is reached, the decision is made and the execution has been initiated. Note that there could be late inhibition after onset of an action (in the example, once you grabbed the pizza, you realize this choice goes against your good resolutions and put it back), but that is notoriously difficult and not very efficient, compared to moderating the choice process in an earlier phase, through selective attention processes[48] (we will return to this idea in Chapter 8).

One assumption of this model is that there is indeed a common currency of choice—the integrated value in Figure 5.2—which has recently been questioned by psychologists, who argue that social goods like health, education or love cannot can be rank-ordered in a common currency.[49] And neuroscientist Kent Berridge, who we encountered in Chapter 3, distinguished the neural processes underlying "wanting" and "liking" to explain why and how a sensitized "wanting" reach could still cause an addicted person to choose a drug use despite not liking it anymore due to experience of the problems that it creates. One possible solution could be to skip the idea of a common currency and to focus on competing goal-directed learned response options per se (pizza or salad), for which evidence is accumulated until a threshold is passed that initiates a response, after which other response tendencies are inhibited.

Hence, then, the vertical axis in Figure 5.2 would not represent a single currency, but the accumulated evidence favoring two competing goal-directed actions (upward: take pizza or downward: take salad), where the action wins, for which the accumulated evidence first passes the threshold.

Ego depletion and decision making

A term that has often been used in recent decades to explain choices for short-term fixes rather than more sensible long-term alternatives is *ego depletion*, indicating a depletion of self-control capacity.[38,50] In an influential model, Roy Baumeister and colleagues proposed that cognitive control processes have a limited amount of "fuel" (sometimes equated with sugar), which might run out at some point, resulting in impulsive decision-making.[51] In a prototypical experiment in this line of research, the participant's self-control capacity is first exhausted. This can be done in many ways, for example, by having people do a tiring task that requires them to constantly go against their habits. An example of such a task is the *Stroop task*, in which you have to name the color of ink while reading the names of other colors (e.g., you read "red" in blue ink and have to say "blue" in response to the color of the ink, while ignoring the meaning of the word which would lead to saying "red"). Compared to a group that had performed a less exhausting task, the depleted group afterwards typically shows a preference for eating unhealthy but tasty snacks (e.g., chocolate rather than an apple). However, recent work has cast doubt on whether ego depletion is a real phenomenon: a large-scale replication-study, in which the standard procedures were tested in various labs according to predetermined procedures, provided little supporting evidence.[52,53]

Another line of recent research has indicated that, to the extent that ego depletion occurs at all, the effect may depend on beliefs people have: if they have the idea that self-control wears out after exhaustion (in accordance with ego depletion), this was indeed confirmed, but when people were convinced of the contrary, that they should actively engage in something else when getting tired of a task, no such exhaustion effect was found.[54] This was confirmed in an experiment in which participants were first convinced of one of the two beliefs, by reading an article that substantiated one of the two perspectives (mental exhaustion or need for variety), as demonstrated by University of Toronto professor of psychology Michael Inzlicht and colleagues.[50] Much like the aforementioned internal struggle between passion and reason, ego depletion seems another idea about how the brain works that is consistent with some intuitions (feelings of exhaustion after doing the same task for a long time), which nevertheless may not give an accurate picture of how things really work in the brain. According to Inzlicht, the exhaustion signal indicates that you are going on too long with an activity, which by definition comes at the expense of other opportunities: if you keep on doing one thing, you may miss opportunities for evolutionarily more important things, such as food, social contacts, etc.[50]

Hence, research has shown that it is often possible *not to* give in to temptation, even when exhausted, as long as you focus on your goals and attractive aspects of the alternative. It should be noted that although many scientists now doubt the existence of *ego depletion*, a recent study did find some evidence in the brain that mental exhaustion is not only psychological in nature, at least in extreme cases. French researchers made one group perform tasks that were designed to cause mental exhaustion for no less than six hours in a brain imaging scanner, while another group was assigned easy tasks in the same scanner. The first group reported more exhaustion and subsequently made more impulsive choices, as the ego-depletion model would predict, and this was related to the glutamate levels in the lateral PFC.[55] So perhaps there is a grain of truth in the ego-depletion model in extreme cases, although in most everyday life examples, the nature of the effect appears to be more psychological: if you think your brain wants you to take an easy fix when tired, chances are that's what you will do, but maybe you can convince yourself that your brain needs variety if that better fits your long-term goals.

Brain changes in addiction bias choice

As we saw in Chapter 3, a number of neuroadaptations or brain changes have been related to the development of addiction: sensitization (becoming hypersensitive to signals that indicate the possibility of taking the addictive drug), negative reinforcement or the "dark side of addiction" (where the drug helps to counteract negative feelings), the development of more or less compulsive habits, and craving related to bodily awareness in the hidden island of addiction (the *insula*). How are these changes compatible with the idea that addiction still involves choice, albeit more biased than without addiction?

The idea is that all these neuroadaptations influence one's choice behavior, based on general (neuro)psychological learning mechanisms. Addictive drugs influence valuation, possibly through selective attention: for signals of reward the curve in Figure 5.2 goes up more steeply. The idea of sensitization is thus easily combined with the general idea of choice and related attentional processes being affected in addiction, as a consequence of learning-based on previous experience of making those choices and their (rewarding) effects.[56–59] It indicates that choosing something other than the addiction option becomes more difficult when there is a salient signal indicating the availability of the drug. Note that the separate "wanting" system from a "liking" system indicates that the biased choice may not be because of increased value on a single currency ("value" is close to liking), but as a response tendency for a quick and sure fix for the current situation. That implies that salient reward signals dominate the attention landscape earlier than goal-directed biasing of attention and bias choice toward the quick fix.[28,35] We saw that individual differences play a role here—the difference between the "sign-trackers" and "goal-trackers"—where the former group can be so distracted by a reward signal that the actual reward is lost (the rats who start to lick the light that signals a reward, which made them forego the reward). These are represented in Figure 5.2, by a steep curve upward toward the threshold associated with the quick fix, driven by the presence of a cue that has previously been established as a signal of short-term reward.

The "dark side of addiction" (negative reinforcement) can also be understood as biasing choice. In this case, it involves an enhanced choice of the drug under the influence of negative feelings, because a person has learned that taking the drug leads to a decrease in negative emotions, in the short run.[60] In this case, the negative emotion becomes part of the signal, along with the actions to take the drug and the expected relaxing effects, with the goal to reduce the negative emotions. In Figure 5.2, this could be represented by a steep curve toward substance use in the context of negative emotions and the availability of the "solution" (the drug or addictive activity, which in the longer term leads to more negative feelings). Individual differences also play a role here; especially people who develop negative emotions relatively easily (for example, due to a genetic predisposition or early trauma) are prone to this mechanism.[61]

Habitual and perhaps compulsive behaviors play a role in addiction. Habitual behavior is triggered by context signals: you can easily teach yourself to have a drink or smoke a joint after work. Most people can change this behavior, but will find that it is difficult to do so, because the old context still triggers the tendency to repeat the old behavior. Therefore, as we saw, a context change can be an opportunity to change an unwanted habit (never smoke in your new car).[62] As mentioned in chapter 4, there is no debate as to whether habitual behavior plays a role in addiction, but there is debate as to whether it leads to *compulsive* behavior, the total lack of choice once the signal is there, for which the evidence has been judged to be meagre, both in laboratory animals and in humans.[60,63] This process can be understood as an increasing difficulty in correcting a decision, once it goes one way (in Figure 5.2, passing the threshold for A, before the top-down moderating effect that steers toward choice B, has been initiated). One could imagine that a general tendency to make quick decisions (impulsivity), would be a predictor of this pattern, and indeed impulsivity was found to predict compulsive drug use in laboratory animals.[64]

Finally, there are indications that addiction may influence self-awareness and body awareness, and the process of decision making, including the ability to mentally simulate the outcomes of different actions.[65–67] If that ability is chronically compromised in the course of addiction, calling it a chronic brain disease may be appropriate. Luckily, so far, research has indicated that these differences should be seen as gradual rather than absolute, with indications that most may at least partly recover after successful abstinence.

In summary, the brain changes that have been described to occur in addiction can be understood as processes by which decision making and the closely related process of attentional prioritization are influenced. Thus, the model of addiction as biased choice can embrace the neurobiological findings of altered brain functioning with a developing addiction, without having to draw the conclusion that addiction is a chronic brain disease in which choice is no longer possible (except perhaps in exceptional cases to which I return below). Nor is the other extreme correct: it does not involve a morally reprehensible choice for the addictive behavior, as the old moral model wanted (chronic drunkenness explained by an exceptional liking of alcohol). In addition, the social and environmental influences that clearly play an important role in risk for addiction can also be modeled to influence choices made. For example, poverty has been shown to facilitate negative affect and

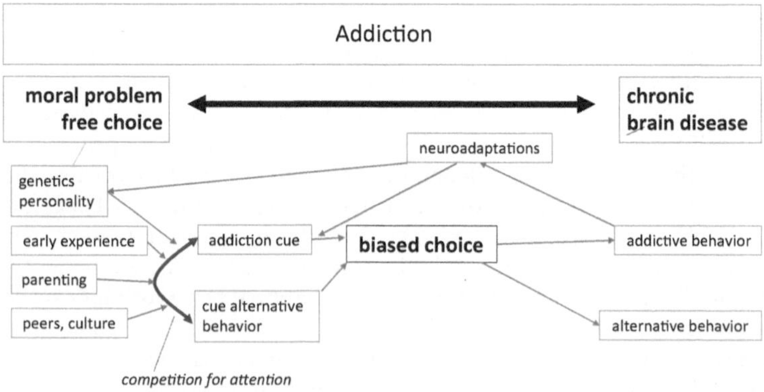

Figure 5.3 Addiction as biased choice incorporates both neuroadaptations (related to the chronic brain disease model) and moral development (personality and early experience). Biased choice is central, with neuroadaptations influencing responses to drug cues as well as personality (e.g., more negative affect, more impulsive responding).

short-term focused decision-making,[19] which would both steer choices toward addictive behaviors. Add the negative psychological effects of discrimination,[68] and lack of perspective,[69] and it is clear that the decision-making processes in addiction take place in an influential social context, and not merely in an isolated brain.

To counter the effect of this bias in choice, one of the most important things to change in addiction is to take more time for relevant decisions; to not give in to the lure of the quick reward. As a consequence, long-term goals have more chance to exert their effects on decision making, which can be trained to some extent in development (Chapter 6) and in therapy (Chapter 7). Moreover, as we will see in Chapter 8, training techniques have been developed to reduce the salience of reward signals in an attempt to make the drug-choice less attractive, and these have improved success of long-term outcomes of addiction treatment.

Choices are made in the brain, so addiction is still a brain disease

A recent defense of the brain disease model of addiction was provided by Markus Heilig and colleagues.[70] Heilig is a Swedish researcher and former director of NIAAA's intramural clinical and translational research program. Heilig and colleagues also concluded that decision making is one of the key problems in addiction. And as decision making takes place in the brain, addiction is a brain disease after all. Interestingly, the "chronic" qualification of this brain disease was sacrificed along the way. In addition, it was emphasized that the brain disease characterization does *not* apply to most people who use more substances than is good for their health, and not even to most people who meet the criteria for an addiction (or in current terminology a substance use disorder), it would only apply to a small group of severely addicted people, in line with the distinction made by the influential American physician Elvin Jellinek in the 1950s: according to him the disease model applies only to severely addicted people, characterized by loss of control.[71] They further argued that the disease label is useful for treatment and that biomedical research has yielded useful treatments. We saw earlier, however, that this claim is debatable: the vast majority of currently used biomedical treatments were developed before the proclamation of addiction as a chronic brain disease.[72]

What to think of this defense? I largely agree with this perspective, which puts biased choice at the center. It is consistent with our "black swan argument" mentioned in Chapter 4: not those people who recovered successfully from an addiction should be considered the proverbial black swans, but the small group of truly chronically addicted people.[73] And in this small group, "collateral damage" plays an important role (e.g., Korsakoff syndrome, which is due to vitamin B deficiency and often, but not always, *indirectly* due to alcoholism). Further, the sting of the argument was taken out when the "chronic" label was abandoned as characterizing the brain disease for the vast majority of addicted people. Nora Volkow did the same in a debate on the brain disease model in Amsterdam—along with Marc Lewis and a number of others, including myself—which can be viewed on YouTube.[74] So far, however, this has not led to changes in the official NIDA doctrine, as can be seen on their website, where addiction is still characterized as a *chronic* brain disease.[75] If disease is defined broadly, such that it includes anyone who is not functioning optimally, then a lot of people have a brain disease, but what does that mean or imply? In the words of Serge Ahmed, a well-known scientist from Bordeaux who does animal research on addiction:

> I finally read "Addiction as a brain disease revised: why it still matters ..." I applaud the effort of trying to save the brain disease model of addiction, as initially advocated by Alan Leshner (Leshner 1.0), from reality. However, Leshner 2.0 has been so much loosened to try to fit reality that it no longer really matters whether addiction is a brain disease or not. There is no question that the brain is involved in addiction, of course, but is it diseased, as the authors postulate? As I see Leshner 2.0, addiction is a pragmatic medical label for a pattern of harmful drug use that is not necessarily chronic relapsing, but instead "spontaneously" remitting most of the time; that is not associated with any individually identifiable brain dysfunction (so far). And, finally, that leaves fundamentally intact an individual's freedom of choice. But despite all these important qualifications, addiction would still be a brain disease. Clearly, as revamped, Leshner 2.0 looks nearly unassailable scientifically. But at the same time, it is also more difficult to distinguish from other competing models that do not postulate that addiction is a brain disease (e.g., the disorder of choice model developed by Gene Heyman over the years). To sum up, Leshner 2.0 is a heroic, albeit desperate attempt to save the original brain disease model of addiction from a scientific crisis that it is traversing since its inception. Leshner 2.0, unlike Leshner 1.0, is alive, but barely recognizable.

This is a nicely worded criticism. Indeed, since almost everyone would agree that all mental processes take place in the brain, mental disorders can be called brain diseases but the question is whether this is helpful or that it can bring a myopia to the brain part of the disorder, while ignoring the important social and developmental aspects. As argued above, and in my recent work with Paul Verschure, I would argue that biased choice is a better label than a brain disease, chronic or not, because it takes away the stigma and leads to a solution (treatment helping to optimize decision making to change behavior) rather than to despair. And, as we will see in the following chapters, prevention and treatment can target decision making in addiction, which can help people to steer their behavior away from addictions.

References

1. Maturana HR, Varela FJ. Autopoiesis and cognition: the realization of the living. Boston, MA: Kluwer; 1980.
2. Edelman GM. Neural Darwinism: the theory of neuronal group selection. Basic Books; 1987.
3. Wiers RW, Verschure PFMJ. Neurale netwerken en ontwikkelingspsychologie: alternatief in ontwikkeling. Tijdschr voor Ontwikkelingspsychologie. 1991;18:123–47.
4. Wiers RW, Verschure PFMJ. Curing the broken brain model of addiction: neurorehabilitation from a systems perspective. Addict Behav [Internet]. 2021;112:106602. Available from: 10.1016/j.addbeh.2020.106602
5. Verschure PFMJ, Wiers RW. Addiction biases choice in the mind, brain, and behavior systems: beyond the brain disease model. In: Evaluating the brain disease model of addiction. Routledge; 2022. pp. 384–404.
6. Seth A. Being you: a new science of consciousness. London: Faber & Faber; 2021.
7. Bouton ME. Context, ambiguity, and unlearning: sources of relapse after behavioral extinction. Biol Psychiatry. 2002;52:976–86.
8. Verschure PFMJ. Distributed adaptive control: a theory of the mind, brain, body nexus. Biol Inspired Cogn Archit. 2012;1:55–72.
9. Verschure PFMJ. Synthetic consciousness: the distributed adaptive control perspective. Philos Trans R Soc B Biol Sci [Internet]. 2016;371:20150448. Available from: http://rstb.royalsocietypublishing.org/lookup/doi/10.1098/rstb.2015.0448
10. Chinn CA, Brewer WF. The role of anomalous data in knowledge acquisition: a theoretical framework and implications for science instruction. Rev Educ Res. 1993;63:1–49.
11. Michotte A. The perception of causality. London: Routledge.
12. Dennett DC. The intentional stance. MIT Press; 1989.
13. Johnson-Laird PN. Mental models and discourse. Trends Cogn Sci. 2001; 5:434–42.
14. Friston K. The free-energy principle: a unified brain theory? Nat Rev Neurosci [Internet]. 2010;11:127–38. Available from: www.ncbi.nlm.nih.gov/pubmed/20068583
15. Harari YN. Sapiens: a brief history of humankind. Random House; 2014.
16. Henrich J. The secret of our success: how culture is driving human evolution, domesticating our species, and making us smarter. Princeton, NJ.: Princeton University press; 2016.
17. Lewis M. The biology of desire: why addiction is not a disease [Internet]. NY: Public Affairs; 2015. 256 p. Available from: https://books.google.com/books?hl=en&lr=&id=CRtpCQAAQBAJ&pgis=1
18. Köpetz CE, Lejuez CW, Wiers RW, Kruglanski AW. Motivation and self-regulation in addiction: a call for convergence. Perspect Psychol Sci [Internet]. 2013 [cited 2013 Mar 2];8:3–24. Available from: http://pps.sagepub.com/lookup/doi/10.1177/1745691612457575

19. Haushofer J, Fehr E. On the psychology of poverty. Science (80–). 2014; 344:862–7.
20. Farrelly MC, Nonnemaker J, Davis KC, Hussin A. The influence of the National Truth campaign on smoking initiation. Am J Prev Med [Internet]. 2009;36:379–84. Available from: 10.1016/j.amepre.2009.01.019
21. Thayer JF, Lane RD. A model of neurovisceral integration in emotion regulation and dysregulation. J Affect Disord. 2000;61:201–16.
22. Kox M, Van Eijk LT, Zwaag J, Van Den Wildenberg J, Sweep FCGJ, Van Der Hoeven JG, et al. Voluntary activation of the sympathetic nervous system and attenuation of the innate immune response in humans. Proc Natl Acad Sci U S A. 2014;111:7379–84.
23. Muzik O, Reilly KT, Diwadkar VA. "Brain over body": a study on the willful regulation of autonomic function during cold exposure. Neuroimage [Internet]. 2018;172:632–41. Available from: 10.1016/j.neuroimage.2018.01.067
24. Duin RJ. Oefeningen Iceman Wim Hof eisen slachtoffers. Het Parool [Internet]. 2016; Available from: www.parool.nl/nieuws/oefeningen-iceman-wim-hof-eisen-slachtoffers~be5fa5d0/
25. Morsella E, Berger CC, Krieger SC. Cognitive and neural components of the phenomenology of agency. Neurocase. 2011;17:209–30.
26. Minsky M. Society of mind. NY: Simon and Schuster; 1986.
27. Heyman GM. Addiction and choice: theory and new data. Front Psychiatry. 2013;4:1–5.
28. Pearson D, Watson P, Albertella L, Le Pelley ME. Attentional economics links value-modulated attentional capture and decision-making. Nat Rev Psychol. 2022;1:320–33.
29. Rangel A, Camerer C, Montague PR. A framework for studying the neurobiology of value-based decision making. Nat Rev Neurosci. 2008; 9:545–56.
30. Hare TA, Camerer CF, Rangel A. Valuation system. Science (80–). 2009; 324:646–9.
31. Rangel A, Hare T. Neural computations associated with goal-directed choice. Curr Opin Neurobiol [Internet]. 2010;20:262–70. Available from: 10.1016/j.conb.2010.03.001
32. Scholz C, Dore BP, Cooper N, Falk EB. Neural valuation of antidrinking campaigns and risky peer influence in daily life. Heal Psychol. 2019; 38:658–67.
33. Garrison KA, DeMartini KS, Corlett PR, Worhunsky PD, Krystal JH, O'Malley SS. Drinking and responses to antidrinking messages among young adults: An fMRI study. Addict Biol. 2021;26.
34. Heatherton TF, Wagner DD. Cognitive neuroscience of self-regulation failure. Trends Cogn Sci [Internet]. 2011;15:132–9. Available from: 10.1016/j.tics.2010.12.005
35. Gladwin TE, Figner B, Crone EA, Wiers RW. Addiction, adolescence, and the integration of control and motivation. Dev Cogn Neurosci [Internet]. 2011 [cited 2013 Feb 28];1:364–76. Available from: www.ncbi.nlm.nih.gov/pubmed/22436562
36. Hazy TE, Frank MJ, O'Reilly RC. Towards an executive without a homunculus: computational models of the prefrontal cortex/basal ganglia system. Philos Trans R Soc Lond B Biol Sci [Internet]. 2007;362:1601–13. Available from: www.ncbi.nlm.nih.gov/pubmed/17428778

37. Hare TA, Malmaud J, Rangel A. Focusing attention on the health aspects of foods changes value signals in vmPFC and improves dietary choice. J Neurosci. 2011;31:11077–87.
38. Berkman ET, Hutcherson CA, Livingston JL, Kahn LE, Inzlicht M. Self-control as value-based choice. Curr Dir Psychol Sci [Internet]. 2017;26:422–8. Available from: 10.1177/0963721417704394
39. Berkman ET. The motivated brain [Internet]. Psychology Today. Available from: www.psychologytoday.com/intl/blog/the-motivated-brain
40. Berkman ET. Value-based choice: an integrative, neuroscience-informed model of health goals. Psychol Heal [Internet]. 2018;33:40–57. Available from: 10.1080/08870446.2017.1316847
41. Awh E, Belopolsky A V., Theeuwes J. Top-down versus bottom-up attentional control: a failed theoretical dichotomy. Trends Cogn Sci [Internet]. 2012;16:437–43. Available from: 10.1016/j.tics.2012.06.010
42. Le Pelley ME, Pearson D, Griffiths O, Beesley T. When goals conflict with values: counterproductive attentional and oculomotor capture by reward-related stimuli. J Exp Psychol Gen. 2015;144:158–71.
43. Anderson BA. Relating value-driven attention to psychopathology. Curr Opin Psychol [Internet]. 2021;39:48–54. Available from: 10.1016/j.copsyc.2020.07.010
44. Nigg JT. On inhibition/disinhibition in developmental psychopathology: views from cognitive and personality psychology and a working inhibition taxonomy. Psychol Bull. 2000;126:220.
45. Williams J, Taylor E. The evolution of hyperactivity, impulsivity and cognitive diversity. J R Soc Interface. 2006;3:399–413.
46. Hare TA, Hakimi S, Rangel A. Activity in dlPFC and its effective connectivity to vmPFC are associated with temporal discounting. Front Neurosci. 2014;8:1–15.
47. Hommel B, Wiers RW. Towards a unitary approach to human action control. Trends Cogn Sci. 2017;21
48. Larsen JK, Hollands GJ. Targeting automatic processes to reduce unhealthy behaviours: a process framework. Health Psychol Rev [Internet]. 2022;16:204–19. Available from: 10.1080/17437199.2021.1876572
49. Walasek L, Brown GDA. Incomparability and incommensurability in choice: no common currency of value? Perspect Psychol Sci. In press.
50. Inzlicht M, Schmeichel BJ, Macrae CN. Why self-control seems (but may not be) limited. Trends Cogn Sci [Internet]. 2014;1–7. Available from: 10.1016/j.tics.2013.12.009
51. Baumeister RF, Bratslavsky E, Muraven M. Ego depletion: is the active self a limited resource? In: Self-regulation and self-control. Routledge; 2018. pp. 24–52.
52. Hagger MS, Chatzisarantis NLD, Alberts H, Anggono CO, Batailler C, Birt AR, et al. A multilab preregistered replication of the ego-depletion effect. Perspect Psychol Sci. 2016;11:546–73.
53. Vohs K, Schmeichel B, Lohmann S, Gronau QF, Finley A, whenyoup I, et al. A multi-site preregistered paradigmatic test of the ego depletion effect. Psychol Sci. 2021; 10.1177/0956797621989733.
54. Job V, Walton GM, Bernecker K, Dweck CS. Beliefs about willpower determine the impact of glucose on self-control. 2013;110:14837–42.
55. Wiehler A, Branzoli F, Adanyeguh I, Mochel F, Pessiglione M. A neuro-metabolic account of why daylong cognitive work alters the control of economic decisions. Curr Biol. 2022; 10.1016/j.cub.2022.07.010.

56. Anderson BA. What is abnormal about addiction-related attentional biases? Drug Alcohol Depend [Internet]. 2016;167:8–14. Available from: 10.1016/j.drugalcdep.2016.08.002
57. Albertella L, Le Pelley ME, Chamberlain SR, Westbrook F, Fontenelle LF, Segrave R, et al. Reward-related attentional capture is associated with severity of addictive and obsessive–compulsive behaviors. Psychol Addict Behav [Internet]. 2019;33:495–502. Available from: 10.1080/13506285.2014.994252
58. Wiers RW, Van Gaal S, Le Pelley ME. Akrasia and addiction: Neurophilosophy and psychological mechanisms. In: J Harbecke, C Herrmann-Pillath (Eds.). Social Neuroeconomics: integrating the neurosciences and the social sciences. London: Routledge; 2020.
59. Field M, Heather N, Murphy JG, Stafford T, Tucker JA, Witkiewitz K. Recovery from addiction: behavioral economics and value-based decision making. Psychol Addict Behav. 2020;34:182–93.
60. Hogarth L. A critical review of habit theory of drug dependence. In: B Verplanken (Ed.). The psychology of habit. Cham: Springer; 2018. pp. 325–41.
61. Cooper ML, Frone MR, Russell M, Mudar P. Drinking to regulate positive and negative emotions: a motivational model of alcohol use. J Pers Soc Psychol [Internet]. 1995;69:990–1005. Available from: www.ncbi.nlm.nih.gov/pubmed/7473043
62. Verplanken B, Walker I, Davis A, Jurasek M. Context change and travel mode choice: combining the habit discontinuity and self-activation hypotheses. J Environ Psychol. 2008;28:121–7.
63. Hogarth L. Addiction is driven by excessive goal-directed drug choice under negative affect: translational critique of habit and compulsion theory. Neuropsychopharmacology [Internet]. 2020; Available from: 10.1038/s41386-020-0600-8
64. Belin D, Mar AC, Dalley JW, Robbins TW, Everitt BJ. High impulsivity predicts the switch to compulsive cocaine-taking. Science (80–). 2008; 320:1352–5.
65. Schoenbaum G, Chang CY, Lucantonio F, Takahashi YK. Thinking outside the box: orbitofrontal cortex, imagination, and how we can treat addiction. Neuropsychopharmacology. 2016;41:2966–76.
66. Moeller SJ, Beebe-Wang N, Woicik PA, Konova AB, Maloney T, Goldstein RZ. Choice to view cocaine images predicts concurrent and prospective drug use in cocaine addiction. Drug Alcohol Depend [Internet]. 2013;130:178–85. Available from: 10.1016/j.drugalcdep.2012.11.001
67. Goldstein RZ, Bechara A, Garavan H, Childress AR, Paulus MP, Volkow ND. The neurocircuitry of impaired insight in drug addiction. Trends Cogn Sci. 2009;13:372–80.
68. Hart CL, Hart MZ. Opioid crisis: another mechanism used to perpetuate American racism. Cult Divers Ethn Minor Psychol. 2019;25:6–11.
69. Sterling P, Platt ML. Why deaths of despair are increasing in the US and not other industrial nations—insights from neuroscience and anthropology. Am J Psychiatry. 2022. doi: 10.1001/jamapsychiatry.2021.4209
70. Heilig M, Mackillop J, Leggio L. Addiction as a brain disease revised: why it still matters, and the need for consilience. Neuropsychopharmacology [Internet]. 2021; Available from: 10.1038/s41386-020-00950-y
71. Jellinek EM. The disease model of addiction. New Haven, CT: Hillhouse Press; 1960.

72. Hall W, Carter A, Forlini C. The brain disease model of addiction: is it supported by the evidence and has it delivered on its promises? The Lancet Psychiatry [Internet]. 2015;2:105–10. Available from: 10.1016/S2215-0366(14)00126-6
73. Fenton T, Wiers RW. Free will, black swans and addiction. Neuroethics. 2017;10.
74. Volkow ND, Lewis M, Van der Wolff M, Bastiaans J, Wiers RW. Addiction brain disease debate Amsterdam [Internet]. 2018. Available from: www.youtube.com/watch?v=05PH-lY-ELs&t=30s
75. VolkowND. What does it mean when we call addiction a brain disorder [Internet]. 2018 [cited 2022 Aug 10]. Available from: https://nida.nih.gov/about-nida/noras-blog/2018/03/what-does-it-mean-when-we-call-addiction-brain-disorder
76. Sterling P. What is health? Allostasis and the evolution of human design. Cambridge, MA: MIT Press; 2020.
77. Heyman GM. Addiction: a disorder of choice. Harvard University Press; 2010.
78. Heather N. Q: Is addiction a brain disease or a moral failing? A: Neither. Neuroethics [Internet]. 2017; Available from: 10.1007/s12152-016-9289-0
79. Bickel WK, Jarmolowicz DP, Mueller ET, Gatchalian KM. The behavioral economics and neuroeconomics of reinforcer pathologies: implications for etiology and treatment of addiction. Curr Psychiatry Rep. 2011;13:406–15.
80. Rigoli F. Reference effects on decision-making elicited by previous rewards. Cognition [Internet]. 2019;192:104034. Available from: 10.1016/j.cognition.2019.104034
81. Festinger L. A theory of cognitive dissonance. Vol. 2. Stanford University Press; 1957.

6 Development, vulnerability and prevention

In the summer of 2021, while I was working on this book, I received the following email:

> I came across your name in a report from 1994. At that time, at the request of the alcohol clinic, I participated in your research into the extent to which addiction is hereditary. Your report has had a great impact on the rest of my life, I would like to share that with you. Not from reprimand or seeking therapy, but more from the perspective of sharing experiences on an equal basis. Perhaps you could also tell me more on the background and results of the research now. I think this could also help me in my acceptance process. I would greatly appreciate it if you could spare an hour of your time so that I can tell you how I came to you then and what effect the report had.

We agreed to meet, more than 25 years later. Chantal turned out to be an athletic-looking woman with an open face. We didn't recognize each other, and I explained that I probably hadn't tested her myself, because an intern did the testing of the children, while remaining "blind" to the background of the child (parent with alcoholism or not), while I interviewed one of her parents. She told me about the difficult time she had had in the period before she participated in our study. Her parents were divorcing at the time, and she (the oldest) had not wanted to move with her father, but also could no longer handle staying with her mother, the parent with the alcohol problem. At the clinic, they had gone through family sessions, where she had been asked to participate in the study. After participation, she had received feedback, which had hit her like a bomb: she had to be careful not to become addicted too, while her little brother was not at risk.

I had read the reports that had been sent at the time (she had sent copies of the originals with her email): one from the child psychiatrist involved and from the medical assistant about her physical health and

DOI: 10.4324/9781032634548-6

development, one from a colleague about her personality, and one from me, about the findings regarding her intelligence, social-emotional development and expectations about the effects of alcohol. She gave further background about her circumstances at the time: she suffered a lot from fear of failure. Her mother felt it was very important for the children to be able to take care of themselves, probably foreseeing that she would not be able to take care of them long, and therefore placed a high value on a good education. So already in elementary school, Chantal and her brother received extra homework assignments from her, to enable them to go to a good school afterwards. She had been diagnosed with dyslexia, so her school career had been difficult. My report stated that she scored above average on performance IQ (perceptual organization and processing, related to math), and slightly below average on verbal IQ, in line with her story. She agreed; she had also had a psychologist friend read the reports, who also had little to say about them. And yet those reports had really upset her. What had happened?

First, the feedback about her personality: Chantal scored high on both sensation seeking and (negative) emotionality, two traits that in different ways somewhat increased the likelihood of developing addiction. I had found that she also scored relatively high on the expectancy that consuming alcohol allows you to relax and forget about your problems for a while, which—coupled with negative emotionality—is a risk factor for developing problem drinking. These findings were, of course, packed with the necessary caution; for example, it stated that this *could be related* to a slightly increased likelihood of developing a problem and that it was therefore advisable to be careful with alcohol.

Things probably went wrong further down the line, because the reports were sent to her parents (in line with the law back then for studies with minors), who subsequently gave a brief summary of them to the children. From that summary, Chantal remembered that she had to be extra careful, because she was like her mother. If she drank or used drugs, before she realized, she would be at risk of becoming a problem drinker or drug user. As a result, she had been very cautious with alcohol and other substances for the rest of her life. She had smoked for a bit, but had quit when she started to feel dependent on it. She had also tried cocaine on occasion, but had immediately stopped, not wanting to follow in her mother's footsteps. She told me that that her mother's last year had been especially terrible. Chantal had hardly been able to reach her, but she knew her mother mostly wandered around the city of Amsterdam drunkenly, and finally died of pneumonia. Looking back now, in the context of her story, the objections to the chronic brain disease model of addiction suddenly sounded a bit academic. Maybe Jelinek and current proponents of the chronic brain disease model of addiction are right that in some people, addiction is indeed a persistent disease that leads to self-destruction. Luckily in most it is not.

Chantal wanted to know what had come out of the research on the heritability of alcohol addiction. I explained that our research was not so much answering the question to what extent addiction is hereditary, because twin studies had already indicated at the time that it was partly genetic. How did that work? You compare twins—when one twin develops an addiction problem, what is the chance that the other twin develops the same problem? Importantly, when this chance is considerably larger when the twins share the same genes, that is, they are monozygotic, than when they are dizygotic, and share half their genes, like other siblings, that points toward a genetic factor in the development of addiction. And indeed, that had been demonstrated in many studies already at the time. In contrast, our study aimed to investigate possible mechanisms underlying the increased risk for addiction in children with an alcohol-dependent parent. How does this work, what are the steps between being born with an above-average risk for addiction and later outcomes, like developing an addiction or not. The idea behind the research was that if we understood these mechanisms better, we might be better able to help these children to prevent this outcome in the future. Our approach had been inspired by the research of Ken Sher from the University of Missouri at Columbia, who became my external PhD advisor, after a memorable visit to Amsterdam in my first year as a PhD student. At the start of my unusual PhD trajectory (which I was setting up with my advisors, who were not experts in addiction), I was given the chance to invite an international scholar that I expected to learn from most, concerning psychological factors in the enhanced risk for addiction in children with an alcohol-dependent parent. That was an easy choice as Ken had just written an excellent book about the topic.[1] I also visited Ken and his family later during my PhD and especially the organization of his research team and the advanced statistical methods to test hypotheses in an optimal way made a great impression. He has remained a dear friend throughout the years.

With Chantal I shared some of our findings and showed her some tests she might remember, such as the door game. The participant opened doors on a computer screen, after which either a smiling or a frowning face would appear. When it was a smiley, the child received a nickel, with a frowny a nickel was taken away. The child could decide when to stop playing the game and when they stopped, they could keep the collected nickels. The game was programmed so that behind the first ten doors there were only smileys (10 wins, 0 losses), behind the next ten doors, there were 9 smileys and one frowny (9 wins, 1 loss), behind the next ten doors 8 smileys and 2 times a frowny, and so on. The maximum number of doors that could be opened was 110, at that point all previously gained nickels were gone again. The maximum win was around 55 opened doors, and remarkably, the control children (with no addiction in the family, nor a diagnosis of ADHD) stopped on average after 55 doors—a nice example of the "wisdom of the crowd". Some of these kids stopped too early, after a couple of losses, missing out on further gains, others went on too long and lost part of their previously gained reward, but as a group they stopped at the optimal point in time. Apparently, as a group we sense at some point that things are going in the wrong direction and that we would be better off quitting.

How did the children with an alcohol-dependent parent fare? On average they went on longer, not as long, however, as children with ADHD who had not family members with an alcohol problem (a contrast group we included).[2] I remember a lively boy of about 8 years old who was totally absorbed in the game and kept telling himself to open one more door and then he would stop, for sure. He kept repeating the phrase: "just one more" to the very end, losing all of his previously won reward, even facing almost only losses (among the last twenty doors 19 were frowning faces with losses). The most remarkable observation was that the boy repeated this behavior during the second session of the game, at the very end of the test session. The idea behind this repetition was to examine whether the children had learned from their earlier experience and would adjust their strategy accordingly. Here it seemed like you could almost foresee the later addiction problems in the behavior during the game.

"So did the boy get addicted?"

"We don't know", I had to answer. Unfortunately, the study had not been continued after we had graduated, the PI moved to a different hospital and that was it. It would not be easy to resume the study, if possible at all, given current stringent privacy rules.

"However, this was only one measure, so yes, based on this measure only, you would guess this boy was more likely than average to develop addiction problems later. But ... so many things can happen afterward. Maybe he found a great mentor at school or at his football club, those things can also make a major difference, research has shown."

Chantal nodded; she vaguely remembered the game, and did not like it so much, but did remember her brother loving it.

I told her about our findings on the development of alcohol expectancies, that they developed from negative to positive in all children once they started drinking and that this was often even more pronounced in children with an alcohol-dependent parent. She recognized this and found this interesting. I explained to her that this shift was likely related to the genetic factor in risk for addiction: when your body reacts favorably to a substance, chances are you repeat taking it, while this chance decreases when you felt bad afterwards. So some of the genetic factors only become relevant once you start using the substance. She nodded. I explained that a favorable reaction should actually be interpreted as a warning signal, but that it is easily misinterpret it as a positive sign: my parent had problems with alcohol, but I take it well.

We talked further about the feedback. She felt that the feedback had intensified her fear of failure and that for a long time she had felt a kind of doom about her, the feeling that it would end badly for her, no matter what. But she was over that now, and she was even helping other people finding their destiny, as a coach. She had taken her life into her own hands. I told her the background of the feedback, that this had first of all been a requirement of the ethics committee in such a comprehensive study: when participation requires a lot of time, personalized feedback was expected. And giving feedback was also an advantage in recruiting the control children. Why would they participate if nothing was the matter with them nor with their parents? Parents enjoyed getting some feedback on their child's personality and IQ, and the children could gain some money and received a present.

The feedback with the children of alcohol-dependent parents was of course more sensitive, and we carefully composed and triple checked our formulations. However, despite our careful formulations, she had received the feedback through the parents, which had resulted in an overly simple summary in her case: "you have to watch out". That is something to consider in future research. I should have realized that it is difficult to properly assess risk and perhaps we should have paid more attention to transmitting the information to the children, although that would not have been easy with the large age-range of participants (6–18). As a grown woman, how did she feel about the risk now? I decided to put it to the test: "Suppose you have a school class of twenty children. Then, on average, one of those children develops an alcohol addiction. Now suppose we take a class that includes only children of alcohol-dependent parents, how many would that be?" She looked at the ceiling.

"All of them?", she replied.

"No, about three or four; the vast majority would *not* develop an addiction problem themselves."

This was an eye-opener. Should we have shared this with Chantal at the time? The fact was that the feedback had affected her further development; she had been very cautious with substances, but she had also been unhappy about it.

I asked her if she wanted to hear a bit more about the genetic part of the story, which she did. I told her about the large number of genes that all determine a very small piece of risk. That there are hundreds if not thousands of genes involved that all affect a very small piece of the genetic part of risk. The risk variant of the gene is generally less common, let's say 1 in 6. So with the genes you get, it is like throwing dice. What is the probability of someone throwing a 6 over and over again? If you throw the dice, say, a hundred times, you expect a six 16 to 17 times. But some people might throw a six 25 times; then they have a somewhat increased risk, but you have to remember that environmental factors also play an important role. Therefore, the summary of the feedback as "you have high risk and your brother does not" was a simplification. This is a gradual scale, with everyone having some risk to develop an addiction, but some a bit more than others.

We talked about the "doom" she had experienced and I told her about the famous geneticist Ken Kendler who had stated that people are uniquely able to "trump their genes".

As we can to some extent imagine the effect of our choices, some children of alcohol-dependent parents decide to never start drinking themselves.[3] This is smart, given that a lot of the important genetic factors involved in the risk to develop addiction are related to how your body reacts to the substance, whether you experience a strong kick and the extent to which you experience negative feelings. Genetic research has shown that your choices are especially important when you have an increased vulnerability: for example, if you do well on alcohol, it may be not such a smart idea to join a fraternity where drinking is a main activity, which is likely to be less of a problem if you do not handle alcohol well: you will have a good reason to not drink too much. Chantal had always been aware of a risk and she now sees that our feedback might have had a beneficial side, because after two wines she knew she had to stop. But the doom idea had also caused her lots of stress and despair. She thanked me for the conversation, which I could assure her, had also been interesting for me. The question remains, how best to share that heightened-risk story with people who are affected themselves. I'm thinking now: warn, but at the same time explicitly avoid a black-and-white interpretation (the school class question) and perhaps learn to recognize signs (e.g., a favorable response to alcohol) and discuss strategies to curb the risk, without conjuring up a doom-and-gloom mindset.

Development, genetics and biased choice

In the previous chapter, I discussed the model of addiction as biased choice, as an alternative to the dichotomy of seeing addiction either as a chronic brain disease or as moral failure. What do we know about the development of addiction and how does it relate to these views? Why do some people develop addiction and others do not? If you ask this, in all likelihood you will get an answer like: it must have something to do with genes and environment. And that's true, as it is for almost all behaviors in which people differ from one another; by now that's almost a dead giveaway. And in addiction, the influence of both aspects is also estimated to be about 50%, with some differences between substances:

the highest genetic contribution is found for hard drugs such as opiates and cocaine, around 70%, while for the most commonly used substances, alcohol, tobacco and cannabis, the estimate is about 50%, and the same is true for pathological gambling.[4]

But what does this mean? That we know exactly which genes play a role and can predict exactly who especially should not take opiates because of high genetic vulnerability? No, it does not. These are global estimates of the contribution of hereditary factors to differences between people, based on twin studies, how often traits cooccur in monozygotic versus dizygotic twins. The idea behind this is that twins grow up in the same environment. If a trait is more common in both individuals in case of identical twins, then genes will play a role, and the extent of that influence can be estimated. Based on this idea, large twin registries have been started in various places around the world, in which thousands of twins have been periodically questioned about all sorts of things, including health behaviors. From these, then, an estimate can be made of the contribution of hereditary factors to behavior. Based on this kind of research, we know that in addiction, by and large, about half of the differences between people have to do with hereditary factors, but how does that work as a child develops?

As mentioned in the interchange with Chantal, in my doctoral studies, I investigated this in children with a parent with alcohol dependence, which were compared with matched controls and with a contrast group of children with ADHD who did not have addiction in the family. ADHD and related traits likely play a role in the increased risk of developing addiction at an early age,[2] with shared genetic vulnerability playing a role.[5] Research has shown that the genetic contribution to the risk of becoming addicted has to do partly with general traits (e.g., personality) and partly with specific reactions to a substance. Personality is an important general predictor: children who are relatively impulsive and who score high on sensation seeking are more likely to start drinking and use other drugs at an early age.[6] Children who are relatively anxious and somber have this to a lesser extent,[7–9] but they are also more likely to develop problems later in life (once they start drinking). They are more likely to teach themselves to drink or use other substances or engage in addictive behaviors to temporarily get rid of their negative feelings, an expectancy Chantal scored high on.[10,11]

Drug-specific genetic effects influence the effect of a drug—some genes influence the extent to which you experience a "kick" after ingestion and others to what extent you experience negative effects later on (the main trouble with drugs, from a learning perspective: what comes first gets a stronger connection in your memory). This is related to the aforementioned negative reaction to alcohol of relatively many people of Asian descent; they have variants of genes that produce enzymes that do not break down alcohol effectively in the stomach (ALDH2 and ADH1B).[12] This is a strong protective factor against developing an alcohol problem. The reverse is also true: if you are naturally very resistant to alcohol and end up in a context where there is a lot of drinking, your risk of alcohol dependence increases.[13] These effects are well documented for alcohol and probably work like this in general: the more a person experiences short-term benefits and suffers less negative effects from a substance, the more likely problematic use is to develop.[4]

In terms of the decision model, then, neuroadaptations take place that encourage repeated use. This applies not only to alcohol, but also to other substances, for example, the variety of nicotine receptors you inherit play a role in the genetic risk of developing tobacco addiction and how difficult it is to quit.[14] The important point here is that these drug-specific genetic effects only manifest themselves when you start using the drug. I might have a huge genetic vulnerability to develop cocaine or heroin addiction, but this risk factor remains dormant as long as I don't take the drug. That is how we can trump our genes. The genetic contribution to starting or not starting a drug is smaller than the genetic contribution to the subsequent course of the relationship with that drug (how much a person takes and whether it leads to addiction), which is understandable because only after someone starts using, substance-specific genetic factors come into play.[15,16]

The puzzle of missing heritability

Note that current genetic research focuses much more on effects of specific genes, rather than the overall estimates of heritability of a certain behavior (based on twin studies). That research has produced an interesting puzzle: that of *missing heritability*. What this boils down to is that more and more specific genes are becoming known to contribute to a specific behavior (e.g., smoking). Those specific genes are all responsible for a very small piece of the puzzle (the "explained variance"), per gene involved rarely more than 1% and more often a fraction of a percent (the aforementioned variants of ALDH2 and ADH1B are outliers, they explain more than other genes).[17,18] They have a strong influence on behavior: if you immediately feel terrible after taking a substance, the chances of becoming addicted to that drug are extremely small. As alcohol use is widespread, chances are that someone will try it one day, making this genetic influence generally relevant.

The puzzle of missing heritability is the following: if we add up all the known small contributions of specific genes in explaining differences between people in a certain trait, for example alcohol addiction, we arrive at about 10%, which is a far cry from the estimates from the twin studies, which arrive at, 50% heritability. What happened to the rest? Early on, the response was usually that this would work itself out once larger samples were taken, but it is now clear that the problem persists even with very large samples of more than a hundred thousand people. The explained variance then grows a few percent, but the gap remains large between the summed contribution of specific genes and the estimated total heritability.[19]

One possible explanation is that the estimates based on twin studies are too high, for example, because the assumed equal environment of the two children is not quite correct.[19] While parents tend to raise children broadly the same, a child has its own micro-environment in a family. For example, if Milan is perceived a little cheekier than Joshua, which could be based on chance (say the boys drew straws who would steal cookies, and Milan subsequently got caught)[i], parents will tend to hold Milan a little shorter, which in turn can create negative feelings in Milan ("Joshua is allowed … and I'm not!"). Thus, child-specific positive or negative spirals of interactions can occur. Other explanations have been proposed on the genetic side: rare genetic factors may contribute large effects that are not easily found in standard genetic genome wide association studies (GWAS, e.g., rare genes with a variable number of repeat structures).[20,21] Finally, part of the explanation may come from interactions between genes and between genes and environment.

Interactions between genes and environment

Importantly, whether risk factors come to expression or not often depends on the environment. One of the most famous examples is the MAOA gene, which was first related to aggressive and dangerous behavior (fights, arson, etc.) by Han Brunner and his team in the Netherlands. They examined a notorious family from the Nijmegen area

i Chance has been identified as the third factor in development, in addition to genes and environment.[90,91] While many people believe that if you could perfectly measure genetic and environmental influences, you should be able to perfectly predict development, this is not true. The reason is that in complex systems, such as the developing human brain in a complex environment, small deviations in early development can have a disproportionate effect on later outcomes, as was shown in simulation studies by Van der Maas and colleagues.[91] The research goes back to efforts to minimize variance (differences between individuals) of biological traits in laboratory rats by standardizing environmental and genetic conditions, which surprisingly failed to reduce variance, from which it was concluded that there is an important third source of variance based on interactions between chance (starting values) and genetic and environmental factors. Hence, the straw Milan drew could hypothetically set a negative spiral in motion, and as we will see later, a random encounter with a stimulating teacher or coach can also set positive spirals into motion.

in which such behavior was common, at least among the men.[22] The gene was found to be on the X chromosome, which explains a high incidence of this behavior in male carriers of the risk variant. Remember from biology, that men have only one X chromosome (the other sex chromosome is Y, in contrast with women who have XX), so the influence of the rare "risk variant" is much greater in men than in women, where a possible effect is typically masked by the gene on the other X chromosome. This makes some women carriers of the risk variant without showing the related symptoms.

Caspi and colleagues showed in a landmark *Science* paper that this gene plays a role in the development of antisocial behavior, but that interaction with the environment was crucial: only in children who had been maltreated in childhood, a strong association was found between the presence of the risk variant of the gene and the development of antisocial behavior later on.[23] These data came from the Dunedin study, named after the city in New Zealand where a cohort of some two thousand children born in the early 1970s was followed. Importantly, the outcome was determined with objective measures, such as police convictions and reports of child abuse.

A year later, the same group published another influential study, on a variant of a serotonin transporter gene that, in combination with stress, increases the risk of depression.[24] Subsequent studies did not always confirm this relationship, but that included the fact that it often did not involve objective measures, such as past stress, but rather a look back at how stressful a person's childhood had been.[25] These studies were very influential, but the field has largely abandoned the search for individual genes that influence the development of mental health problems: currently the collective influence of sets of "risk genes" are studied, based on large genome-wide association studies (GWAS).[26] However, this research is still in its infancy. Few replicated findings have yet emerged from it, which is also due to uncertainty about which risk genes can now be reasonably summed without losing information.[27] In conclusion, there is no doubt that genes influence behavior, including choices that can result in addiction, but it involves a complex interplay between many genes with a small influence and environmental factors with a role of chance.

Orchids and dandelions or …

Regarding the relationship between genetic and environmental factors, in recent years another model has received much attention in psychology: that of the proverbial dandelions and orchids, or the model of *differential susceptibility* by University of California's Jay Belsky and colleagues,[28] and popularized by Tom Boyce.[29] The idea of this model is that many of the gene-environment interactions that influence individual differences in vulnerability to mental health problems affect the degree of sensitivity to environmental factors. Thus, when a child with high genetic sensitivity to environmental factors is placed in a poor environment, his development is more negative than for other children, as we saw in the study by Caspi and colleagues: after child maltreatment, the likelihood of convictions increased dramatically in genetically vulnerable children. The model of differential sensitivity also highlights the other side of the coin: the same sensitive children would also be more reactive to a positive environment and to therapy.[30] Indeed, there is evidence that the latter is true.[31] As Belsky nicely put it: some children are more sensitive to their environment than others, *for better and for worse.*[28] In his book, Tom Boyce relates this idea to his own history, where he describes himself as the dandelion (as about 80% of the population) and his sister as the orchid. Their parents were very critical and fighting a lot, by which he was not affected a great deal, but his sister was, resulting in mental health problems that ended in suicide. From the orchid dandelion perspective, she might have thrived even more than he did, when she had been raised in a nurturing environment.

Now what does this have to do with dandelions and orchids? An orchid is very sensitive and dies easily (especially on my windowsill), but produces the most beautiful flowers under good conditions; dandelions, on the other hand, grow just about anywhere—a strip of soil between two paving stones is enough—and always produce the same, pretty nice flowers. Thus, according to this model, there are also some children who are very sensitive (the proverbial orchids), who have the poorest outcomes in bad circumstances, but the best outcomes ones under good conditions, and other children (the proverbial dandelions) who more or less imperturbably follow their life paths unless conditions get too harsh. The idea of differential susceptibility is interesting and attractive, but the empirical underpinnings are not strong as yet: sometimes findings are made that are consistent with theory, but often not.[27,32]

As my dear friend Ron Dahl from Berkeley pointed out, the inconsistent findings may be because it seems counterintuitive that this mechanism takes place at the level of the individual: that some individuals are very sensitive to *all sorts* of environmental influences and others not. An evolutionary more likely scenario could be that sensitivity to environmental influences differs by trait. So that individuals who are likely to develop impulsive and aggressive behaviors in some environments not necessarily also are the same individuals who are most sensitive to develop posttraumatic stress syndrome after trauma or who develop most positively in a nurturing environment. This could relate to some of the phenomena we saw in the development of addiction: some genes make people very sensitive to the effects of a *specific* substance (e.g., a type of nicotine receptors), which does not influence risk to develop another addiction (e.g., alcoholism), for which some other substance-specific genes are relevant. Developmental timing plays an important role as well, as we saw in chapter 4: when substance use begins in adolescence, it becomes more difficult to discontinue it in adulthood. And early use of cannabis increases the vulnerability for later psychosis and other mental health problems in genetically sensitive individuals,[33] illustrating that genetic vulnerabilities interact not only with the environment but also with development.

Evolution and addiction

One of the questions that often arises when discussing the genetic side of addiction is how it is possible that there is a genetic influence, since addiction increases your risk of disease and early death and thus provides no evolutionary advantage. As described, there are broadly two types of genes that play a role in susceptibility to addiction: genes that influence brain or bodily reactions to the substance and genes that influence general personality traits, which in turn cause an increased risk of starting addictive substances early (sensation seeking and impulsivity) or having difficulty getting off once you start (predisposition to strong negative feelings of anxiety and hopelessness).

As for the first type of genetic influences, there is evidence that taking a drug may have had a selection advantage under certain circumstances.[34] Evolutionary psychologists argue that humans and psychotropic plants evolved together. The use of psychoactive substances such as khat, coca, tobacco and the betel nut go back more than ten thousand years. These substances were generally chewed for their energy-boosting qualities rather than to get "high", similar to the way we use coffee and tea today. Furthermore, some substances were selected for pain relief or medicinal effects. The psychoactive ingredients of these plants have evolved over hundreds of millions of years as defensive chemicals that closely resemble mammalian neurotransmitters.[34] So it is no coincidence that these substances affect our brains. For important neurotransmitters in the brain, such as dopamine, serotonin and adrenaline, we actually need nutrients, some of which can be obtained from psychoactive plants. Humans developed methods to consume the plants, either mechanically (long chewing) or with behavior (drying or cooking). The reason was that the substances from these plants had positive effects in the low natural dose, although you had to get used to the often bitter taste first, related to the defensive function of the plants involved.[34] We still experience the same when first encountering psychoactive substances: the first cigarette is downright nasty for almost everyone, causing headaches, sore throats and nausea.[35] So why do many start smoking?

It must be because of other factors, especially in the social environment, such as joining the group (also a strong evolutionary determined need). And eventually after some persistence, rewarding brain mechanisms are activated.[36]

This adaptive evolutionary explanation differs from the variant commonly linked to addiction as a chronic brain disease. The idea there is that drugs *hijack* evolutionarily adaptive motivational brain mechanisms,[37] and from that approach, the use of psychoactive substances is bad, because we don't want our motivational system to be hijacked. Whereas we normally find things attractive that are good for our chances of survival (and opportunities to reproduce), addictive substances act directly on the underlying brain mechanisms, with the result that they make repeated use of the same substance attractive, for example, by dopamine activation in response to an addictive substance leading to an attentional bias for cues of the substance and a tendency to approach a cue signaling the substance (sensitization; see Chapter 3).

The question to this evolutionary explanation is: why don't *most* people who use addictive substances become addicted? The adaptive evolutionary account states that we have co-evolved with certain plants and that many people benefit from the use of these substances, but that a proportion of people develop problems with them, especially when the dose used is much stronger than the naturally occurring dose, as with distilled alcohol and cocaine. With alcohol, distilling first led to social problems as a result of drinking it. Before that, in the European Middle ages, drinking light alcoholic beer was a protective factor for health, since water was often unhealthy.[38] To illustrate the difference between the original coca leaves, still chewed in South America, and cocaine, guess how many kilograms of coca leaves are needed to produce 1 gram of cocaine.[ii]

Expectancies

As discussed with Chantal, in humans an additional factor plays a role in the risk for addiction: we can become aware of an increased risk for addiction, for example, because family members are addicted. If your grandfather and your father had an alcohol problem, you are probably told at some point that you have to be careful with booze. When starting my doctoral research on risk factors for alcohol addiction in children

ii 17 kilograms! According to records from a coca museum in Peru. Hence, chewing coca leaves or drinking coca tea made from the leaves is not comparable to using cocaine. The recent opiate crisis in the US is attributed in part to the availability of increasingly potent artificial opiates.

with an alcohol-dependent parent, I began by doing a literature review that showed that an important psychological influence were expected effects of alcohol, or the degree to which one expected positive and negative effects from drinking, as investigated by Sandra Brown and Mark Goldman, at the University of South Florida.[39] How much an individual drinks is predicted by the extent to which someone more strongly endorses positive alcohol expectancies, like alcohol makes you sociable, you have more fun after drinking and alcohol helps you relax. In contrast, the more negative expectancies a person endorses—such as that alcohol makes you tired, sluggish and gives you a hangover—the less someone drinks.[40,41]

The question now was how that would be in children with an alcohol-dependent parent, compared to other children. From the literature on alcohol expectancies, one would think that they would have stronger positive and weaker negative expectancies, because they respond more favorable to alcohol because of genetic factors. At that time, I lived in a kind of courtyard next to Amsterdam's Oosterpark and below me lived the street elder, Madam Bouquet, who was never shy of an opinion: "No of course these children don't have positive expectations, they see before their eyes what misery alcohol causes!"

Who was right, the Amsterdam neighbor or the international research literature? It turned out to depend on age and experience. Children of elementary school age indeed predominantly endorsed negative alcohol expectancies, and this was even more true for the children of alcohol-dependent parents.[42] So in this age group, Madam Bouquet was right and she was happy about that ("You see? Told you!"). But in adolescence, positive expectations became stronger, especially once drinking started—a general trend that was confirmed in a large recent American study.[43] Interestingly, this trend was seen even more strongly among the children of alcohol-dependent parents, because once they started drinking they made more positive judgments, especially about the effects of drinking a lot of alcohol.[42]

This is likely related to genetic differences. We know that children of alcohol-dependent parents on average respond better to alcohol: they experience both the stimulating effects immediately after intake more strongly on average than others[44] and the later negative effects less strongly.[13] The latter differences have been found to have a strong predictive value for who developed alcohol dependence in subsequent years.[13] So it is risky to be able to stand alcohol well in a society where alcohol is never far away. Years later this would be illustrated dramatically by a tennis buddy of mine, who had a father and a grandfather with a drinking problem and had himself, in agreement with the literature, a very high tolerance of alcohol. We played on a competition team together, with beers after all matches were done.

The pace of drinking was typically a little too fast for me, but he thought it was just too slow, so he regularly took an in-between beer, which appeared rather diagnostic to me. Later he lost his driver's license, by crashing into a police car from behind, when it told him to stop.

Children with an alcohol-dependent parent first see mainly the misery of alcohol abuse, which makes them (on average) judge alcohol even more negatively than other children. But when they are older and start drinking themselves, they experience more positive effects from it and relatively few (short-term) negative effects. They then adjust their expectations, and to a greater extent than other children, and that in turn is a danger of developing an alcohol problem. But this does not apply to all children of alcohol-dependent parents: some are aware of the risk and for that reason decide not to drink alcohol at all. This is the "trumping your genes" effect, discussed with Chantal, as described by Ken Kendler, famous psychiatrist and geneticist from the Virginia Institute for Psychiatric and Behavioral Genetics: people can to some extent trump their genetic risk by their behavior (not drinking). This also ties into another theme in this book: people can indeed use their conscious thought processes to influence their behavior if they imagine the future scenarios associated with either choice, and with philosopher Woodward, Kendler described this as a convincing example of "downward causation".[3] This could be related to intelligence, which has been found in many studies as a protective factor against developing addiction,[14] which of course does not mean that intelligent people cannot get addicted.

Resilience

One interesting question is why some children develop against the odds. Emmy Werner and Ruth Smith were among the first researchers study resilience, focusing on predictors of *positive* outcomes despite negative circumstances. They examined a large group of vulnerable children born in 1955 in Kauai, one of Hawaii's islands. Of about 700 children, one-third had been born into difficult circumstances: into poor families with many problems, including parents with addiction or other mental health problems, and the children often had experienced birth problems. Of these vulnerable children, two-thirds developed psychiatric problems and problems in school. Werner and Smith studied extensively what the characteristics of the resilient children were who did well and developed into healthy adults, despite these difficult beginnings.

Personality and its early precursor, temperament, played an important role: children who did well later, were often social as young children as well as rather independent, going their own way and only calling for help when necessary. They were generally good-humored and affectionate; in short, pleasant children to have around. The resilient children had been able to find an alternative person to attach themselves to when the parents were less able to do so. This could be a grandfather or grandmother or another family member, but also, for example, a teacher or caregiver. The study also emphasizes the importance of a good and engaged teacher: *all* resilient children could name at least one teacher who listened to them and challenged them in a positive way.[45] They relatively often did well in school and had something they derived pride from, such as a hobby in which they excelled. As adolescents, they scored remarkably high on autonomy and had a relatively positive self-concept, as well as the idea that they had taken control of their lives.[45–47]

Many of these characteristics have later also been found in other studies of resilient children who do well despite a difficult start.[45] You could summarize it this way: a number of factors in their early childhood were setting them up for positive trajectories, such as a pleasant temperament and intelligence, and they were able to establish a positive attachment relationship with at least one person, often someone other than a parent. The resulting relatively autonomous child did well in school, which encouraged further positive development. Resilient children often have a talent for choosing stimulating environments for their further development, positively affecting their future. Hence, going back to the debate on the role of free will in Chapter 2, the "naive" idea (according to hard determinists, proclaiming free will an illusion), that we can influence our destiny with our choices, seems to be a crucial beneficial factor in the positive development of resilient children. Related, resilient children can "trump their genes", for example, by not starting drug use and thus not developing addiction, despite a genetic vulnerability and a difficult start. And they may have had some luck in finding a positive bonding figure, which we know is important for social and emotional development since the seminal work of Bowlby.[48–50]

"Respect!"

Research by Werner and others indicated that teachers play a role in children's positive outcomes despite adversity, what we now call resilience. What might they have done to achieve this? Recent research points to some key elements: they listened to them, respected them and challenged them in a positive way. These are key elements in effective interventions for adolescents. Previous research had shown that general classroom education, for example about healthy eating or anti-bullying, often showed a (small) effect in elementary school children, but not in adolescents.[51] David Yeager from the University of Texas, Ron Dahl (Berkeley, expert on adolescent development) and Carol Dweck (Stanford, best known for the effects of *mindset*, about which more in a bit) analyzed data on effects of health interventions in children and adolescents, controlling for a variety of other possible explanations. They found indeed that some interventions that do well with elementary school children often do not work well with adolescents, and sometimes even make things worse, a so-called iatrogenic effect. What could be the reason? They developed a theory on the cause of this phenomenon and methods to positively influence adolescent development.

Central to their analysis is autonomy and *respect*. Everyone has a need for respect, but at puberty this need is stronger under the influence of the sex hormone testosterone, which strongly rises in puberty in both boys and girls (indeed, more in boys). Fundamental research has shown that testosterone makes people more sensitive to learning what is important for gaining status in the social group. When that is aggression, then testosterone levels are related to aggression, but when that is social behavior, then it is actually related to social behavior.[52] One of the authors, my friend Ron Dahl, tells a story of early adolescent Buddhist monks in training who compete vigorously for being the kindest and most social. Hence, whatever is highly valued in an individual's (sub) culture, gets more important in puberty. We can also conclude that testosterone is not the "aggression hormone" as it is sometimes portrayed; it depends on whether aggression is rated as good or bad for social status in a person's context. An experiment also nicely demonstrates the effect of respect on adolescent behavior: when approached with respect, they drank much more of a bad-tasting "drug" (in reality, a harmless bitter substance) than when told to do so, and this was especially true for adolescents whose testosterone levels had been temporarily raised with a nasal spray. An adolescent with high testosterone levels does not want to be told what to do; they want respect and only then are willing to do anything. What the authors then show is that many general interventions do not relate well to this; indeed, when adolescents are told at length what they already know (that snacking or drugs or bullying are bad), this can be explained a lack of respect for what they already know, i.e., as condescension ("they treat us like toddlers, why should I listen to this any further?"), undermining the message and sometimes even backfiring.

How can this be done better? Maybe by responding to the need for respect. For example, interventions have been developed against smoking that provide information about strategies used by the tobacco industry to manipulate young people. Interestingly, as the junk food industry has adopted some techniques from the tobacco industry, interventions have now been developed to make young people aware of the manipulation strategies used to promote eating of junk food. The goal of these industries is to get young people addicted to their products, ironically often by linking the product to independence and freedom.

The intervention aims to change the image of the person who does not smoke or eat junk food from that of a good nerd who listens (too) closely to his or her parents, to that of a freedom fighter who is at the forefront of the fight against the manipulating multinationals. The "Truth" anti-smoking campaign[iii] is successful and has already kept millions of Americans from smoking.[53]

An intervention based on the same principles to made adolescents more aware of manipulative junk food marketing and how that did not align with their own values of social justice and independence of adult control. This was done by explaining the manipulative techniques used by food marketing companies, that disproportionally target vulnerable populations like children and poor people. One of the exercises the adolescents did was making junk food ads true, by drawing or writing over the ads, using graffiti-like techniques, to express rebelliousness against adult-imposed injustice. In contrast to a traditional classroom intervention, focusing on future health effects of current food choices, the new value-alignment intervention not only reduced adolescents' automatically activated positive attitudes for junk food, the intervention also changed their actual eating behavior[iv] during the rest of the school year (3 months).[54] This is important because often interventions change attitudes or intentions but not actual behavior. Moreover, effective low-cost classroom interventions have a huge potential, as they can reach many individuals and therefore have effects at the population level, as the prototypical introduction of obligatory seatbelts in cars demonstrated (enormous reduction in fatal car accidents). Often, however, classroom interventions do not work, both in prevention of substance use and obesity, which has been related to a lack of relevance for the adolescents' values. For that reason and given the promising results, the value-aligned approach could be a more effective alternative.

An intervention reminiscent of what some teachers appeared to do spontaneously with resilient children is to give so-called "wise feedback". This involves giving positive-critical comments and responses, conveying

iii See www.thetruth.com. The brilliantly evil marketing invention of linking an addictive drug to freedom had famously been invented by Edward Bernays, who in the late 1920s devised a campaign to get women to smoke, by linking smoking to emancipation. An emancipated modern woman smoked like a man, which he staged by paying emancipated women to light a cigarette during an Easter parade in New York, as a "torch of freedom". This generated much publicity and many smoking women in the years that followed and as a consequence many premature deaths; given that an estimated 40 to 50% of smokers die from smoking-related diseases.

iv The effects on eating behavior were stronger in boys, likely because in girls the traditional intervention also had some effect, through relating healthy eating to the cultural ideal to be thin.

that you take the child or adolescent seriously, as well as that you trust them to be able to cope with the required level, which is often explicitly added: "I am giving you this feedback because I have high expectations of you". Interestingly, this approach was particularly effective with youth from a minority group (African American students) and within that group especially with those who had previously felt disrespected. In one study, positive-critical feedback on an essay led to a halving of disciplinary actions the following year.[51,55]

A third type of intervention addresses theories people have about traits, such as personality and intelligence, what has been called "mindset", by Carol Dweck. Many believe traits are set in stone, influenced in part by information about the strong genetic influence on these traits. However. research has shown that people can develop and that these traits can change over time. Carol Dweck has demonstrated that a so-called growth mindset has a positive effect on a range of developmental outcomes.[56] For example, children who grew up in poor circumstances—a predictor of relatively poor educational outcomes—could compensate for this background if they had a growth mindset compared to when they had a fixed mindset of immutable traits'.[57]

Mindset turned out to be also relevant to interventions with adolescents: gaining knowledge about personal growth eased the impact of negative experiences. For example, when you arrive at a new school and are not invited to a classmate's party, you can easily create the idea that you are a *loser* with low social status. If you believe in the theory that this is an immutable trait (once a *loser*, always a *loser*), then such a negative event becomes very influential; it is an indication that you will have to continue as a *loser* in school for years to come. In an experiment, those who learned about personal growth were found to exhibit less aggressive behavior than those who had received traditional intervention or no intervention.[51,58] A very recent *Nature* article by David Yeager and colleagues found that a brief intervention aimed at promoting a growth mindset and a positive interpretation of stress helped young people avoid mental health problems, during the COVID crisis.[59]

We can conclude that it is important for positive development that people learn to set goals, and also to be approached by others as a goal-oriented individual (respect!). This ability starts at an early age, in infancy. Adele Diamond from the University of British Columbia and her team have shown that social games can help develop goal-oriented behavior.[60] This trains so-called "executive functions" that enable goal-oriented behavior to achieve long-term goals, but it is clear that the social context plays a crucial role. Training executive functions with specific computer programs in a solitary way has been done a lot in children with ADHD, who on average show lower scores on these control functions.[61] However, the results were rather disappointing: the children became better and better at the task in which they were trained, but these gains did not translate well into progress in another task and not into positive effects on behavior in daily life, which was the whole point of the training. Hence, the learning showed no generalization (a topic that will return in Chapter 8).[62,63] Perhaps that's why everyday social games work better, such as those that require you to hold back your impulses and games that require you to imagine yourself in a different role.

Education

Education can also contribute to the development of self-control and related positive outcomes. For example, a beneficial effect of Montessori education has been shown in a rare experimental study in education science (rare because we don't normally randomize people to schools). But in the American city of Milwaukee, Wisconsin, this was done through a lottery for children who attended public education. In the American context, this is related to poorer socioeconomic conditions: children of wealthier parents tend to be sent to the better private schools. The study is unique because almost all other studies compare outcomes between school types where parents had made their own choice of school. As a result, any differences could be related not only to the type of education, but also to the type of parents (and their genetic and social background). Because of its uniqueness, the outcomes of this study were published in the journal *Science*.[64] In Montessori schools, children can to a certain extent decide for themselves what they want to work on at a certain time, as long as the weekly assignments are completed. In addition, cooperation is encouraged, even between children of different ages, and much instruction is given in small groups. What did this approach yield?

The children assigned by lot to Montessori schools did better on a whole series of tests than the children in the control group, both on school-related skills, such as reading and math, and on social behavior and on various tests measuring the aforementioned executive functions, which enable goal-directed behavior. They also had better developed ideas about fairness and justice. These differences were found throughout elementary school age. The results are important because they show that education that encourages goal-oriented and social behavior in young children has positive outcomes. Note that there are more teaching methods than Montessori alone that use similar methods, but so this is one of the few truly experimental studies that clearly showed the effects.

Another approach is to implement a program specifically aimed at rewarding positive behaviors, regardless of the type of education. One example is an intervention called the *good behavior game*. Children set their own goals and work in groups, and positive behavior is consistently rewarded at different levels (the individual, group and class). The group level rewards yield a strong social motivation to do well and be appreciated by peers. The result is a positive constructive work atmosphere that benefits children and reduces aggression. A Dutch version of this program was even found to reduce the likelihood of starting smoking and drinking in high school, years later.[65]

I personally witnessed a related program developed by Jim Swanson from the University of California at Irvine, which was developed for children with high scores of ADHD and related problems. I had met him through my PhD thesis advisor, Joe Sergeant, an international expert in the field of ADHD. He invited me to experience the program in practice, and it was indeed an experience: although they included only "wild kids" into the program (children with ADHD or related behavioral problems), you could hear a pin drop when you walked around. The kids were concentrating on their schoolwork and using it to collect reward tokens, both for themselves and their group, but also for the class as a whole (just like the task game).

One social skills training session involved very wild games, so much so that I wondered if that wouldn't get out of hand. Swanson told me the background:

> In the beginning, we did this skills training, and they seemed to be doing pretty well, but then they would play dodgeball in the break, and you'd see the kids derailed in no time. After one of these occasions, a supervisor afterwards said: "That's it, we don't play dodgeball anymore." However, after further discussions in the staff, it was decided to keep the wild games, because it was the perfect exercise for the real world.

In these games, you could learn to deal with injustices. Even when someone throws you out in a bad way, say too hard—not unthinkable—you have to remain a *good sport*. You accept your loss and get on. If you don't, you not only lose points, but you forfeit to the group the chance to win pizza-points. And the others don't like that: with a *yell* they urge you to accept that you are out. Again, the social context of the learning is crucial. Learning to accept that sometimes things can get tough, rather than impulsively beating around the bush, is further rewarded at other moments that can easily lead to frustration, such as when your computer time runs out for the day, just as you were about to find a treasure. Parents are also trained to reward the children when they control themselves in the face of perceived injustice and do not freak out, in order to promote learning to deal with frustration at home. Teachers from the children's original school were also invited to visit to learn about the method. The results of the program were good, although hardly better than when combined with medication.[66,67]

While this method shows promise for difficult or busy children in elementary school, it is not easily translatable to middle school. As we have seen, such a mainly reward-oriented approach is not as effective after elementary school ("they treat us like kids"), but it can lay the foundation for later positive development. In high school, it is better to focus interventions on opportunities for the young person to develop positively in a way that commands respect from peers.[51,68] This can lead to positive development, for example, young people becoming committed to change or exploring new frontiers in music or science, but unfortunately, it can also lead to negative development: that can be the case when status is taken from the position in the hallway. Therefore, it is important that positive development is encouraged from this perspective, which means taking into account the wishes and goals of the young person.

Prevention of addiction

When looking at interventions in middle school that aim to prevent addiction, there are several approaches. The most widely used is the universal approach: this involves educating children about the dangers of smoking, alcohol and drugs. Although this is widely used (yes, we do something to prevent alcohol and drug problems!), unfortunately, much research shows that this approach hardly yields benefits if at all.[69,70] More interactive programs generally do slightly better than educational programs alone (respect!), and as we saw new universal approaches that appeal to adolescents' own values show more promise (the truth approach to counter manipulation by tobacco and fast food companies).

While most universal interventions have no effects, it is not the case that "if it does not help it does not harm". Prevention costs money, so if it does not help, it does harm to some extent. But it can be worse: adverse or iatrogenic effects of well-intended preventive interventions occur with some regularity.[71–74] A famous example comes from research on effects of summer camps for youth at high risk of developing behavioral problems. The children were encouraged to participate in a variety of positive, social activities during the summer camp. Although the intention was to reduce the likelihood of behavioral problems and later crime, these outcomes were the exact opposite: they were found to increase, and most strikingly the more so, the more summer camps someone had participated in.[71] How could this happen?

The late Arizona State University professor of psychology Tom Dishion devoted his research career to unraveling the underlying mechanism of these negative effects of peer influence, which he called *deviance training*. He showed that when you put high-risk youth together, chances are that a dynamic develops in which they push each other to great heights in terms of undesirable behavior (as defined by adults), which is likely to garner respect from peers, but was not of the adults who designed the intervention or ruled the camp. These often appeared to be subtle interactions outside the actual training, occurring, for example, while they were sitting in the waiting room to join a program to learn to behave better or when they were on the bus home and ridiculed everything they were taught. The same mechanism (deviance training) probably also causes the effects of spending time in a juvenile prison to often backfire: it can be a training ground for a later criminal career.

Back to general alcohol and drug prevention. Until recently, most school-based prevention programs focused only on students and they showed little or no effect. What if the parents would be targeted as well? The reason for exploring this was that parental rule setting regarding adolescent alcohol and drug use was shown to have an impact, contrary to what many parents believe, especially in Europe—something several studies have now shown.[75–77] Setting clear rules (for example, no smoking and no drinking under the age of 18) was found to have a positive effect, while many parents think that "it will only stimulate them to do it" (as I also often hear as a reaction when I tell about this finding). Of course, it is important to use an open communication style (i.e., talk about it together and discuss the background of the rules, which goes along with the importance of "respect" at this age).

There was one caveat concerning the interpretation of these studies: they involved a relationship (a correlation), indicating that children of parents who set clear rules about alcohol started drinking later in life than children of parents who did not. Because this was not an experiment, the conclusion was not unequivocal: one could think of other potential explanations for this correlation. Perhaps parents who set clear rules are smarter, or have better self-control themselves than parents who do not set clear rules. They may have passed those traits on to their children (through genes and upbringing), then the rules are irrelevant in the explanation. How could you prove the impact of these rules? The answer may look familiar by now: by doing an experiment! If you randomly assign children to a group in which parents receive training in alcohol rule-setting, you can investigate whether it makes any difference. And sure enough, it did.

The starting point was a universal intervention, which had shown little effect on its own, but was nevertheless widely used at the start of secondary education in the Netherlands, when children are in early puberty, around 12 years of age.[69] The study added parent evenings to random classes in different schools, in which parents were taught to set specific rules about alcohol consumption and learned why that is important for their child, for example for better brain development and lower risk of later addiction. Four experimental groups were formed: a group who received no intervention at all (control group), a group who received only the standard intervention for the teen, a group in which only the parents received an intervention at parent night, and a group in which both parents and teens received the intervention. The latter group did markedly better on several outcomes, even years later: they started drinking later in life and when they started, they drank less.[78,79] Hence, the ineffective universal school intervention,[v] did become effective when the parent evening intervention about rule setting was added. Interestingly, just doing the parent evening was not enough: only the group in which parent and child had received the intervention did better.

The finding is of practical relevance: as noted earlier *effective* universal interventions have a great potential for public health. The findings are also important theoretically because it shows unequivocally that parental rule-setting has a real effect and thus cannot be explained by traits of parents doing it spontaneously. Finally, the study was interesting in terms of the mechanism: it was found that the stricter rule setting by the parents caused an *increase* in self-control in the adolescent, and that increase in turn predicted that the adolescent drank less at later measurement.[80] This indicates that rule setting can help develop self-control, whether in games in preschoolers,[60] in elementary school (good behavior game)[65] and in middle school (universal alcohol and drug prevention, when a parent component is added).[80] It becomes increasingly important that the children themselves support the rules in connection with their increasing need for autonomy and respect. While the finding that rule-setting has a positive effect on self-control in children, this finding does not come in isolation, there is more evidence that a predictable environment fosters self-control and the ability to maintain goals over a long time, which has been related to the developmental context of the predictive brain.[81] Conversely, growing up in an unpredictable chaotic household has a negative impact on the development of self-control and goal-directed action,[82] while it may have a positive effect on the ability to switch (another executive control function).[81]

The interventions described above, which involve educating an entire class (and if possible, including the parents) about alcohol and drugs, are general or universal. An alternative is to target the intervention specifically to youth with an increased risk of developing addiction. In doing so, you can select in two ways: on risk factors or on early signs of

v which was confirmed here: no difference between teen only intervention and no intervention. Ironically, the teen only version is still the one that is implemented widely.

the problem behavior itself. In targeted prevention, you select young people who are statistically at increased risk of developing a problem, for example, the previously discussed children with an alcohol-dependent parent, whom you could teach, for example, that a good reaction to alcohol is a sign of increased risk rather than that alcohol's not all that bad. In this strategy, stigmatization is a potential problem: it is not nice to be selected because of a problem of your parents, as Chantal, our ex-participant, had made clear.

Patricia Conrod, professor of psychology at the University of Montreal, came up with a more acceptable alternative: select on personality. We know from many previous studies that four traits are predictive of later problems with alcohol and drugs (again in the statistical sense, not in the sense that the outcome definitely occurs). Two related traits are impulsivity and sensation seeking, and two other related traits are sensitivity to anxiety and hopelessness. The path to excessive substance use is different for children with those traits: impulsive and sensation seeking children want to try things out and seek kicks, while children with an enhanced risk to develop anxiety and depression are generally not at the forefront of experimentation. The latter, however, may later in life teach themselves that substance use helps them to manage their negative emotions. What Conrod and colleagues' method boils down to is that you give all children in the classroom a short personality test, which they also get feedback on. Kids like that, because they like to learn about their personality and about who they "really are".[vi]

Children who scored high on one of the four traits that predict later problems (impulsivity, sensation seeking, anxiety and hopelessness) were invited to participate in a series of group sessions, during which they learned that people have different personal needs and that the key is to find a good fulfillment of needs for themselves. If you score high on sensation-seeking, then alcohol and drugs can be exciting, but perhaps

vi A brief aside from my college days: on the big celebratory event, at the time called Queen's Day and now King's Day in the Netherlands, the challenge was to come up with something with which you could earn money during the day in order to party later that night. We did several unsuccessful trials, until a friend and I, freshmen in psychology, put up an old tent in the Vondelpark, with a slogan on it: *Learn who you are, in our tent* (which rhymes in Dutch: *wil je weten wie je bent: kom in onze tent*). There we told visitors a funny short story, and at the end, visitors were asked to rank the characters in terms of likability, after which we gave them the key to unravel their own character (the test reportedly came from a real job application procedure). All day there were lines in front of our tent: who doesn't want to know who they "really" are. In retrospect, this may be less surprising (but that's true of many things, prediction is way easier when it concerns the past): the billion-dollar industry of astrology is also based on it, without scientific foundation.

there are other things that can be exciting as well, such as kite surfing or mountain climbing. And the advantage of those alternatives is that they help you achieve other goals, on which excessive alcohol and drug use actually have a negative effect. If you want to climb or kitesurf, you shouldn't start out with a hangover. And so positive developmental spirals can emerge instead of negative ones, at least on paper. The question, of course, is whether this is how it works in practice.

Conrod and colleagues showed in several large studies in the UK, Canada and Australia that this approach indeed has a positive effect regarding alcohol, especially among sensation seekers.[83] The intervention also reduced the use of marijuana and cocaine[84] and even shows long-term positive effects, up to two years after the (brief) intervention.[85] Thereby, it was interesting that the positive effect on the young people with anxious and gloomy feelings arose in the longer term, which you would also expect from the hypothesized mechanism (starting late, but then running the risk of escalation). I was involved in a test in the Netherlands, conducted as part of the doctoral research of Jeroen Lammers, who unfortunately died at a young age. We did find some effects, but they were modest in terms of excessive drinking[86] and related to education level, with stronger effects occurring in adolescents at lower education levels.[87] The latter is encouraging because a low level of education is also a high risk factor of a less healthy development. The idea behind the intervention is good and has already produced positive effects in several countries, but the question is how to optimize the effects in practice.

The last form of prevention, indicated prevention, targets individuals who experience emerging problems, in this case, for example, young people who suddenly show little interest in school, make an absent or sleepy impression and whose grades deteriorate. In many cases, excessive substance use plays a role in this, nowadays often combined with excessive gaming. The problem for parents is that on the one hand they know they have to let go of their children in this phase, but at the same time they see that the child is not doing well, and then letting go becomes difficult. When should you let go and let your child become wise through experience and when should you intervene because the situation becomes too extreme and threatening? There is no set recipe, but the general principle of "Respect!" applies: it often works better to find an entrance through the young person's ambitions, rather than to impose stricter rules that lead to more resistance.[vii]

vii Hence, clear rule-setting (with some explanation) works before the adolescent starts to use, but not anymore after use has started, then a respectful dialogue would seem more appropriate.

The aforementioned technique of motivational interviewing is a method in which you do not try to convince someone to change their substance use, aim is to rather invite someone in a conversation to come to that conclusion themselves. For example, talking to heavy drinking students about what they want to achieve in their studies, or perhaps further in life. The late Canadian psychologist Alan Marlatt applied this method in a study with heavy-drinking students and found positive effects, after a single motivational interview session: the heavy-drinking students who had received such a motivational interview by trained counselors still drank less two years later than the equally heavy-drinking students who had not received such a counseling session (determined by chance).[88]

In a related method, Ricky Greenwald developed a "film script" method to positively influence young people with behavioral problems, along with addiction problems.[89] It uses techniques from motivational interviewing, which means approaching the young person with respect and empathy. A possible future is discussed: what will they be doing in ten years? I gave treatments for a while in the context of Cognitive Behavioral Therapy training and tried this intervention out, which was fun to do, especially with "difficult" youngsters, who were *sick and tired* of all the well-meaning advice and who wanted to find their own way, but had enjoyed psychoactive substances a bit too much along the way, causing them to get stuck.

I tried the film script intervention with a girl of about 13, who was marijuana dependent and did not go to school anymore. After a stiff start, she was willing to go along with developing a film script about her future and began to fantasize that in ten years she would own a clothing store. Questions I asked her in connection with an imaginary movie script included, "Tell me more about your life now?", "What do you do?", "How do you live?". The imaginary movie script had to be worked out as visually as possible, after all we were going to develop a movie script. The effect is that she vividly imagined herself as a successful young clothing store owner. We then wondered together how she got there, further developing her film script. What were crucial events and choices that had led to her store? We also briefly discussed a less rosy scenario and she was clear: she would be an addict and wander the streets of Amsterdam, without her own place to stay. How could she work toward the clothing business? Maybe she had to start looking at those tedious economics books again, because she had to be able to keep her accounts later. And languages, of course, the customers will not all speak Dutch! And maybe even mathematics … because that could be useful for that accounting. So, not too much marijuana blowing, because then she would not study anything for sure … She came to these conclusions herself, whereas she would have no doubt gone against those if I (or a parent or a teacher) had chewed them out to her, no matter how well-meaning.

This particular "movie-method" has been examined in a few small studies, mostly with youth in detention; in that context, it can be called promising. I describe the method here not only because of my own positive experience with it (as a researcher, I know that you have to be careful with positive clinical experiences), but because it fits well with the general theme of this chapter: try to positively influence young people's motivation, tap into their existing values and creative potential. The key question to young people with problem behavior is "Where do you want to go?" And for many of them, doing something fun often works better than just talking about problems.

What can we conclude about the developmental psychological side of addiction and other *akrasia* problems? Some people, more than others, tend to make impulsive decisions, which they often regret later, because in doing so they have gone against something they do not really want. There is a hereditary side to this, but upbringing and school also play a key role. Reward-based programs can help children to behave less impulsively and it is important that children learn to accept rules and deal with frustrations, something that can be well practiced, for example, in the context of a sports. In order not to go for the easy short-term solution, it can help to imagine the future, which may be stimulated with reading aloud, self-reading, drama and other creative subjects. And in adolescents the strategy to single out how tobacco or fast food industry manipulates them to act against their own values has shown promise. Teachers also play an important role. Virtually everyone who showed resilience after a rough start and developed positively, could name a teacher who stimulated them, perhaps letting them dream for a moment of a different future and giving them the message that you can actually get there, if you just put your best effort into it. It can also be helpful to single out high-risk children to encourage positive development given their personality (Conrod's programs). You can also inform and warn children with a specific risk (e.g., children with an addicted parent), that a favorable response to the drug is actually a sign of additional risk. The lesson learned from Chantal was that we do need to be careful about feeding back risk information and perhaps encourage positive development above all else.

References

1. Sher KJ. Children of alcoholics: a critical appraisal of theory and research. University of Chicago Press; 1991.
2. Wiers RW, Gunning WBW, Sergeant JAJ. Is a mild deficit in executive functions in boys related to childhood ADHD or to parental multigenerational alcoholism? J Abnorm Child … [Internet]. 1998 [cited 2013 Apr 5];26:415–30. Available from: http://link.springer.com/article/10.1023/A:1022643617017

3. Kendler KS, Woodward J. Top-down causation in psychiatric disorders: a clinical-philosophical inquiry. Psychol Med. 2021;51:1783–8.
4. Goldman D, Oroszi G, Ducci F. The genetics of addictions: uncovering the genes. Nat Rev Genet [Internet]. 2005;6:521–32. Available from: www.ncbi.nlm.nih.gov/pubmed/15995696
5. Treur JL, Demontis D, Smith GD, Sallis H, Richardson TG, Wiers RW, et al. Investigating causality between liability to ADHD and substance use, and liability to substance use and ADHD risk, using Mendelian randomization. Addict Biol. 2021;26:e12849.
6. Nees F, Tzschoppe J, Patrick CJ, Vollstädt-Klein S, Steiner S, Poustka L, et al. Determinants of early alcohol use in healthy adolescents: the differential contribution of neuroimaging and psychological factors. Neuropsychopharmacology. 2012;37:986–95.
7. Stewart SH, McGonnell M, Wekerle C, Adlaf E. Associations of personality with alcohol use behaviour and alcohol problems in adolescents receiving child welfare services. Int J Ment Health Addict. 2011;9:492–506.
8. Cerdá M, Bordelois PM, Keyes KM, Galea S, Koenen KC, Pardini D. Cumulative and recent psychiatric symptoms as predictors of substance use onset: does timing matter? Addiction. 2013;108:2119–28.
9. Peeters M, Monshouwer K, van de Schoot R, Janssen T, Vollebergh WA, Wiers RW. Personality and the prediction of high-risk trajectories of alcohol use during adolescence. J Stud Alcohol Drugs. 2014;75.
10. Conrod PJ, Pihl RO, Stewart SH, Dongier M. Validation of a system of classifying female substance abusers on the basis of personality and motivational risk factors for substance abuse. Psychol Addict Behav. 2000;14:243.
11. Kuss DJ, Louws J, Wiers RW. Online gaming addiction? Motives predict addictive play behavior in massively multiplayer online role-playing games. Cyberpsychol Behav Soc Netw [Internet]. 2012 [cited 2013 Mar 6];15:480–5. Available from: www.ncbi.nlm.nih.gov/pubmed/22974351
12. Luczak SE, Glatt SJ, Wall TJ. Meta-analyses of ALDH2 and ADH1B with alcohol dependence in Asians. Psychol Bull. 2006;132:607.
13. Schuckit MA, Smith TL. An 8-year follow-up of 450 sons of alcoholic and control subjects. Arch Gen Psychiatry. 1996;53:202–10.
14. Treur JL, Munafò MR, Logtenberg E, Wiers RW, Verweij KJH. Using Mendelian randomization analysis to better understand the relationship between mental health and substance use: a systematic review. Psychol Med.
15. Vink JM, Willemsen G, Boomsma DI. Heritability of smoking initiation and nicotine dependence. Behav Genet. 2005;35:397–406.
16. Broms U, Silventoinen K, Madden PAF, Heath AC, Kaprio J. Genetic architecture of smoking behavior: a study of Finnish adult twins. Twin Res Hum Genet. 2006;9:64–72.
17. Kendler KS. "A gene for …": the nature of gene action in psychiatric disorders. Am J Psychiatry. 2005;162:1243–52.
18. Walters RK, Polimanti R, Johnson EC, McClintick JN, Adams MJ, Adkins AE, et al. Transancestral GWAS of alcohol dependence reveals common genetic underpinnings with psychiatric disorders. Nat Neurosci. 2018;21:1656–69.
19. Young AI. Solving the missing heritability problem. PLoS Genet. 2019; 15:1–7.
20. Gymrek M, Goren A. Missing heritability may be hiding in repeats. Science (80–). 2021;373:1440–1.
21. Mukamel RE, Handsaker RE, Sherman MA, Barton AR, Zheng Y, McCarroll SA, et al. Protein-coding repeat polymorphisms strongly shape diverse human phenotypes. Science (80–). 2021;373:1499–505.

22. Brunner HG, Nelen M, Breakefield XO, Ropers HH, Van Oost BA. Abnormal behavior associated with a point mutation in the structural gene for monoamine oxidase A. Science (80–). 1993;262:578–80.
23. Caspi A, McCray J, Moffitt TE, Mill J, Martin J, Craig IW, et al. Role of genotype in the cycle of violence in maltreated children. Science (80–). 2002;297:851–4.
24. Caspi A, Sugden K, Moffitt TE, Taylor A, Craig IW, Harrington HL, et al. Influence of life stress on depression: moderation by a polymorphism in the 5-HTT gene. Science (80–). 2003;301:386–9.
25. Caspi A, Hariri AR, Holmes A, Uher R, Moffitt TE. Genetic sensitivity to the environment. Am J Psychiatry [Internet]. 2010;167:509–27. Available from: http://ezproxy-prd.bodleian.ox.ac.uk:3179/doi/pdf/10.1176/appi.ajp.2010.09101452
26. Belsky DW. Translating polygenic analysis for prevention: from who to how. Circ Cardiovasc Genet. 2017;10:1–3.
27. Pasman JA, Verweij KJH, Vink JM. Systematic review of polygenic gene–environment interaction in tobacco, alcohol, and cannabis use. Behav Genet [Internet]. 2019;49:349–65. Available from: 10.1007/s10519-019-09958-7
28. Belsky J, Bakermans-Kranenburg MJ, Van Ijzendoorn MH. For better and for worse: differential susceptibility to environmental influences. Curr Dir Psychol Sci. 2007;16:300–4.
29. Boyce WT. The orchid and the dandelion. Monument, CO: Bluebird; 2019.
30. Belsky J, Pluess M. Beyond diathesis stress: differential susceptibility to environmental influences. Psychol Bull. 2009;135:885–908.
31. van Ijzendoorn MH, Bakermans-Kranenburg MJ. Genetic differential susceptibility on trial: Meta-analytic support from randomized controlled experiments. Dev Psychopathol [Internet]. 2015;27:151–62. Available from: http://journals.cambridge.org/abstract_S0954579414001369
32. Fischer K, Weeland J, Leijten P, van den Akker A, Overbeek G. Current and future perspectives on children's genetic- and endophenotype-based differential susceptibility to parenting. J Child Fam Stud. 2020;29:773–9.
33. Sideli L, Quigley H, La Cascia C, Murray RM. Cannabis use and the risk for psychosis and affective disorders. J Dual Diagn [Internet]. 2020;16:22–42. Available from: 10.1080/15504263.2019.1674991
34. Sullivan RJ, Hagen EH. Psychotropic substance-seeking: evolutionary pathology or adaptation? Addiction. 2002;97:389–400.
35. Hirschman RS, Leventhal H, Glynn K. The development of smoking behavior: conceptualization and supportive cross-sectional survey data 1. J Appl Soc Psychol. 1984;14:184–206.
36. Laviolette SR, Van Der Kooy D. The neurobiology of nicotine addiction: bridging the gap from molecules to behaviour. Nat Rev Neurosci. 2004;5:55–65.
37. Nesse RM, Berridge KC. Psychoactive drug use in evolutionary perspective. Science (80–). 1997;278:63–6.
38. Porter R. The drinking man's disease: the "pre-history" of alcoholism in Georgian Britain. Br J Addict. 1985;80:385–96.
39. Brown SA, Goldman MS, Inn A, Anderson LR. Expectations of reinforcement from alcohol: their domain and relation to drinking patterns. J Consult Clin Psychol. 1980;48:419–26.
40. Wiers RW, Hoogeveen KJ, Sergeant JA, Gunning WB. High- and low-dose alcohol-related expectancies and the differential associations with drinking in male and female adolescents and young adults. Addiction [Internet]. 1997 [cited 2013 Apr 5];92:871–88. Available from: http://doi.wiley.com/10.1111/j.1360-0443.1997.tb02956.x

41. Goldman MS, Brown SA, Christiansen BA. Expectancy theory-thinking about drinking. In: H. Blane and KE Leonard (Eds.), editor. Psychological theories of drinking and alcoholism. NY: Guilford; 1987. pp. 181–226.
42. Wiers RW, Gunning WB, Sergeant JA. Do young children of alcoholics hold more positive or negative alcohol- related expectancies than controls? Alcohol Clin Exp Res. 1998;22:1855–63.
43. Padovano HT, Janssen T, Sokolovsky A, Jackson KM. The altered course of learning: how alcohol outcome expectancies are shaped by first drinking experiences. Psychol Sci. 2020;31:1573–84.
44. Conrod PJ, Peterson JB, Pihl RO, Mankowski S. Biphasic effects of alcohol on heart rate are influenced by alcoholic family history and rate of alcohol ingestion. Alcohol Clin Exp Res. 1997;21:140–9.
45. Werner EE. Vulnerable but invincible: high-risk children from birth to adulthood. Acta Paediatr Int J Paediatr Suppl. 1997;86:103–5.
46. Werner EE, Smith RS. Vulnerable, but invincible. NY: Adams, Bannister, Cox.; 1989.
47. Werner EE. Vulnerability and resiliency in children at risk for delinquency: a longitudinal study from birth to young adulthood. In: Burchard JD, Burchard SN, editors. Vermont conference on the primary prevention of psychopathology. Vol 10. Thousand Oaks, CA: Sage; 1987. p. 16–43.
48. Bowlby J. Attachment and loss, vol. 1: attachment. NY: Basic Books; 1969.
49. Bowlby J. Attachment and loss, vol. 2: separation-anxiety and anger. NY: Basic Books; 1973.
50. Bowlby J. Attachment and loss, vol. 3: loss-sadness and depression. NY: Basic Books; 1980.
51. Yeager DS, Dahl RE, Dweck CS. Why interventions to influence adolescent behavior often fail but could succeed. Perspect Psychol Sci. 2018;13:101–22.
52. Dreher JC, Dunne S, Pazderska A, Frodl T, Nolan JJ, O'Doherty JP. Testosterone causes both prosocial and antisocial status-enhancing behaviors in human males. Proc Natl Acad Sci U S A. 2016;113:11633–8.
53. Farrelly MC, Nonnemaker J, Davis KC, Hussin A. The influence of the national Truth campaign on smoking initiation. Am J Prev Med [Internet]. 2009;36:379–84. Available from: 10.1016/j.amepre.2009.01.019
54. Bryan CJ, Yeager DS, Hinojosa CP. A values-alignment intervention protects adolescents from the effects of food marketing. Nat Hum Behav [Internet]. 2019;3:596–603. Available from: 10.1038/s41562-019-0586-6
55. Yeager DS, Purdie-Vaughns V, Hooper SY, Cohen GL. Loss of institutional trust among racial and ethnic minority adolescents: a consequence of procedural injustice and a cause of life-span outcomes. Child Dev. 2017; 88:658–76.
56. Dweck C. Mindset-updated edition: changing the way you think to fulfil your potential. Hachette UK; 2017.
57. Claro S, Paunesku D, Dweck CS. Growth mindset tempers the effects of poverty on academic achievement. Proc Natl Acad Sci USA. 2016; 113:8664–8.
58. Yeager DS, Trzesniewski KH, Dweck CS. An implicit theories of personality intervention reduces adolescent aggression in response to victimization and exclusion. Child Dev. 2013;84:970–88.
59. Yeager DS, Bryan CJ, Gross JJ, Murray JS, Cobb DK, Santos PHF, et al. A synergistic mindsets intervention protects adolescents from stress. Nature. 2022.

60. Diamond A, Lee K. Interventions shown to aid executive function development in children 4 to 12 years old. Science (80–) [Internet]. 2011;333:959–64. Available from: www.pubmedcentral.nih.gov/articlerender.fcgi?artid=3159917&tool=pmcentrez&rendertype=abstract
61. Klingberg T. Training and plasticity of working memory. Trends Cogn Sci [Internet]. 2010;14:317–24. Available from: 10.1016/j.tics.2010.05.002
62. Sonuga-Barke EJS, Brandeis D, Cortese S, Daley D, Ferrin M, Holtmann M, et al. Nonpharmacological interventions for ADHD: systematic review and meta-analyses of randomized controlled trials of dietary and psychological treatments. Am J Psychiatry [Internet]. 2013;170:275–89. Available from: http://journals.psychiatryonline.org/article.aspx?articleID=1566975
63. Dovis S, Van Der Oord S, Wiers RWRW, Prins PJMPJM. Improving executive functioning in children with ADHD: training multiple executive functions within the context of a computer game. a randomized double-blind placebo controlled trial. PLoS One. 2015;10:1–30.
64. Lillard A, Else-Quest N. The early years: evaluating Montessori education. Science (80–). 2006;313:1893–4.
65. van Lier PAC, Huizink A, Crijnen A. Impact of a preventive intervention targeting childhood disruptive behavior problems on tobacco and alcohol initiation from age 10 to 13 years. Drug Alcohol Depend. 2009;100: 228–233.
66. Swanson JM, Kraemer HC, Hinshaw SP, Arnold LE, Conners CK, Abikoff HB, et al. Clinical relevance of the primary findings of the MTA: success rates based on severity of ADHD and ODD symptoms at the end of treatment. J Am Acad Child Adolesc Psychiatry [Internet]. 2001;40:168–79. Available from: 10.1097/00004583-200102000-00011
67. Jensen PS. A 14-month randomized clinical trial of treatment strategies for attention-deficit/hyperactivity disorder. Arch Gen Psychiatry. 1999; 56:1073–86.
68. Crone EA, Fuligni AJ. Self and others in adolescence. Annu Rev Psychol. 2020;71:447–69.
69. Cuijpers P, Jonkers R, De Weerdt I, De Jong A. The effects of drug abuse prevention at school: the "Healthy School and Drugs" project. Addiction. 2002;97:67–73.
70. Foxcroft DR, Tsertsvadze A. Universal alcohol misuse prevention programmes for children and adolescents: Cochrane systematic reviews. Perspect Public Health. 2012;132:128–34.
71. Dishion TJ, McCord J, Poulin F. When interventions harm. Am Psychol. 1999;54:755–64.
72. Werch CE, Owen DM. Iatrogenic effects of alcohol and drug prevention programs. J Stud Alcohol. 2002;63:581–90.
73. Moos RH. Iatrogenic effects of psychosocial interventions for substance use disorders: prevalence, predictors, prevention. Addiction. 2005;100: 595–604.
74. Faggiano F, Allara E, Giannotta F, Molinar R, Sumnall H, Wiers R, et al. Europe needs a central, transparent, and evidence-based approval process for behavioural prevention interventions. PLoS Med. 2014;11:1–6.
75. Van Der Vorst H, Engels RCME, Meeus W, Deković M. The impact of alcohol-specific rules, parental norms about early drinking and parental alcohol use on adolescents' drinking behavior. J Child Psychol Psychiatry. 2006;47:1299–306.

76. Mares SHW, Lichtwarck-Aschoff A, Burk WJ, van der Vorst H, Engels RCME. Parental alcohol-specific rules and alcohol use from early adolescence to young adulthood. J child Psychol psychiatry. 2012;53:798–805.
77. Carver H, Elliott L, Kennedy C, Hanley J. Parent–child connectedness and communication in relation to alcohol, tobacco and drug use in adolescence: an integrative review of the literature. Drugs Educ Prev policy. 2017; 24:119–33.
78. Koning IM, Vollebergh WAM, Smit F, Verdurmen JEE, Eijnden RJJM, Van Den Bogt TFM, et al. Preventing heavy alcohol use in adolescents (PAS): cluster randomized trial of a parent and student intervention offered separately and simultaneously. 2009;1669–78.
79. Koning IM, Verdurmen JEE, Engels RCME, van den Eijnden RJJM, Vollebergh WAM. Differential impact of a Dutch alcohol prevention program targeting adolescents and parents separately and simultaneously: low self-control and lenient parenting at baseline predict effectiveness. Prev Sci. 2012;13:278–87.
80. Koning IM, Maric M, MacKinnon D, Vollebergh WAM. Effects of a combined parent-student alcohol prevention program on intermediate factors and adolescents' drinking behavior: A sequential mediation model. J Consult Clin Psychol. 2015;83:719–27.
81. Munakata Y, Placido D, Zhuang W. What's Next? Advances and Challenges in Understanding How Environmental Predictability Shapes The Development Of Cognitive Control. Curr Dir Psychol Sci. 2023;32(6):431–8.
82. Andrews K, Atkinson L, Harris M, Gonzalez A. Examining the effects of household chaos on child executive functions: A meta-analysis. Psychol Bull. 2021;147:16–32.
83. Conrod PJ, Castellanos N, Mackie C. Personality-targeted interventions delay the growth of adolescent drinking and binge drinking. J Child Psychol Psychiatry Allied Discip. 2008;49:181–90.
84. Conrod PJ, Castellanos-Ryan N, Strang J. Brief, personality-targeted coping skills interventions and survival as a non-drug user over a 2-year period during adolescence. Arch Gen Psychiatry. 2010;67:85–93.
85. Conrod PJ, Castellanos-Ryan N, Mackie C. Long-term effects of a personality-targeted intervention to reduce alcohol use in adolescents. J Consult Clin Psychol [Internet]. 2011;79:296–306. Available from: http://doi.apa.org/getdoi.cfm?doi=10.1037/a0022997
86. Lammers Ferry Conrod, Patricia Engels, Rutger Wiers, Reinout W. Kleinjan, Marloes J, Lammers J, Goossens F, Conrod P, Engels R, Wiers RW, et al. Effectiveness of a selective intervention program targeting personality risk factors for alcohol misuse among young adolescents: results of a cluster randomized controlled trial. Addiction [Internet]. 2015;110:1101–9. Available from: 10.1111/add.12952%5Cnhttps://acces.bibl.ulaval.ca/login?url=https://search.ebscohost.com/login.aspx?direct=true&db=pbh&AN=103339941&lang=fr&site=ehost-live
87. Lammers J, Goossens F, Conrod P, Engels R, Wiers RW, Kleinjan M. Effectiveness of a selective alcohol prevention program targeting personality risk factors: results of interaction analyses. Addict Behav. 2017;71.
88. Marlatt GA, Baer JS, Kivlahan DR, Dimeff LA, Larimer ME, Quigley LA, et al. Screening and brief intervention for high-risk college student drinkers: results from a 2-year follow-up assessment. J Consult Clin Psychol. 1998;66:604.

89. Greenwald R. Treating problem behaviors: a trauma-informed approach. NY: Taylor & Francis; 2009.
90. Molenaar PCM, Boomsma DI, Dolan C V. A third source of developmental differences. Behav Genet. 1993;23:519–24.
91. Kan KJ, Ploeger A, Raijmakers MEJ, Dolan C V., Van Der Maas HLJ. Nonlinear epigenetic variance: review and simulations. Dev Sci. 2010;13:11–27.

7 Pills or talk therapy?

I am sitting across from a man in his seventies, Johan, who has been addicted to alcohol for a long time, basically since his divorce thirty years earlier, and who also had sleep problems as long as he can remember, probably related to the many nightshifts he has worked. He had always run his own business and was still active. Over the years, he developed a deadly exhausting nightly ritual: he took sleeping pills and drank some alcohol, fell asleep, slept for a few hours, woke up, got up to pee, took another sleeping pill, and slept for a while, until he woke up again to go to the bathroom, and so on until he couldn't sleep at all anymore and got up to do some work. During the day he was always tired and was unproductive. He drank every night to get to sleep and met criteria for alcohol dependence. How could I best help him? Exercise during the day and no more work at night seemed like a good start, and maybe other ways could be found to make him fall asleep? Or should he deal with his alcohol addiction first? Fortunately, I would be able to discuss all this with my supervisor later that week. I felt very young, although I was an old intern, but the client could have been my dad.

Oh dear, there was the next one already: a nice young guy, Bas, still a student—a smooth talker with side jobs in the cultural sector, but … he could be evicted from his house any moment, because of debts, due to his use of coke. Once he had drunk, he "had to" take coke, so in a way, the problems were really because of the alcohol. He also smoked, which made him feel like having a drink at night. Where to start? Work on the coke first and then on the other substances, or deal with everything at once? Or would that be too much of a good thing, causing him to drop out? Following the rules of motivational interviewing, I put this decision in his hands, although, after asking permission, I did give him information about the long-term effects of the various substances. Bas was eager to learn, and after a few sessions he came to the conclusion that he actually needed to quit all those substances, because the smoking led to drinking (and of course had

DOI: 10.4324/9781032634548-7

negative effects on his health), and the drinking led to coke use, and all of that eventually led to debts and eviction.

In 2008, I had returned to Amsterdam, after working at the universities of Maastricht and Nijmegen, to become professor of Developmental Psychopathology at the University of Amsterdam's department of psychology, back to my Alma Mater. There was one minor issue: the department was known for its excellent research with advanced methods, but many students wanted to be taught primarily in clinical developmental psychology. My own addiction research had become increasingly more clinically relevant, as we will see in the next chapter, but I had no experience in treatment myself. I therefore decided to pursue training as a cognitive behavioral therapist and started seeing clients as part of that process.

Psychological treatment

Treating addiction is not theory-neutral. The definition of addiction as a chronic brain disease leads to different treatment strategies than the older idea of a moral problem. And what treatment implications does the new model of addiction as biased choice have? In the moral model, addiction is seen as a sign of a poorly developed sense of morality. Since drinking is done voluntarily, it would be based on a choice—the drunk apparently likes drinking very much, as the moral model explained excessive drinking until the nineteenth century.[1] The logical recommendation from this model is to educate people better, to prevent addiction, and—if they use too much—to punish them.

Theodore Dalrymple, a retired British psychiatrist and writer, can be seen as a contemporary representative of the moral model. He stated that the Chinese dictator Mao Zedong was the most effective practitioner of treating addicted people: he allegedly gave patients the choice of continuing to use and getting shot, or to stop and stay alive, with the result that all addicted people stopped. Dalrymple's statement can be seen as a provocative way of opposing the chronic brain disease model of addiction where free will is lost, which according to him led to an industry of addiction treatment that costs lots of money, but benefits no one except people who are part of the treatment industry.[i] If you assume that addiction is either a chronic brain disease or a moral problem and you do not believe in the story of a chronic brain disease that would cause addicted people to use compulsively, as can be "disproven" by giving them the choice between the bullet and refraining from use, then

i The title of one of his books is *Junk Medicine: Doctors, Lies and the Addiction Bureaucracy.*[90]

the moral model remains and reeducation is required. As described in Chapter 5, I believe this is a false dichotomy because there is an alternative: addiction as biased choice. This is why the conclusion is wrong: from the fact that even severely addicted patients in many cases can still make a choice other than taking the drug (as Carl Hart had shown in more humane experiment with many severely addicted people choosing food vouchers over their drug),[2] you cannot conclude that they are morally unsound if they do choose the drug again.

The model of addiction as a chronic brain disease opposed hard punishment: as patients suffered from a brain disease, they should be treated rather than punished. The logical approach from the chronic-brain disease model is to repair the addicted brain, such as with medication or other techniques like brain stimulation. From this perspective, like the AA, the logic behind treatment is "once addicted, always addicted", therefore abstinence is the only solution. The model creates clarity to the severely addicted patient: the addictive drug should never be used again, because your brain remains addicted and therefore vulnerable for relapse ("Hi, I am Monica and I am an alcoholic").

An interesting question is how effective AA and related 12-step methods like the Minnesota model are—the most widely used treatment for alcohol addiction in the US, and also widely used in other parts of the world. As we saw in the first chapter, the method is based on the experiences of its founders, Dr. Bob (Smith) and Bill Wilson, and initially developed as a self-help movement: people who experience that they have lost control over their alcohol use are welcome to join the anonymous self-help groups (which now exist for numerous other addictions or problematic behaviors as well). The approach is spiritual and has Christian roots, but the spiritual interpretation can be filled in differently than in a Christian way, when desired. What dominates is the idea of the addict as being powerless, who have to renounce alcohol or their other addictive behavior and contemplate on their sins and repair them where possible on a voluntary basis (this approach is sometimes confused with the confrontational approach, which has psychoanalytic roots).[3]

It is interesting to note that the AA movement is based on the lived experience of its founders rather than on scientific theorizing. That's not to say it can't work: perhaps Wilson and Smith had a brilliant idea about treating addiction based on their own experiences. In fact, in recent years, there has been increasing interest in involving experts by experience in treatment. It should be noted, however, that experts by experience relatively often adhere to the disease model of addiction and are less inclined to follow a client if they have a goal other than total abstinence, which might not always be optimal.[4] What do we know about the effectiveness of AA-based therapy?

In the 1990s, a large study was conducted on the effectiveness of the three most widely used forms of therapy at the time, the 12-steps method (the first three steps of AA and onward referral to AA self-help groups), cognitive behavioral therapy (CBT) and motivational interviewing. As briefly introduced earlier, motivational interviewing is a non-confrontational method in which a therapist or counselor explores goals and values of the client and how their addictive behavior interferes with achieving these goals. The idea is that the central issue in addiction is motivational, once there is a strong motivation to change (either through therapy or through a natural event),[5] most clients will be able to overcome their addiction with minimal further help. CBT assesses thought processes of clients and how they maintain the addictive behavior. For example, if the client has the strong idea that drinking or smoking pot is the one way to fall asleep, this idea is challenged, and the client is invited to do an experiment to challenge this idea (e.g., not drink or smoke before going to bed for a week and graph sleeping).[ii] About a thousand patients were randomly assigned to one of these three therapies (AA, CBT or motivational interviewing). The project was called "match" because the idea was that a certain type of patient was likely to be better off with a specific treatment if there was a match. Lots of hypotheses were proposed concerning optimal matching, but almost all of them had to be rejected based on the outcomes. The overall outcome was rather sobering: irrespective of therapy, after one year about half of those treated had relapsed, and after three years it was 70%.[6,7]

Even though most matching hypotheses were rejected, some were confirmed. For example, patients who scored high on anger appeared to do better with motivational interviewing, which was found both after one and after three years.[iii] As discussed earlier, moving with the client rather than seeking confrontation is an important principle in motivational interviewing, which thus apparently works relatively well with anger and resistance. This makes sense: telling angry people what to do generally only makes them angrier. The point is to help them determine what they would like to do with their lives, only then can you see if you can help them do that (the film script method discussed in the previous chapter was also developed from this perspective). A second matching hypothesis that was supported was that alcohol-dependent patients with a social network in which there were many heavy drinkers were better off with the 12-steps method. That requires surrender to a new identity and

ii This is not the place for extensive introductions, but numerous books have been written on both topics, and the treatment manuals used in project match can be downloaded.

iii This matching result needs to be interpret with caution, given the many possible matching hypotheses that were examined.

absolute abstinence, which apparently works well precisely in this difficult social context to return to after treatment. The 12-steps also worked slightly better than the other two therapies in terms of the outcome of total abstinence. A recent meta-analysis of research on the effectiveness of AA and the 12-step method to date also yielded slightly better abstinence outcomes than other treatments.[8] While this looks positive, the other side of the same coin is that this approach is also more likely to lead to full relapse if abstinence is not sustained, which seems to indicate more of an all-or-nothing outcome than for other treatments.[9] In cases of successful abstinence, work can be done to build a new identity as a non-drinker, but if you drink again, your interpretation is that your addicted brain has taken over again, leaving you helpless and there you go again …

In CBT and motivational interviewing,[iv] the difference between a small slip or mistake (a *lapse*: using once) and relapse (using again for several days in a row) is emphasized. From this perspective, a mistake is interpreted as a learning experience: I thought I had alcohol under control, but apparently, I underestimated the triggering factors in this context. What can I learn from this? What would be another way to handle this situation in the future? In the 12-step context, a more catastrophic interpretation is obvious: you failed because you drank again, confirming the motto once an alcoholic always an alcoholic. The perspective of a *lapse* as a learning experience is more in line with the model of addiction as biased choice, in which the practitioner tries to help people make better choices in light of their long-term goals, which are activated using motivational interviewing. People then learn techniques for recognizing difficult situations and dealing with them in a different way, such as saying no and having an alternative ready (part of CBT).[10,11]

The overall treatment outcomes of the various standard psychosocial treatments thus differ little from one another (new variations follow in the next chapter), and there is much room for improvement, given that most people who receive treatment eventually relapse.[7] The latter should be seen in a broader context, as discussed in Chapter 4, most people who meet criteria at some point in their lives manage to overcome their addiction *without* professional help; thus, they do not enter treatment. For many of them, addiction is linked to a particular stage of life. Young adults drink and use other substances the most, and in most of them this decreases again when they enter a stage of life where they get more responsibilities, related to a job, a partner or a child (a process known as

iv Nowadays motivational interviewing and CBT are often combined: first work on motivation to change, then employ CBT techniques to help the actual change.[10,91]

"maturing out").[12,13] Hence, most people who suffer from addiction problems for a while can redirect themselves, perhaps aided by a minimal intervention, like a serious warning from the general practitioner, which can be enough to make people quit smoking.[14]

Another low-threshold way to get help is with online interventions (e-health). The contents of such interventions is similar to what happens in face-to-to face treatment—elements from CBT lend themselves to this—and its effects are similar to "real" therapy, both for lighter and for more severe problems.[15] However, dropout is a major issue, with many participants dropping out prematurely; many people need some guidance to stay motivated to tackle their problems.[15,16] This can be done by a counselor, but maybe also with smart chatbots, as we and others have started to investigate.[17,18]

Addiction alongside other problems

Although most people who have been struggling with addiction problems for a while manage to overcome them with no or minimal help, there is a substantial minority who does not. They seek help, often not until about ten years after their problems began (especially men, as women typically escalate quicker).[19] By that time, new problems have almost always appeared, for example in relationships or at work, so that a situation has developed where something really needs to be done. Some of the people who have long-term addiction problems are referred to specialized treatment. The group that ends up there often has many additional problems, such as depression, which fortunately disappears in many cases after detoxification.[20,21] There are also many who struggle with anxiety or personality problems in addition to their addiction, which do not disappear by themselves, once the addiction has been tackled. Research is being done on the optimal way to address this type of combined problem ("comorbidity"). The general idea is that it is good to deal with the drug first, because usually it does not work well to learn new skills when under the influence of substances. Then—preferably quickly—the additional problems should also be addressed, because they are often a reason to use. It is therefore important to develop new ways to learn to deal with those other problems, without having to be referred to another mental health treatment center (with a waiting list) as is now often the case.

In recent years, there has been a lot of focus on treating the most common second diagnosis besides alcohol addiction: cigarette smoking, or tobacco use disorder in current terminology—not insignificant when you consider that one-third to one-half of people with an alcohol or drug problem eventually die from the effects of smoking.[22] This is first of all because persons addicted to alcohol or drugs are much more likely to smoke than others; in addiction clinics, the rate is sometimes as high as 80%, and smoking is one of the most efficient ways to get deadly diseases. On top of that, there is also evidence that using multiple substances at the same time increases the risk of getting some cancers more than if you were to add up the risks of both.[13] For a long time the idea in treatment centers was that patients should be allowed to continue their smoking, because it was hard enough to quit alcohol. In recent years, however, also out of practical considerations following inside smoking bans, this view has changed, and rehab from smoking and drinking is often combined, with good outcomes.[23] This also makes sense from a relapse prevention perspective, because use of one substance often triggers use of the other.

A better life expectancy and greater chance of successfully treating alcohol addiction may be good reasons to quit smoking as well, but many addicted people have the idea that smoking helps them think clearly. The question is whether this is true. The short answer is "no".[24,25] A large study was done at the Amsterdam University Medical Center, on cognitive processes that could play a role in the development of schizophrenia, one of the most serious psychiatric disorders. For this, over a thousand patients were studied, and an equally large group of siblings of the patients, and another group with a partially overlapping risk profile, without the disorder, and a fourth group of over five hundred healthy volunteers. In all groups, cognitive functioning became *worse* when people started smoking cigarettes. This finding is consistent with the finding that in identical twins, one of whom starts smoking and the other does not, attention functions become worse in the smoker.[26] Furthermore, in both the patient group and their siblings, symptoms related to schizophrenia increased in smokers compared to non-smokers.[25] Thus, the conclusion is that smoking is actually bad for thinking. The follow-up question is why so many people think they will think more clearly when they smoke, when the survey data consistently show the opposite. The reason is probably that the average ability to concentrate goes down when a person becomes a regular smoker, but recovers briefly immediately after smoking (see Figure 4.1), creating the illusion that smoking improves mood and makes one think clearly.

We can conclude that there is reasonably effective "talk therapy"[v] for addiction, depending on how you look at it (the well-known and fitting half empty or half full glass): about half of the people relapse within a year and not many differences are found between the three commonly used therapies (motivational interviewing, CBT and AA-based 12-steps

v Note that the term "talk therapy" is a bit misleading, especially for cognitive behavior therapy (CBT), where patients have to do homework.

treatment).[7] At the same time, we must remember that this is a specific group: most people who become addicted to something at some point succeed in changing it again without professional help.[27,28]

Drugs and pills

From the disease model of addiction, it makes sense to search for a drug against this brain disease. The word "drug" is interesting in this context, as in fact many illegal drugs once entered the market as pharmaceutical drugs. For example, Bayer introduced heroin as a medicine for severe coughing by the end of the nineteenth century, only to be forbidden again in the 1914 Harrison Act.[29] Medications for addiction broadly follow one of three different strategies: the drug strengthens the negative effects, reduces the desire for the positive effects (craving) or replaces the drug itself (e.g., nicotine patches). An example of the first is one of the best-known drugs for alcohol addiction: disulfiram. Disulfiram blocks the breakdown of alcohol in the stomach, similar to what happens naturally to some of the people with Asian background: they quickly become poisoned because of the inefficient breakdown of the alcohol, followed by vomiting and feeling miserable. The difference is that this genetic variant *prevents* alcohol problems, because the negative effects occur immediately after the initiation of drinking, thus preventing positive learning experiences and related neuroadaptations and positive expectations. It's different for people with an alcohol problem: they have a more positive learning history with drinking, therefore alcohol-cues will trigger craving, making it likely that they will drink anyway after taking the medication, and that not only leads to feeling sick but can also result in serious medical complications. However, the drug can be effective when properly supervised and can sometimes prevent drinking in patients motivated to quit.[30]

The second class of drugs, focuses on reducing craving or the strong desire to use the drug (or perform the addictive behavior). A commonly used drug in the treatment of both alcohol and opiate addiction is naltrexone. It blocks a particular type of opioid receptor (the mu-type) in the brain, which plays a role in the rewarding effects of alcohol and in craving. It is proven effective for both addictions, although its effect is not large. The effect-size in these types of studies is often indicated by the number of patients you need to treat to cure someone ("number needed to treat"). For this drug, that is estimated to be twelve based on a meta-analysis,[31] meaning that if you treat twelve people with alcohol addiction with naltrexone, one gets better who would not have been cured without the drug.

The follow-up question is, of course, who this person is. If we know this beforehand, we can give medication to the person who is likely to benefit from it, an approach called personalized medicine. There were clear ideas about a candidates in this example: there is a gene associated with mu-opioid receptor function (OPRM1), which was also shown to be associated with stronger craving for various substances when its availability is signaled, for example, when someone smells a drink.[32,33] Strong craving for alcohol is related to relatively strong brain responses in areas associated with reward after a sip of alcohol[34,35] and with the automatic tendency to approach alcohol, as we will see in the next chapter.[36]

In clinical studies that assessed patients' genotype, it was found that alcohol dependent patients with a relatively rare g-allele in this gene (about 15% of Caucasian people) responded better to this drug than people without a g-allele. Hence, there was a clear genetic matching hypothesis, related to the mechanism of action: alcohol dependent patients with a g-allele in this gene should get this medication. Unfortunately, a large study in which this outcome was predicted in advance, did not show the expected effect.[37] A recent meta-analysis summarizing all the research on genetic matching and effects of naltrexone also found little support for genetic matching.[38] This disappointing finding is in line with the general move away from single-gene prediction discussed in the previous chapter. Note that recent research has demonstrated that reward drinkers can be identified using questionnaires and that this predicts a relatively good response to naltrexone,[39,40] probably based on many genes involved.

Recently, another drug was approved that works slightly differently[vi] (on the so-called "kappa" opioid receptors): nalmefene. It was marketed for people who want to drink less, but do not wish to stop drinking altogether; to do this, they take an occasional tablet. That's a commercially interesting target group, because most people with a drinking problem want exactly that. There have been a number of clinical studies on the effectivity of nalmefene, in which small positive effects have been reported. However, the main finding in these studies was that everyone reduced, whether they received the real drug or placebo, but the people who reduced with the real drug reduced slightly more than those who were given placebo.[41,42] There is still debate about the evidence base,[43] and the drug has now been approved by the European medical authorities, but not by the American.

A final drug approved for the treatment of alcohol addiction is acamprosate. It targets other neurotransmitters that play a role in the effects of alcohol: GABA and glutamate. The exact mechanism is not yet completely clear, but there are indications that it mainly acts on the tendency to drink to get rid of negative feelings ("the dark side of

vi both on the "mu" opioid receptors like naltrexone and on the "kappa" opioid receptors.

addiction"). A logical prediction was therefore that this drug would mainly help people who drink to get rid of their negative feelings. Again, this assumption was not supported by research; it also appears to be difficult to predict for whom acamprosate works.[44] The drug's effectiveness is about as strong (or weak) as that of naltrexone: you need about 12 patients to cure one of them (a statistically small effect).[31]

For the treatment of alcohol addiction, there is another drug that came in the public eye, as French medical doctor Olivier Ameisen described how he treated his own addiction with baclofen (a GABA-b agonist). Baclofen had been used for decades against muscle spasms.[45,46] As an MD, he could search the research literature and found that a higher dose of the same drug decreased alcohol use in addicted rats. Might that be something for him? He had already unsuccessfully followed the 12-step program and had tried the available medications in vain. Maybe a high dose of baclofen could help him? As a doctor, he could get hold of the drug …

He decided to self-administer incrementally higher doses, to test if this would make his craving for alcohol disappear, when the drug was taken at a dose he could handle. He experienced a total reduction of his craving for alcohol at about ten times the standard dose and wrote a case *report* about his findings.[45] This was an unusual case report: typically a physician or researcher describes something interesting that happened to a patient, from which other MDs can learn. In this case, researcher and patient were one and the same. He subsequently wrote a book about his miracle cure, which received lots of publicity.[46] As a result, the drug became widely used in France, even though no placebo-controlled study had shown efficacy. A problem in setting up a clinical trial was that the drug was off patents because it had already been marketed for its use for muscle spasms. For that reason, there was no more money to be made from it for the pharmaceutical industry, so it was not interesting to put money into it.[vii]

Sometime in 2010, when Olivier Ameisen's book was published in the Netherlands, he visited our country to talk about his book and his miracle cure. A new pill for alcoholism that was as cheap as aspirin! A promising additional finding was that baclofen strained the liver much less than other alcohol medications or alcohol, which is clearly beneficial for medication against alcohol addiction.[47] During this period, I received

vii There is some research on a variant of baclofen (R-baclofen; baclofen consists of two chemical variants, S- and R-baclofen), which seem to have different effects. In animal studies, it has shown some positive results, both in autism-like behavior and alcohol addiction. Additional benefit for the pharmaceutical industry: this variant is not yet off patent.

a call from a friend who worked as a psychiatrist in an addiction clinic at the time. He asked me what a placebo-controlled study with baclofen would cost and if I would be interested in leading such a study. That certainly seemed interesting, but where was the money to come from, since the pharmaceutical industry would not be interested to sponsor, as they would not be able to gain money from it? Turned out he had treated a patient with a high dose of baclofen (a psychiatrist can prescribe a registered drug for another use "off-label", or on his responsibility, just like Ameisen had done for himself). The patient was a multimillionaire and was willing to act as a sponsor of an efficacy study. This provided a rather unique form of research funding.

The tricky thing with research for external sponsors is that they logically want value for money, in this case that we would demonstrate that baclofen was indeed the new miracle drug for (alcohol) addiction. But your mission as a scientist is to critically examine such claims. Hence, you have to do good placebo-controlled research. We deliberated about this and arranged the financial side of the study through the Amsterdam University Fund, so that our independence would be guaranteed. With the sponsor, we agreed to publish the results, whether favorable or unfavorable. I also involved the most experienced Dutch medical addiction researcher, Wim van de Brink. He was skeptical beforehand, but also found it interesting to participate, both regarding the trial and the unique sponsoring. We organized a randomized controlled trial with several clinics (a laborious task for PhD candidate Esther Berhara and assistants: in each participating clinic employees had to be trained to do everything exactly according to protocol).

We devised a placebo-controlled design, in which one group would continue to receive a placebo, one group would remain on the standard low dose of baclofen (30 mg), and one group would be dosed higher and higher, as long as craving persisted and the side effects (such as drowsiness and nausea) did not become too strong, based on Ameisen's description of his own search for an optimal dose. This was all done blind, that is, craving and possible side effects were measured every week in all participants, after which a decision was made whether to increase the number of pills or not. As a result: some patients who continued to experience cravings for alcohol took increasing amounts of placebo pills. We hypothesized that a high dose of baclofen would work better than a low dose, with the further assumption that this would be especially true for anxious people with an alcohol problem (based on Ameisen's book where he described that he took alcohol primarily to overcome anxieties and the pharmaceutical profile of baclofen).

A study like this takes years: first there is the preparation, including medical-ethical approval, then getting placebos produced according to the very stringent rules of the game and getting the various clinics involved and instructed, and then finding patients willing to participate. It was a big project that attracted a lot of attention. For example, a piece about our study appeared in the scientific journal *Science*.[48]

The anonymous sponsor was naturally very curious about how things were going, and every year we were summoned to his beautiful canal house to fill him in on the progress of the study over a good glass of wine (apparently he had switched to controlled drinking). This was about the numbers of participants, not about outcomes, because that could only be done once the study was completed. What would come out? The excitement grew. Meanwhile, a French study without a control group reported good effects of a high dose of baclofen: half of the participants had gone from high to low risk and remained so, even after two years.[49] And just before we published our results, a first small placebo-controlled study of effects of high-dose baclofen (180 mg) came out that found a better outcome for baclofen than for placebo, that is, a higher percentage of people achieved abstinence and maintained it longer.[50] But only 56 people with alcohol addiction were involved, divided into two groups, so the favorable effect was a surprise. What was the outcome of our larger study?

The first surprise was that very few people in the high-dose group ended up on the maximum dose of 150 mg (9 out of 58 patients); for most, satiety had already occurred, they no longer craved for alcohol or were too bothered by side effects (indeed, there were more of side-effects in the high-dose medication group). Did high-dose baclofen help them stay abstinent? That was the second surprise: no more than either the low dose or the placebo. So the result was negative, which we published, as agreed upon beforehand.[51]

There was criticism, of course: the dose administered would not have been high enough (the French uncontrolled study went up to 300 mg per day, like Ameisen had done himself), but given that few people reached this dose due to side-effects, this did not seem a strong argument. We also did not find support for the hypothesis that baclofen works mainly in anxious people with an alcohol problem.[52] We did find one unexpected effect: one of the participants in the experimental group had a severe stutter, which disappeared like snow in the sun after baclofen. After he stopped taking it, the stuttering returned, and when he returned to baclofen later (he responded well to it, also in terms of alcohol consumption), the stuttering stopped again. We wrote a case report about this unexpected finding.[53] Perhaps baclofen is not a panacea for addiction, maybe it is for stuttering![viii]

viii Which, of course, would then have to be investigated further with a well-controlled study. Given the previous use of baclofen as a muscle relaxant, it is not a totally surprising finding, in retrospect.

What can we conclude about the effects of baclofen in alcohol addiction? A later Australian study found an effect both for a low (30 mg) and for slightly higher (75 mg) doses compared to placebo.[54] A meta-analysis taking the effects of all controlled studies together, found a statistically small effect (as for other medications), but remarkably, it was better for a low dose than for a high dose.[55] This conclusion goes against Ameisen's contention that only a high dose of baclofen would help against alcohol addiction, a belief that is still strongly held in France. Ameisen himself did not live to see these unexpected conclusions (he died in 2013). A recent meta-analysis also concluded that there was a small effect after taking baclofen relative to placebo with—as we predicted but did not find—stronger effects for anxious people with an alcohol problem.[52] The drug does not directly reduce anxiety, but the anxiety-reducing effects of alcohol seem to become less strong, which could reduce the appeal for people who drink to overcome their anxiety. Besides baclofen, there are a number of other *off-label* medications for which promising effects have been found, for example topiramate,[56] but even those need to be critically examined in some good clinical trials and approved before they can be marketed.

Substitution: nicotine for the smoker and heroin for heroin-dependent people

The last form of medication is substitution—by the drug itself (for example, nicotine patches for someone who wants to quit smoking) or by a drug similar to the addictive drug, which reduces the craving for it but is less bad for health (for example, methadone or buprenorphine instead of heroin).[57] The most commonly used substitute medication is undoubtedly nicotine, which is readily available in the form of gum, patches, tablets and nasal sprays. It helps with smoking cessation, as a large meta-analysis showed, although again the effect is statistically small.[58] It should be remembered that a cigarette contains more than a thousand active substances, and research has shown that the combination of nicotine with one of those many other substances—acetaldehyde—is much more addictive than nicotine alone.[59] On top of that, many other substances in tobacco are carcinogenic. This is the reason why it makes little sense to call an addiction to cigarettes "nicotine addiction", as is often done in research, tobacco addiction (or tobacco use disorder in current DSM terminology) is more appropriate. Therefore it could be regarded as a harm-reduction strategy, when tobacco smoking is replaced by taking nicotine, whether in the form of chewing gum or perhaps even in the form of an e-cigarette.

The latter is a hot topic of controversy in the world of addiction and health research. E-cigarettes appear to help inveterate smokers, replacing the deadly smoking of tobacco with e-cigarette vaping. The long-term health effect of this replacement is not yet clear, but most experts agree that they are in all likelihood less severe than those caused by smoking tobacco, with its many carcinogenic ingredients. A British study found evidence that e-cigarettes can help inveterate smokers quit, with better effects than nicotine gum and other nicotine substitutes.[60] A logical reason may be that they are a better substitute in the social context in which many people smoke, especially when e-cigarettes are allowed in social settings. This is the case in England: if you step into a pub, the air sometimes seems to be old-fashioned blue with smoke, which turns out to be water vapor, which has the pleasant side effect that your clothes don't smell terrible afterwards (not to mention the effects on your lungs).

A recent meta-analysis of all studies to date, in which e-cigarettes were used for smoking cessation, found a positive effect with a similar (statistically small) effect as other nicotine replacement drugs.[61] Whereas quitting smoking with an e-cigarette is considered a good option in England, it is viewed very suspiciously in the US, and in many countries in Europe, partly because of its unclear long-term effect and partly because e-smoking could be a stepping stone to cigarette smoking for young people.[62] In fact, a direct relationship between vaporizing and smoking (the e-cigarette makes you smoke) is often made, but that is too premature: it may also be that a trait (e.g., impulsivity) predicts both trying e-cigarettes and real cigarettes (and other substances in adolescence).[62] One solution to prevent the stepping-stone toward tobacco smoking, might be to sell the e-cigarette only as a medical device to smokers who want to quit. With Martin and his partner from the Chapter 2, whom I helped to quit smoking, the replacement with an e-cigarette helped well, Martin can now smoke an e-cigarette in his nice patio after a gathering with music and friends.

Can we also find a replacement for alcohol? David Nutt thinks we can. He is a professor of neuropsychopharmacology at Imperial College London, and he is known for his independent views on drug harms. For example, he wrote an editorial in which he stated that equasy is more dangerous than taking ecstasy, in terms of brain damage.[63] What is equasy? It is a made-up word for horse riding; brain damage due to horse riding (and falling off) is far more prevalent per exposure compared with taking ecstasy. His point was that people take risks and that an unbiased assessment of the risks should be made. He did so in a *Lancet* paper, ranking all the drugs, both for harm to the individual and for society, and alcohol and tobacco ranked high, higher than some forbidden fruits like cannabis and LSD.[64] These controversies cost him his appointment as the government's Advisory Council on the Misuse of Drugs. I know him from our joint participation in an aforementioned European project, where we concluded that the most important thing in addiction is excessive use, because this takes away the stigma associated with addiction and points to a solution (use less), rather than to pessimism and despair associated with the chronically addicted brain.[65] Nutt has long worked on trying to develop an alternative to alcohol that will provide a tipsy buzz and some of the relaxing qualities of alcohol, without the hangovers, brain damage and associated health issues. He created a spin-off firm that is now producing Alcarelle. Maybe in 10 years from now, we can order an Alcarelle in the bar and smoke an e-cigarette with it, with much less harm to our health than the originals.

In a way, the perfect replacement for an addictive drug is … the drug itself. Nicotine alone, even when vaped, is not quite the same thing as smoking a cigarette,[66] likely related to the combined effects of the many ingredients of tobacco. For severe heroin addiction, replacement therapy has been common, where patients receive methadone or buprenorphine. Here the same problem emerges: the replacement is not quite the real thing, so many heroin addicted people on replacement therapy take additional heroin. What if you were to provide the real thing instead? Research has been conducted in several countries on the effects of providing heroin treatment to long-term heroin addicted people. The idea behind this treatment, which may seem surprising at first glance, is that many of the problems experienced by heroin addicted people have to do with the illegal status of the drug, and the related high costs. If long-term addicted people no longer have to hunt for their expensive drug, this should reduce their stress and improve their quality of life. In the Netherlands, heroin became popular in the 1970s; the number of addicted people rose to some 30,000. Since the 1980s it has been a fairly stable group (the average age increases by almost a year each year).[67] Most of these people receive methadone regularly and sometimes attempt rehab. More than three-quarters also use additional heroin and cocaine occasionally. And most are not doing well in terms of their mental health and social conditions; they are a marginalized group. Initial experiments in England and Switzerland in the 1990s on the effects of heroin dispensing had shown promising effects: participants' mental health improved. However, these studies did not have good control groups.[67]

A large controlled study on the effects of heroin distribution was initiated in the Netherlands in 1998. Nearly six hundred long-term addicted people participated. They had tried in vain to get off the heroin and regularly attended methadone dispensing centers. Participants used additional heroin almost daily, they can be described as "therapy-resistant" heroin-addicted people. Participants were randomly assigned to a group that received heroin in addition to methadone and a group that did not. A group was also added that did not receive heroin for the first six months but did for the second six months. People to whom heroin was dispensed received it in their preferred manner (injecting or smoking). In addition to methadone (and thus heroin in some groups), all participants were offered psychosocial support. A positive response was defined in advance as a substantial improvement in at least one domain (physical or mental health or social functioning) and no increase in the use of other substances, such as cocaine.

The outcomes were very positive: the group that received heroin did better in all domains, with a large difference (23%, NNT 4). That is, one out of every four people who received heroin improved significantly, representing a much larger effect than the medication effects discussed earlier in alcohol addiction (a smaller number needed to treat indicates a larger treatment effect). There were no differences in medical complications between the two groups. Although heroin provision obviously costs quite some money, an interesting finding was the treatment was cost-effective: the people receiving heroin needed less care for (mental) health problems and caused less harm to get money for heroin. A follow-up study on the effects of long-term heroin provision (four years) found that the percentage of people who no longer had serious social, physical or mental health problems had increased from 30% to 80%. There was also a gradual increase in the number of people who had completely recovered in terms of health and were no longer using other illicit drugs.

The beneficial effects seem to be primarily related to the elimination of stress, as some of the interviewed participants indicated:

> Well, I liked it, yes. You have more security. That's very important. That you don't have that fear anymore: "How am I going to get money or drugs, today?" That's something you otherwise wake up with every morning.

And the money saved can be spent on useful things, which can facilitate the return to a normal life:

> Since I've been here, I've spent between seven, eight hundred guilders [about US$350] on books. I bought clothes. I bought stuff for my computer. You see, it's stuff that I used to spend on heroin and that I can now spend on other things.

And another participant:

> I have changed my way of life, nowadays. ... Before, life was just too fast, you know, now I want to live my life more slowly.[67]

There were also seven patients who stopped taking part in the heroin administration and switched back to abstinence-oriented treatment.

Most of them fell back to methadone treatment; quitting completely did not occur, according to Peter Blanken, the lead author of the research, in response to an email. This is, of course, relevant for the discussion on addiction as a chronic brain disease. Chronic opiate addiction is perhaps the clearest example of a form of addiction for which the chronic brain disease model makes sense (although Lewis pointed to successfully discontinued exceptions),[68] which is also evidenced by long-term outcomes: of a group of nearly six hundred heroin users in the 1960s, 33 years later about half were found to have died and the rest still had many mental health problems and many were still using heroin and/or other substances, with some 15% recovered (mostly early after the initial measurement).[69,70] Thus, with heroin addiction, there is a possibility to quit, especially early in the process, but after long-term addiction, there is a world to be gained with substitution treatment aimed at counteracting negative health effects of being addicted, by providing an alternative or, in some cases, by providing the drug itself, to alleviate the stress surrounding the acquisition. Heroin provision should be part of treatment repertoire, based on these results, but is politically difficult, especially for those who think about addiction from the moral model. In some countries, it has become part of regular treatment for the group of therapy-resistant heroin addicted people.

"Replacement therapy" has also been applied to alcohol addiction, especially in Canada.[71] This has found positive effects on the mental and physical health of the participants. In Amsterdam, a project ran for some time in which alcohol was provided to people chronically addicted to alcohol in the Oosterpark (the park I lived next to when doing my PhD), which attracted the world press.[72] In this "Beer for Work" program, addicted participants received a hot meal, a small wage of 10 euros and five beers, which they could consume during the day, in exchange for working three days a week, primarily cleaning the park and its surroundings. The project caught on: the participants had a day job and drank less than usual. These projects can be considered a successful outcome of the approach to addiction as a chronic brain disease: they provide a better quality of life for long-term addicted people. For this therapy-resistant group, the alternative is despair, often leading to suicide or overdose ("deaths of despair").[73]

Regarding the latter: Dutch journalist Marcel Langedijk described the gripping story of his brother Mark's euthanasia, who suffered for a long time from anxiety, depression and alcohol addiction, and after 21 unsuccessful rehab attempts decided he wanted to step out of life. The story about his euthanasia made the world press, linking it to the Dutch euthanasia policy: *in the Netherlands they are now euthanizing their alcoholics*.[74] The difficult question remains whether a treatment might still have been possible for Mark that could have helped, or an acceptance-oriented approach, in line with the replacement therapies discussed above: accept that substance use is part of your life and try to make the best out of it. We will never know, but we must realize that a focus on the success stories of people who have overcome severe addiction, should not blind us to the fact that the battle is unwinnable for some. For that group of people in particular, controlled use of the drug to which they are addicted can provide a solution, after which a more stable life emerges, perhaps with opportunities to redirect life for the better. For this small group of long-term addicted people, the term "chronic brain disease" does appear appropriate. The problem is that this term is applied much more broadly, namely to anyone with a diagnosis of addiction (or in current terminology substance use disorder), the vast majority of whom appear to be able to stop or reduce with little or no help.[75]

Pills *and* talk therapy?

As we saw, addiction can be treated with varieties of "talk therapy" and there are some varieties of medication that help some people with addiction problems. A logical follow-up question is how the combination works: pills *and* "talk therapy". This was investigated in the large American Combine project, the successor to project Match described earlier. In project Combine, the effects of two anti-craving medications—naltrexone and acamprosate—were compared (a participant could receive the real version of either drug or placebo), which was combined with the effects of a general form of "talk therapy", combining motivational interviewing with cognitive behavioral therapy and, if desired, AA self-help groups. More than 1,300 alcohol-dependent patients were assigned to one of as many as nine experimental groups (of either drug real or placebo, with or without further therapy).[ix]

Naltrexone was found to have an effect, as did "talk therapy", but perhaps surprisingly, the combination of both showed no added value. All patients also received minimal counseling ("medical management"), which was apparently sufficient to find the medication effect. A recent article systematically summarized the literature on "pills and talk therapy". The majority of 28 studies examined whether medication had added value to psychotherapy, which was the case in about half of the studies (ten out of nineteen). Other studies examined the added effect of psychotherapy as add-on to medication, and there an additional effect

ix That adds up to 8 groups: 2 (naltrexone, real or placebo) × 2 (acamprosate, real or placebo) × 2 (talk therapy or not) = 8 groups. The ninth group received no pills at all, only talk therapy, to investigate the placebo effect.

was found in one-third of the studies (three out of nine). The authors concluded that in many cases pharmacotherapy has an added effect to therapy, but that the reverse is not necessarily true. Thus, combining pills and talk therapy does not necessarily produce a better outcome than either of the two separately, and effects remain modest.

Brain stimulation

Finally, based on the brain disease model, there has been much recent interest in brain stimulation: if the addicted brain malfunctions, perhaps stimulation could revitalize it. There are three methods by which this can be done. In two of these methods, the skull is stimulated from the outside (non-invasive brain stimulation), while in the third method an electrode is placed deep inside the brain after surgery, which can then provide stimulation in a specific region (typically it is placed in the deep brain structures related to motivation). For external stimulation, electricity can be used, that is *transcranial direct current stimulation* (tDCS) or a magnetic field *transcranial magnetic stimulation* (TMS). Note that these types of stimulation are very different from electroshock, because that involves a high current surge with the aim of "resetting" the brain, for example, in chronic depression.[x] In contrast, tDCS uses such a weak current (usually 2 mA) that participants hardly feel it; they only feel a brief tingling sensation when the device is turned on. This sensation is used in the placebo condition, in which the current is turned on briefly at the beginning (creating a similar brief itch) and then turned off again, while in the active condition the current typically stays on for some 15–20 minutes. There is some evidence that tDCS can reduce craving in the short term, both those for alcohol and for cannabis.[76,77]

With former postdoc Thomas Gladwin and PhD student Tess den Uyl, I conducted a series of studies on the effects of tDCS. We began by doing a series of basic studies in volunteers,[78] followed by clinical studies in which tDCS was added to the treatment of alcohol addiction.[79,80] We found some evidence for a potential positive effect, but it added little to the effects of cognitive training alone (discussed in the next chapter). A number of previous studies had used non-invasive neurostimulation to treat addiction. Still other studies examined whether there was an added effect in addition to medication or psychotherapy. The results have recently been summarized as a cautious indication of a possible positive

x Electroshock therapy understandably has a bad reputation, influenced in part by such films as *One Flew Over the Cuckoo's Nest* (1975). Still, a proportion of chronically depressed patients do recover from depression through its use. There are promising methods for predicting for whom it might work, based on brain scans.[92]

effect; promising findings have emerged from the research, but they are rather inconsistent, and large controlled clinical trials would be needed to reach more solid conclusions.[81,82] The variant with alternating magnetic fields (rTMS) has the advantage that it can provide more precise stimulation of certain brain areas (tDCS runs a current between two electrodes placed on the skull, which results in a rather global stimulation, typically of frontal cortical areas). However, the increased precision comes with higher costs: you first need (expensive) brain scanning to target the stimulation, which is fine in a medical research context, but makes it less accessible in a clinical context. While arguably promising in addiction, the method has proved effective in treating chronic depression.

Finally, one can use invasive deep brain stimulation. This has been used successfully in some progressive brain diseases, such as Parkinson's, and severe psychiatric disorders, such as obsessive-compulsive disorder.[83,84] Perhaps it could also be of use in the small group of severely addicted people with a chronic addiction as a last resort, like heroin delivery to heroin addicted people. It requires brain surgery, which is not without risks, but if it makes someone's life bearable again, this could be a useful intervention. As is often the case in science, research into the possible effects of deep brain stimulation in addiction began with a chance finding: a patient who received a brain implant for severe panic and depression was suddenly able to stay off the alcohol. Meanwhile, research into the effects of deep brain stimulation was conducted in a few individuals with a therapy-resistant form of alcoholism, and two of the five patients achieved long-term abstinence, while the others successfully reduced their drinking.[81,82] Conducting the big clinical trials to study efficacy has proven difficult if not impossible, because few chronically addicted patients want to participate.

Conclusions

What has the chronic brain disease model brought us in terms of treating addictions? A number of drugs have been developed that can help treat addiction, but their effect is statistically small (you need to treat about a dozen of patients to cure one). Note that this small effect size is not an exception in medicine; the effect of medication in psychiatry is not smaller than in most other areas of medicine.[85] The effect of the "miracle drug" baclofen also proved rather disappointing; at best there is an indication of a similarly small effect. In addition, methods have been developed to stimulate the brain directly, which did show some promise, but this line of research is still in its infancy and big clinical trials still need to be done. The chronic brain disease model can also be related to substitution therapy, with the ultimate substitute being the drug itself (heroin for heroin addicted people). This is part of a humane approach for the small group of therapy-resistant long-term addicted people and is used in some countries, with proven positive effects on physical and mental health. For this small group, the chronic brain disease model does seem to apply and substitution therapy can be considered a valuable consequence of the model.

In the US, the number of opiate addicted people, is much higher than in other similarly developed countries, mainly due to the use of painkillers.[73] In the US, nearly 100,000 people die of overdose every year. In a recent article on this opiate crisis, Nora Volkow (the aforementioned director of NIDA) wrote that we need to move away from the black-and-white thinking that only abstinence is a good outcome of treatment, and that cutting back can also yield gains—not only with opiates, but also with other drugs.[86] This is an important departure from the focus on total abstinence that dominated in the US since the rise of AA. The opiate crisis also shows that it is important to look beyond the addicted brain: opiate overdose deaths are relatively frequent in Americans who are struggling economically and socially (Hillary Clinton's famous "deplorables"); poor Americans in former industrial areas, who no longer see a future perspective, leading to despair and declining life expectancy ("deaths of despair").[87–89] This is consistent with the idea that offering an alternative perspective is one of the key ingredients in addiction treatment. Recovery starts with being able to imagine a better life, which you can then work toward with a variety of techniques. Without perspective, any treatment becomes difficult and the short-term fix of the addiction remains alluring.

In the next chapter, I will show what alternatives have been developed beyond pills and talk therapy that are consistent with the idea that biased choice is central in addiction.

References

1. Levine HG. The discovery of addiction: changing conceptions of habitual drunkenness in America. J Stud Alcohol. 1978;39:143–74.
2. Hart CL, Haney M, Foltin RW, Fischman MW. Alternative reinforcers differentially modify cocaine self-administration by humans. Behav Pharmacol. 2000;11:87–91.
3. Miller WR, Kurtz E. Models of alcoholism used in treatment: contrasting AA and other perspectives with which it is often confused. J Stud Alcohol. 1994;55:159–66.
4. Moyers TB, Miller WR. Therapists' conceptualizations of alcoholism: measurement and implications for treatment decisions. Psychol Addict Behav. 1993;7:238–45.
5. Miller WR. Rediscovering fire: small interventions, large effects. Psychol Addict Behav. 2000;14:6.
6. Allen J, Anton RF, Babor TF, Carbonari J, Carroll KM, Connors GJ, et al. Matching alcoholism treatments to client heterogeneity: Project MATCH three-year drinking outcomes. Alcohol Clin Exp Res. 1998;22:1300–11.

7. Cutler RB, Fishbain D a. Are alcoholism treatments effective? The Project MATCH data. BMC Public Health [Internet]. 2005 [cited 2013 Jun 28];5:75. Available from: www.pubmedcentral.nih.gov/articlerender.fcgi?artid=1185549&tool=pmcentrez&rendertype=abstract
8. Kelly JF, Abry A, Ferri M, Humphreys K. Alcoholics Anonymous and 12-step facilitation treatments for alcohol use disorder: a distillation of a 2020 Cochrane review for clinicians and policy makers. Alcohol Alcohol. 2020; 55:641–51.
9. Peele S. A scientific life on the edge: my lonely quest to change how we see addiction. NY: Broadway Books; 2021.
10. Merkx MJM. Individuele cognitieve gedragstherapie bij middelengebruik en gokken. In: GM Schippers, AM Smeerdijk, MJM Merkx, (Eds.). Handboek cognitieve gedragstherapie bij middelengebruik en gokken. Amersfoort: Resultaten Scoren.; 2014. pp. 105–264.
11. Kadden R, Carroll KM, Donovan D, Cooney N, Monti P, Abrams D, et al. Cognitive-behavioral coping skills therapy manual [Internet]. Vol. 3. 1994. Available from: https://pubs.niaaa.nih.gov/publications/projectmatch/match03.pdf
12. Littlefield AK, Sher KJ, Wood PK. Is "maturing out" of problematic alcohol involvement related to personality change? J Abnorm Psychol. 2009;118:360–74.
13. Tucker JA, Chandler SD, Witkiewitz K. Epidemiology of recovery from alcohol use disorder. Alcohol Res Curr Rev. 2020;40.
14. Bartsch AL, Härter M, Niedrich J, Brütt AL, Buchholz A. A systematic literature review of self-reported smoking cessation counseling by primary care physicians. PLoS One. 2016;11:1–18.
15. Riper H, Hoogendoorn A, Cuijpers P, Karyotaki E, Boumparis N, Mira A, et al. Effectiveness and moderators of Internet interventions for adult hazardous and harmful drinking in general and primary care populations: an individual patient data meta-analysis. PLOS Med. 2018;1–26.
16. Koelen JA, Vonk A, Klein A, de Koning L, Vonk P, de Vet S, et al. Man vs. machine: a meta-analysis on the added value of human support in text-based internet treatments ("e-therapy") for mental disorders. Clin Psychol Rev. 2022;102179.
17. He L, Basar E, Wiers RW, Antheunis ML, Krahmer E. Can chatbots help to motivate smoking cessation? A study on the effectiveness of motivational interviewing on engagement and therapeutic alliance. BMC Public Health [Internet]. 2022;22:1–14. Available from: 10.1186/s12889-022-13115-x
18. Olano-Espinosa E, Avila-Tomas JF, Minue-Lorenzo C, Matilla-Pardo B, Serrano MES, Martinez-Suberviola FJ, et al. Effectiveness of a conversational chatbot (Dejal@bot) for the adult population to quit smoking: pragmatic, multicenter, controlled, randomized clinical trial in primary care. JMIR mHealth uHealth. 2022;10:1–15.
19. Becker JB. Sex differences in addiction. Dialogues Clin Neurosci. 2016;18:395–402.
20. Brown SA, Schuckit MA. Changes in depression among abstinent alcoholics. J Stud Alcohol. 1988;49:412–7.
21. Brown SA, Inaba RK, Gillin JC, Schuckit MA, Stewart MA, Irwin MR. Alcoholism and affective disorder: clinical course of depressive symptoms. Am J Psychiatry. 1995;152:45–52.
22. Callaghan RC, Gatley JM, Sykes J, Taylor L. The prominence of smoking-related mortality among individuals with alcohol- or drug-use disorders. Drug Alcohol Rev. 2018;37:97–105.

23. McKelvey K, Thrul J, Ramo D. Impact of quitting smoking and smoking cessation treatment on substance use outcomes: an updated and narrative review. Addict Behav [Internet]. 2017;65:161–70. Available from: 10.1016/j.addbeh.2016.10.012
24. Vermeulen JM, Schirmbeck F, Blankers M, Van Tricht M, Bruggeman R, Van Den Brink W, et al. Association between smoking behavior and cognitive functioning in patients with psychosis, siblings, and healthy control subjects: results from a prospective 6-year follow-up study. Am J Psychiatry. 2018;175:1121–8.
25. Vermeulen J, Schirmbeck F, Blankers M, van Tricht M, van den Brink W, de Haan L, et al. Smoking, symptoms, and quality of life in patients with psychosis, siblings, and healthy controls: a prospective, longitudinal cohort study. The Lancet Psychiatry. 2019;6:25–34.
26. Treur JL, Willemsen G, Bartels M, Geels LM, Van Beek JHDA, Huppertz C, et al. Smoking during adolescence as a risk factor for attention problems. Biol Psychiatry [Internet]. 2015;78:656–63. Available from: 10.1016/j.biopsych.2014.06.019
27. Heyman GM. Addiction: a disorder of choice. Harvard University Press; 2010.
28. Heyman GM. Addiction and choice: theory and new data. Front Psychiatry. 2013;4:1–5.
29. Sneader W. Department of medical history: the discovery of heroin. Med Hist. 1998;352:1697–9.
30. Skinner MD, Lahmek P, Pham H, Aubin HJ. Disulfiram efficacy in the treatment of alcohol dependence: a meta-analysis. PLoS One. 2014;9:e87366.
31. Jonas DE, Amick HR, Feltner C, Bobashev G, Thomas K, Wines R, et al. Pharmacotherapy for adults with alcohol use disorders in outpatient settings: a systematic review and meta-analysis. JAMA—J Am Med Assoc. 2014; 311:1889–900.
32. Van Den Wildenberg E, Wiers RW, Dessers J, Janssen RGJH, Lambrichs EH, Smeets HJM, et al. A functional polymorphism of the μ-opioid receptor gene (OPRM1) influences cue-induced craving for alcohol in male heavy drinkers. Alcohol Clin Exp Res [Internet]. 2007 [cited 2013 Mar 11];31:1–10. Available from: www.ncbi.nlm.nih.gov/pubmed/17207095
33. van der Zwaluw CS, van den Wildenberg E, Wiers RW, Franke B, Buitelaar J, Scholte RHJ, et al. Polymorphisms in the mu-opioid receptor gene (OPRM1) and the implications for alcohol dependence in humans. Pharmacogenomics [Internet]. 2007;8:1427–36. Available from: www.ncbi.nlm.nih.gov/pubmed/17979515
34. Filbey FM, Ray L, Smolen A, Claus ED, Audette A, Hutchison KE. Differential neural response to alcohol priming and alcohol taste cues is associated with DRD4 VNTR and OPRM1 genotypes. Alcohol Clin Exp Res. 2008;32:1113–23.
35. Korucuoglu O, Gladwin TE, Baas F, Mocking RJT, Ruhé HG, Groot PFC, et al. Neural response to alcohol taste cues in youth: effects of the OPRM1 gene. Addict Biol. 2017;22:1562–75.
36. Wiers RW, Rinck M, Dictus M, Van Den Wildenberg E. Relatively strong automatic appetitive action-tendencies in male carriers of the OPRM1 G-allele. Genes, Brain Behav [Internet]. 2009 [cited 2013 Mar 9];8:101–6. Available from: www.ncbi.nlm.nih.gov/pubmed/19016889
37. Oslin DW, Leong SH, Lynch KG, Berrettini W, O'Brien CP, Gordon AJ, et al. Naltrexone vs placebo for the treatment of alcohol dependence: a randomized clinical trial. JAMA Psychiatry. 2015;72:430–7.

38. Hartwell EE, Feinn R, Morris PE, Gelernter J, Krystal J, Arias AJ, et al. Systematic review and meta-analysis of the moderating effect of rs1799971 in OPRM1, the mu-opioid receptor gene, on response to naltrexone treatment of alcohol use disorder. Addiction. 2020;115:1426–37.
39. Mann K, Roos CR, Hoffmann S, Nakovics H, Leménager T, Heinz A, et al. Precision medicine in alcohol dependence: a controlled trial testing pharmacotherapy response among reward and relief drinking phenotypes. Neuropsychopharmacology [Internet]. 2018;43:891–9. Available from: 10.1038/npp.2017.282
40. Roos CR, Bold KW, Witkiewitz K, Leeman RF, DeMartini KS, Fucito LM, et al. Reward drinking and naltrexone treatment response among young adult heavy drinkers. Addiction. 2021;116:2360–71.
41. Mann K, Torup L, Sørensen P, Gual A, Swift R, Walker B, et al. Nalmefene for the management of alcohol dependence: review on its pharmacology, mechanism of action and meta-analysis on its clinical efficacy. Eur Neuropsychopharmacol. 2016;26:1941–9.
42. van den Brink W, Strang J, Gual A, Sørensen P, Jensen TJ, Mann K. Safety and tolerability of as-needed nalmefene in the treatment of alcohol dependence: results from the Phase III clinical programme. Expert Opin Drug Saf. 2015;14:495–504.
43. Fitzgerald N, Angus K, Elders A, de Andrade M, Raistrick D, Heather N, et al. Weak evidence on nalmefene creates dilemmas for clinicians and poses questions for regulators and researchers. Addiction. 2016;111:1477–87.
44. Verheul R, Lehert P, Geerlings PJ, Koeter MWJ, Van Den Brink W. Predictors of acamprosate efficacy: results from a pooled analysis of seven European trials including 1485 alcohol-dependent patients. Psychopharmacology (Berl). 2005;178:167–73.
45. Ameisen O. Complete and prolonged suppression of symptoms and consequences of alcohol-dependence using high-dose baclofen: a self-case report of a physician. Alcohol Alcohol [Internet]. 2005;40:147–50. Available from: www.embase.com/search/results?subaction=viewrecord&from=export&id=L40347343%0Ahttp://dx.doi.org/10.1093/alcalc/agh130%0Ahttp://sfx.library.uu.nl/utrecht?sid=EMBASE&issn=07350414&id=doi:10.1093%2Falcalc%2Fagh130&atitle=Complete+and+prolonged+suppres
46. Ameisen O. Heal thyself: a doctor at the peak of his medical career, destroyed by alcohol: and the personal miracle that brought him back. NY: Sarah Crichton Books; 2010.
47. Addolorato G, Leggio L, Ferrulli A, Cardone S, Vonghia L, Mirijello A, et al. Effectiveness and safety of baclofen for maintenance of alcohol abstinence in alcohol-dependent patients with liver cirrhosis: randomised, double-blind controlled study. Lancet. 2007;370:1915–22.
48. Enserink M. Anonymous alcoholic bankrolls trial of controversial therapy. Science (80–). 2011;332:653.
49. De Beaurepaire R. Suppression of alcohol dependence using baclofen: a 2-year observational study of 100 patients. Front Psychiatry. 2012;3:1–7.
50. Mueller CA, Geisel O, Pelz P, Higl V, Kr??ger J, Stickel A, et al. High-dose baclofen for the treatment of alcohol dependence (BACLAD study): a randomized, placebo-controlled trial. Eur Neuropsychopharmacol [Internet]. 2015;25:1167–77. Available from: 10.1016/j.euroneuro.2015.04.002
51. Beraha EM, Salemink E, Goudriaan AE, Bakker A, de Jong D, Smits N, et al. Efficacy and safety of high-dose baclofen for the treatment of alcohol dependence: a multicentre, randomised, double-blind controlled trial. Eur Neuropsychopharmacol. 2016;26.

52. Agabio R, Baldwin DS, Amaro H, Leggio L, Sinclair JMA. The influence of anxiety symptoms on clinical outcomes during baclofen treatment of alcohol use disorder: a systematic review and meta-analysis. Neurosci Biobehav Rev [Internet]. 2021;125:296–313. Available from: 10.1016/j.neubiorev.2020.12.030
53. Beraha E, Bodewits P, Van Den Brink W, Wiers R. Speaking fluently with baclofen? BMJ Case Rep. 2017;2017.
54. Morley KC, Baillie A, Fraser I, Furneaux-Bate A, Dore G, Roberts M, et al. Baclofen in the treatment of alcohol dependence with or without liver disease: multisite, randomised, double-blind, placebo-controlled trial. Br J Psychiatry. 2018;212:362–9.
55. Pierce M, Sutterland A, Beraha EM, Morley K, van den Brink W. Efficacy, tolerability, and safety of low-dose and high-dose baclofen in the treatment of alcohol dependence: a systematic review and meta-analysis. Eur Neuropsychopharmacol [Internet]. 2018;28:795–806. Available from: 10.1016/j.euroneuro.2018.03.017
56. Reus VI, Fochtmann LJ, Bukstein O, Eyler AE, Hilty DM, Horvitz-Lennon M, et al. The American Psychiatric Association practice guideline for the pharmacological treatment of patients with alcohol use disorder. Am J Psychiatry. 2018;175:86–90.
57. Heidebrecht F, MacLeod MB, Dawkins L. Predictors of heroin abstinence in opiate substitution therapy in heroin-only users and dual users of heroin and crack. Addict Behav [Internet]. 2018;77:210–6. Available from: 10.1016/j.addbeh.2017.10.013
58. Hartmann-Boyce J, Chepkin SC, Ye W, Bullen C, Lancaster T. Nicotine replacement therapy versus control for smoking cessation. Cochrane Database Syst Rev. 2018;2018.
59. Belluzzi JD, Wang R, Leslie FM. Acetaldehyde enhances acquisition of nicotine self-administration in adolescent rats. Neuropsychopharmacology. 2005;30:705–12.
60. Brown J, Beard E, Kotz D, Michie S, West R. Real-world effectiveness of e-cigarettes when used to aid smoking cessation: a cross-sectional population study. Addiction. 2014;109:1531–40.
61. Wang RJ, Bhadriraju S, Glantz SA. E-cigarette use and adult cigarette smoking cessation: a meta-analysis. Am J Public Health. 2021;111:230–46.
62. Chan GCK, Stjepanović D, Lim C, Sun T, Shanmuga Anandan A, Connor JP, et al. Gateway or common liability? A systematic review and meta-analysis of studies of adolescent e-cigarette use and future smoking initiation. Addiction. 2021;116:743–56.
63. Nutt DJ. Equasy: an overlooked addiction with implications for the current debate on drug harms. J Psychopharmacol. 2009;23:3–5.
64. Nutt DJ, King LA, Phillips LD. Drug harms in the UK: A multicriteria decision analysis. Lancet. 2010;376:1558–65.
65. Rehm J, Marmet S, Anderson P, Gual A, Kraus L, Nutt DJJ, et al. Defining substance use disorders: do we really need more than heavy use? Alcohol Alcohol [Internet]. 2013 [cited 2014 Jul 13];48:633–40. Available from: www.ncbi.nlm.nih.gov/pubmed/23926213
66. West R, Cox S. Nicotine addiction: how well has it stood up to three more decades of research? The 1988 US Surgeon General's report. Addiction. 2022;117:2346–50.
67. Blanken P, van den Brink W, Hendriks VM, Huijsman IA, Klous MG, Rook EJ, et al. Heroin-assisted treatment in the Netherlands: history, findings, and international context. Eur Neuropsychopharmacol [Internet]. 2010;20:S105–58. Available from: 10.1016/S0924-977X(10)70001-8

68. Lewis M. The biology of desire: why addiction is not a disease [Internet]. NY: Public Affairs; 2015. Available from: https://books.google.com/books?hl=en&lr=&id=CRtpCQAAQBAJ&pgis=1
69. Hser Y-I, Hoffman V, Grella CE, Anglin MD. A 33-year follow-up of narcotics addicts. Arch Gen Psychiatry. 2001;58:503–8.
70. Hser YI, Huang D, Chou CP, Anglin MD. Trajectories of heroin addiction: growth mixture modeling results based on a 33-year follow-up study. Eval Rev. 2007;31:548–63.
71. Stockwell T, Zhao J, Pauly B, Chow C, Vallance K, Wettlaufer A, et al. Trajectories of alcohol use and related harms for managed alcohol program participants over 12 months compared with local controls: a quasi-experimental study. Alcohol Alcohol. 2021;56:651–9.
72. Alcoholisten uit oost trekken aandacht wereldpers [Internet]. de Brug. 2013. Available from: https://debrugkrant.nl/alcoholisten-uit-oost-trekken-aandacht-wereldpers/
73. Sterling P, Platt ML. Why deaths of despair are increasing in the US and not other industrial nations—insights from neuroscience and anthropology. Am J Psychiatry. 2022;
74. Wiegman M. Broer Marcel Langedijk koos voor de dood de easy way out dat was het ergste verwijt [Internet]. Parool. 2017. Available from: www.parool.nl/nieuws/broer-marcel-langedijk-koos-voor-de-dood-de-easy-way-out-dat-was-het-ergste-verwijt~b98d6125/
75. Fenton T, Wiers RW. Free will, black swans and addiction. Neuroethics. 2017;10.
76. Boggio PS, Sultani N, Fecteau S, Merabet L, Mecca T, Pascual-Leone A, et al. Prefrontal cortex modulation using transcranial DC stimulation reduces alcohol craving: a double-blind, sham-controlled study. Drug Alcohol Depend. 2008;92:55–60.
77. Boggio PS, Zaghi S, Villani AB, Fecteau S, Pascual-Leone A, Fregni F. Modulation of risk-taking in marijuana users by transcranial direct current stimulation (tDCS) of the dorsolateral prefrontal cortex (DLPFC). Drug Alcohol Depend [Internet]. 2010;112:220–5. Available from: 10.1016/j.drugalcdep.2010.06.019
78. Greenwald AG, Mcghee DE, Schwartz JLK. Measuring individual differences in implicit cognition: the Implicit Association Test. J Pers Soc Psychol. 1998;74:1464–80.
79. den Uyl TE, Gladwin TE, Lindenmeyer J, Wiers RW. A clinical trial with combined transcranial direct current stimulation and alcohol attentional retraining. Alcohol Clin Exp Res. 2018;42(10):1961–9.
80. den Uyl TE, Gladwin TE, Rinck M, Lindenmeyer J, Wiers RW. A clinical trial with combined transcranial direct current stimulation and alcohol approach bias retraining. Addict Biol. 2017;22:1–9.
81. Luigjes J, Segrave R, de Joode N, Figee M, Denys D. Efficacy of invasive and non-invasive brain modulation interventions for addiction. Neuropsychol. Rev. 2019;29:116–38.
82. Maatoug R, Bihan K, Duriez P, Podevin P, Silveira-Reis-Brito L, Benyamina A, et al. Non-invasive and invasive brain stimulation in alcohol use disorders: a critical review of selected human evidence and methodological considerations to guide future research. Compr Psychiatry. 2021;109.
83. Denys D, Mantione M, Figee M, Van Den Munckhof P, Koerselman F, Westenberg H, et al. Deep brain stimulation of the nucleus accumbens for

treatment-refractory obsessive-compulsive disorder. Arch Gen Psychiatry. 2010;67:1061–8.
84. Graat I, Figee M, Denys D. The application of deep brain stimulation in the treatment of psychiatric disorders. Int Rev Psychiatry. 2017;29:178–90.
85. Leucht S, Hierl S, Kissling W, Dold M, Davis JM. Putting the efficacy of psychiatric and general medicine medication into perspective: review of meta-analyses. Br J Psychiatry. 2012;200:97–106.
86. Volkow ND. Making addiction treatment more realistic and pragmatic: the perfect should not be the enemy of the good. Health Affairs Forefront [Internet]. 2022; Available from: www.healthaffairs.org/do/10.1377/forefront.20211221.691862/full/
87. Case A, Deaton A. Rising morbidity and mortality in midlife among white non-Hispanic Americans in the 21st century. Proc Natl Acad Sci USA. 2015;112:15078–83.
88. Quinones S. Dreamland: the true tale of America's opiate epidemic. Bloomsbury Publishing USA; 2015.
89. Sterling P. What is health? Allostasis and the evolution of human design. Cambridge, MA: MIT Press; 2020.
90. Dalrymple T. Junk medicine: doctors, lies and the addiction bureaucracy. Harriman House Petersfield; 2007.
91. Moyers TB, Houck J. Combining motivational interviewing with cognitive-behavioral treatments for substance abuse: lessons from the COMBINE research project. Cogn Behav Pract [Internet]. 2011;18:38–45. Available from: 10.1016/j.cbpra.2009.09.005
92. Van Waarde JA, Scholte HS, Van Oudheusden LJB, Verwey B, Denys D, Van Wingen GA. A functional MRI marker may predict the outcome of electroconvulsive therapy in severe and treatment-resistant depression. Mol Psychiatry. 2015;20:609–14.

8 Improving choice

Reward alternatives, cognitive training and mindfulness

Charlie was a little bit late, as he had been the first time. Would he show up at all? He participated in a study testing a new training method we had developed, that had shown positive effects as add-on in the treatment of alcohol dependence, now adjusted to help adolescents quit smoking. Many adolescents, like Charlie, pick up smoking to be part of the cool group, thinking they can easily quit whenever they want. This might be true, but the data show that many don't and that's the group that typically has a hard time to quit later on. That is why we set up the study, in a collaboration with Suchitra Krishnan-Sarin, from Yale University, Connecticut. We combined the "talk therapy" they developed (a combination of motivational interviewing and cognitive behavior therapy, CBT), with a smoking-adapted version of the training, either in the active version or in the placebo-version.

There he was, he sat down and we continued our conversation. I had a double role in this study: lead investigator of the Dutch site of this binational study, and on our side as one of the counselors for the talk therapy part, to practice my skills (it was at the time I was still training to become CBT therapist). We talked about his upcoming quit attempt, went through all the preparations and the reasons why he wanted to quit, which he had summarized on a little note in his phone sleeve: *Make my mother proud of me. Saving up for a moped. Smell better for the girls.* All sounded good, and he had no more questions about the preparations, for his quit attempt, next Saturday. What was left was the computerized training we had developed and the reward for participating in the session. He turned to me: "I get €5 for the session, right?" I nodded. "What if you give me only €2.50 and we skip the training part?" I had to laugh. Clearly, I passed as a trusted counselor and how could he know that I had designed the training with my collaborators? We needed to make the training more attractive for youth, this had not been a problem with the adult patients with alcoholism.

DOI: 10.4324/9781032634548-8

From the model of addiction as biased choice, what could you do to help people who are addicted? The answer seems obvious: help them make better choices. The big question, of course, is how to do this. In part, strategies developed in existing therapies may help, such as getting long-term goals clear (part of motivational interviewing) and avoiding overly risky situations, which is part of AA-inspired treatment and the same strategy can also be used in the first phase after quitting as part of a CBT approach. Perhaps, in addition to these strategies, relevant decision processes could also be influenced more directly. That is what several recently developed intervention strategies are aiming at.

Rewarding positive behavior

The most basic way to influence choice is to reward the desired alternative behavior, which is known as *contingency management* in the context of addiction treatment. It amounts to consistently rewarding the behavior you are striving for, based on Skinner's laws of "operant conditioning".[i] For example, people addicted to cocaine were consistently rewarded if they produced a clean pee during their visit.[1–3] Several variations were developed, where you always get an (increasing) reward, or you get a lottery ticket with a variable reward after the desired behavior.[4–6] This method is effective: rewarding desired behavior works. The only caveat is that the effects generally disappear rather quickly after the rewarding has stopped: three months later, there is still a bit of an effect left, but after six months no more, as a meta-analysis of the studies applying contingency management in the context of addiction treatment concluded.[7]

More promisingly, recent research demonstrated that combining this approach with a group training to quit smoking in the workplace, showed more long-term positive effects: after one year, 41% had not resumed smoking, using this combined method, which is exceptionally high and much higher than the 26% who had received the group training alone.[8] The combination of simple rewards and social processes make this approach more successful in the long run, at least in smoking cessation (and perhaps also in other addictions: there is evidence that social support is an important ingredient in AA-based treatment[9]).

A related method is the *Community Reinforcement Approach* (CRA),[10] which emphasizes the importance of alternative social rewards. CRA emphasizes changing environmental factors: if a person feels better at

i Operant conditioning, or systematically rewarding desired behavior (which can be as small as a gesture in the right direction) is also the basis of the good behavior game, which successfully delayed later substance use, discussed in Chapter 6.

work, in family and with friends, then the appeal of addiction is reduced, thus making it easier to stay off alcohol and drugs. This approach is conceptually similar to the animal studies discussed in Chapter 4, in which it was found that playing with peers almost always outweighed taking an addictive drug alone.[11,12] A systematic review indicated that CRA is an effective complement to treatment to reduce drinking, and in cocaine addiction it works well in combination with direct rewarding of positive behavior.[10]

We can conclude that rewarding good behavior helps, especially when done in a social context—not only with children, but also with adults who want to quit their addiction. This form of reward is effective from which we can tentatively conclude that relevant choice processes in addiction are probably influenced, especially in a social context. We just don't know exactly how it works; choice processes are not directly addressed, which is what happens in cognitive training.

Cognitive training

In cognitive training, two broad approaches can be distinguished: training of general cognitive processes, such as working memory training and training aimed at changing impulsive responses to cues related to the problem (e.g., the tendency to approach alcohol). In Chapter 6, we saw that general training is useful for the development of self-control in children, if it is offered in the form of fun games[13] and rewarded self-control training (good behavior game) also has positive effects in the longer term: when children are in secondary school they start smoking and drinking later.[14]

Could such training of general "executive" or "cognitive control" functions contribute to recovery from addiction? These functions are crucial for goal-directed behavior, which I compared with sailing in Chapter 2, one must keep focused on the buoy in the distance, even when the wind is difficult and there are waves and potentially seductively singing sirens to be ignored. When someone is addicted, it is crucial for sustained recovery that these functions recover. In Chapter 4 we saw that in most cases there is at least partial recovery of executive functions after prolonged abstinence. It is therefore an interesting and clinically important question to what extent this recovery can be enhanced by targeted training.

Training general functions: working memory training in addiction

A fair amount of research has been conducted in recent years on the effect of working memory training in addiction. The rationale behind this type of training is clearcut: relatively weak scores on working memory and related executive control functions pose a risk for addiction and other *akrasia problems*, that is, falling for immediate temptation, even when at the expense of long-term goals.[15–17] In these studies, a randomly selected group of addicted participants receives "brain training", usually in the form of computerized puzzles that progressively increase in difficulty,[18–21] while another randomly selected group receives no such training or a version so easy that no training effects can be expected ("placebo training"). This type of training has been compared to training in the gym: one group receives a personalized training with increasing levels of difficulty, based on their performance, while in the placebo training, always the same light weight is lifted. A lot of this type of research has been done in children with ADHD. In that domain, the conclusion was that brain training led to the children getting better and better at the trained game, with sometimes still a small training effect on similar tasks, but disappointingly, in most cases no effect on their behavior in everyday life was found, either at school or at home, which was the clinical purpose of the training.[22] In short: practice makes perfect in the trained game itself, but there is little or no relevant generalization or transfer of the gains achieved: the children could not apply what they had learned outside the context of the training game.[22]

What were the findings of this kind of training in addiction? Similar to the findings in children with ADHD, addicted participants got better at the trained game, but no effect on recovery from addiction has not been reported in any of the studies published.[21] This does not imply that all results were negative: many of the studies did find effects on other cognitive functions, so there was some transfer, just no effects on the ultimate goal (remaining abstinent). For example, a study on people addicted to stimulants (cocaine, amphetamine) showed that working memory training leads not only to better working memory, but also to a decrease in cognitive impulsivity.[18] That was measured with a choice task, in which participants made a series of choices between a small reward that you would get immediately (say, $1) or a larger one at a later time (say, $5 a week later, or $10 a year later). This is called delay discounting, and has been related to addiction, as Warren Bickel from Virginia Tech and others have demonstrated in many studies.[23] People who are more prone to addiction (including children with ADHD), on average, dislike waiting for rewards; they often prefer an immediate small reward to waiting for a bigger reward in the future.

This phenomenon was first described by Edmund Sonuga-Barke, a British researcher who switched to psychology after a degree in economics. Up to that point, the story was that many children with ADHD are so impulsive that they simply could not wait for a bigger reward and therefore immediately opted for a small one. Edmund realized that time is also an economic good (if you consistently choose the small reward, you finish the task in less time) and showed in a series of studies that children with ADHD were able to choose a delayed large reward when choosing the small reward no longer saved time.[24,25] Hence, it wasn't that children with ADHD *could* not wait; they just hated it and tried to avoid it. For this reason, a decrease in cognitive impulsivity after working memory training in people with addiction, could be good news for the likelihood of recovery, although that has yet to be demonstrated.[26]

We found in the same period that the working memory training in problem drinkers did indeed improve after training over the internet (25 sessions), compared with that of participants randomized to the group undergoing placebo training (continued light weights in the gym metaphor: no increasing difficulty).[27] This was related to a reduction in alcohol consumption in some of the participants—in those who had relatively strong positive associations with alcohol (measured with a variety of the Implicit Association Test; see Figure 1.1 in Chapter 1). One might therefore tentatively conclude that in this group, who probably often drink "on autopilot", working memory training gives more control over their decision to drink or not.

A recent study in alcohol dependent participants showed that, in addition to the expected improvement on the task used for training, an effect was found on *episodic future thinking*, which stands for being able to make a concrete picture of things you would like or need to do in the future. This is an important cognitive function in recovery, where people want to change course in life and need to look for other work, a new home or a new partner. How to do all that? If you can't make a concrete plan for that, chances are that little will come of it. So again, a nice generalized effect of the training, but no effect on the addiction outcome itself. This may have to do with the fact that training was not related to treatment. Perhaps there are opportunities for this if the enhanced general ability to consider the consequences of choices for the future is linked to where a person would like to go and what problems a person would need to address after treatment.[26] The problem of testing such a clinically interesting combination is that it is impossible to do this in a "blind" way, as the methodological state of the art requires.[ii] Given the clinical relevance of episodic future thinking, recently, Warren Bickel

ii Note that there are some alternative designs nowadays, in which single participants are measured intensively for a long time, then at a randomly chosen moment an intervention is given, followed by an evaluation of the effect.[171] These single cases can subsequently be combined using special meta-analytical techniques.[172]

and colleagues developed methods to directly train this ability, with promising first findings in non-clinical groups.[28]

Another form of training, called goal-management training, does combine general training with personally relevant goals. It was tested is a small study with people addicted to multiple substances, which yielded positive effects in combination with mindfulness training (discussed later).[29] A promising outcome was that, unlike effects of computerized working memory training, in this training, acquired skills were found to translate to everyday life.[30] Finally, there is a general positive side to these types of training: feedback is provided, which shows that you are making progress, which is motivating for the confidence in recovery.[31] You are not just talking about how you should do things differently in the future, you are actively working on your recovery yourself! In that sense, this kind of training is indeed somewhat like physical training in the gym or running, which makes you feel better and more energetic. In fact, there is also some evidence that physical training may contribute to recovery, especially with depression[32] and perhaps also with addictions.[33]

Cognitive bias modification: introduction

The second form of cognitive training focuses on *cognitive biases*. Different cognitive biases are distinguished: first, signals of reward (including the opportunity to engage in an addictive behavior) attract attention, as we saw in Chapter 3. This is called an attentional bias. Second, the same cue can evoke the action tendency to approach it ("approach bias"). Third, addiction-related cues can automatically trigger memories of expected outcomes (expectancies). Attentional bias and approach bias are related to sensitization effects found in animal studies (discussed in Chapter 3) and individual differences in salience attribution to cues of reward (sign-tracking, the rats that approached the cue at the expense of the actual reward).[34] During the past decades, various techniques have been developed to measure these biases in people and more recently, these original assessment instruments have been modified with the goal to directly change the targeted cognitive biases. The latter was done first to investigate the relationship between the bias and the addiction problem, as an experimental way to test a causal effect. Note that these cognitive biases are not exclusive to addiction, they also play a role in other common mental disorders, such as anxiety and depression.[35] It was first developed in anxiety, let's have a look there before turning to addiction.

Colin MacLeod is a famous researcher of Scottish origin who has long lived and worked in Perth, Western Australia. As a child he used to stand in the Scottish rain at bus stops, looking at posters of sunny beaches in Australia asking you to come over (immigration into

Australia was still encouraged back then), and he resolved to do so when he was grown up. After receiving his PhD in England, he put his money where his mouth was and moved to Perth, a city known not only for its beautiful beaches, but also as the most isolated city in the world. And that was nice, because besides doing research (mainly on attentional processes in anxiety) he really likes adventure, falsifying the idea that researchers in psychology end up investigating their own issues (or it should be lack of fear in his case).

I visited Colin and his lab a number of times, and on one of those lab visits I was lucky enough to join a trip to the Australian version of the Grand Canyon, over a day's drive, mostly on dirt roads. Of course, there were deadly spiders and snakes in the wild campsite at the top of the canyon, not to mention the dingoes we heard howling in the distance at night. We visited a beautiful coral reef where you could snorkel right from the shore, unlike the Great Barrier Reef, where you first have to boat to. And because it's in the *middle of nowhere*, it was less affected yet. Conditions were ideal: you could walk a short distance over the rocks against the current and then lower yourself into the water, letting the current carry you along, while observing this incredible underwater world, with sea turtles, rays and, of course, sharks, fortunately only harmless reef sharks. However, if you were to flow too far, enchanted by the beauty of the underwater world, you would enter a current, after which you would be thrown over the edge of the reef into the deep ocean, where less innocent sharks would cheer your arrival.

Back to the research. During his research in the 1980s, Colin had already developed a method to measure attentional bias, the so-called dot-probe task. The idea behind this assessment method was elegant and simple: you briefly show two things on a computer screen at the same time, for example, two words or two pictures,[iii] and then you examine what people are looking at. You do this by replacing one of the two pictures with a probe (a symbol) that someone has to respond to, such as an arrow pointing up or down. For example, you see a glass of tea on the left and a glass of beer on the right, and then after half a second an arrow appears in one of the two places and your task is to indicate whether the arrow pointed up or down. If you are faster on average to do this when it replaces the alcohol picture, apparently alcohol catches your eye, indicating an attentional bias for alcohol.[36] And chances are you like to drink alcohol. Note that this task has a poor reliability, which means that the measurement is unstable: if you measure the same person twice, chances are you get a different result.[37] For this

iii I further use the word "pictures" because they are most commonly used in research on attentional processes in addiction, while in anxiety research words are used more often.

reason, a new variety of the test has been developed recently, the dual probe task, which uses two simultaneous videos competing for attention, that shows a much higher reliability, which we, in a collaborative project, successfully adapted for use in alcohol research using ads (alcohol versus soft drinks).[38,39]

Colin and other researchers of cognitive biases in anxiety had found that the more anxious a person is, the more anxiety-provoking words and pictures attract their attention. But is that cause or effect? To investigate this, he devised an experiment in which participants (students who were not very anxious) were randomly assigned to one of two groups. Everyone started with the task as described. Neutral and threatening words were presented at the same time, followed by the probe,[iv] behind one of the two words, which happened equally often, as in the standard assessment method (then you can calculate if a person is quicker to react when the probe replaces the threat word compared with the neutral word). However, after a while this changed: in one group the dots now always appeared behind the threatening words, in the other group always behind the neutral words. Thus, both groups were now trained—either to focus their attention on the threatening words or away from them. This had the corresponding effect on the attention bias for threat: it became stronger in the group trained toward the threat and weaker for the group trained away from it. After this manipulation, students were asked to solve difficult (unsolvable) anagrams and were allowed to stop whenever they wanted. The group trained toward the threat pictures became more stressed than the group trained away from the threat pictures and gave up sooner.[40] The experiment was repeated with similar results, providing strong evidence that attentional bias toward threat does indeed play a causal role in anxiety and stress.

It is important to realize that this was not a clinical study: the participants were students who did not seek help for anxiety problems (in fact, truly anxious students were not allowed to participate), but volunteers who received a small reward or course credit for participation. This type of *proof of principle* study allows researchers to experimentally investigate mechanisms that may be related to mental disorders in healthy volunteers, the so-called "experimental psychopathology" approach. This is a first step in intervention development.[41] Once it has been demonstrated in this way that a process (here, attentional bias for threat) is indeed causally related to symptoms of anxiety disorders, the logical next question is whether such a manipulation of attention could also help people with an

iv In this case the probe consisted of one or two dots; task of participants was to indicate if they saw one or two.

anxiety problem. That is the next step in the experimental approach to intervention development.[41]

MacLeod and his colleagues did a follow-up study with students from Singapore who would be moving to Perth to study—a stressful move to a new unknown country to study, as previous research had shown. Would it help students if they trained in advance to divert their attention away from threat, as in the earlier experiment? Prospective students were randomly assigned to a group that received real training, while another group received placebo training (continued assessment for the same number of trials, which does not train attention). The participants were asked to train every day for two weeks before moving to Perth. The group that had received the real training was less anxious during the first weeks in Perth, compared to the group that had received placebo training, which showed the usual increase in anxiety.[42]

The subsequent first small studies with clinical groups also produced promising results. In people who were to be treated for anxiety disorders (often while on the waiting list for treatment), anxiety decreased when they had entered the active training group, as opposed to those who had received the placebo training.[43,44] These promising results were followed by extensive studies of the effects of training on the Internet. That is a logical step, since this type of training involves doing computerized tasks, so why make people come to the lab or clinic? However logical, those Internet studies showed *no* effects across the board; the bias often did not change, nor did anxiety decrease more in the group that had received real training compared to the group that had received placebo training.[45,46] An initial meta-analysis that analyzed the effects of all the studies up to that point concluded that there is little music in this method of treating clinical anxiety and depression.[47]

Colin and colleagues showed that there was indeed a clear pattern in the data: when the attention bias was successfully changed, effects on anxiety were also observed, and when this was not the case (and thus there was a failure of experimental manipulation, which seemed to be the case in many of the Internet studies), then not.[48] A later meta-analysis, including only studies done in a clinical context, found an effect in which attentional bias training decreased anxiety symptoms.[49] Discussions continue about the effectiveness of attention training for anxiety,[50,51] and the pattern of findings resembles that in addiction, to which we now return.

The initial experimental study with students by MacLeod and colleagues in anxiety had impressed me and we began attempts to manipulate attention to alcohol in students, as did an English colleague, Matt Field. In several studies, students were randomly assigned to a group trained to attend toward alcohol or away from it. The setup was based on MacLeod's research: two images appeared simultaneously on the screen, one showing an alcoholic drink and one showing a non-alcoholic drink. After a while, a probe appeared in one of the two places (at the location of the alcohol picture or the alternative) to which they had to respond (the arrow pointing up or down). In the measurement version of the task, the arrow appeared as often at the place of the alcohol or at the place of the non-alcoholic drink. In the training toward alcohol, after some time the arrows appeared always at the place of the alcohol and in the other group always at the place of the non-alcoholic drinks.[52–55] Results showed that the attentional bias for alcohol could be successfully changed: it increased in the group trained toward the alcohol and decreased in the group trained away from the alcohol. At the same time, there was little evidence for generalization: there was no effect for "untrained pictures", that is, pictures that had not been used during training: they still attracted attention.[53,54] Would that change if we trained people more often?

With my then PhD student Tim Schoenmakers, I conducted the first clinical randomized controlled trial (RCT) on the effects of attentional bias modification as add-on to treatment for alcohol addiction; patients received either real training (consistently away from alcohol) or placebo-training.[v] The results were promising: after five training sessions including new alcohol pictures each session, attentional bias for alcohol decreased, this time both for trained and for untrained pictures.[56] It seemed that the training mainly prevented an increase in attentional bias that was found in the placebo-trained group, but not in the trained group. Such an increase in attentional bias had also been noted in a previous study among alcohol dependent patients in treatment who had not received training.[57] In addition, clinical outcomes were better in the group that had received the real attentional bias modification training as add on to their treatment: they recovered faster and were allowed to go home sooner (which was judged by "blind" clinicians who did not know whether the patient had received real or placebo training). Patients who had been trained also relapsed later.

These were promising results, but they involved a limited number of participants—as with the first clinical studies of the effects of attentional training for anxiety—so results had to be interpreted with caution. Interestingly, a later large study (discussed below as it also involves a different type of training),[58] found similar results: an increase in attentional bias in the control group, which was prevented by the

v One earlier study had been published with a different version of attentional retraining, but no control group was included.[173] In our study a variety of the IAT was used as control training, in which patients sorted the same pictures of alcoholic and non-alcoholic drinks as were used in the active training, which controls for exposure to these pictures.

attentional training in the experimental group. Apparently, an *increase* in attentional bias after abstinence is what happens in many alcohol-addicted people during abstinence. This is not helpful if you have just been discharged from the clinic and on the first street corner see a sign of beer above the entrance to a pub: it still attracts strong attention like a seductive siren.

Meanwhile, I had begun investigating another cognitive bias with my colleague Mike Rinck, from Radboud University Nijmegen: the action tendency to approach alcohol-related cues or approach bias. With his partner Eni Becker, Mike had developed a task to measure action tendencies using a computer and a joystick.[59] Action tendencies are basic motivational processes, in all living creatures that can move, from the single cell amoeba to man, two basic action tendencies can be distinguished: a tendency to approach attractive things and a tendency to avoid threats or disgusting things. Mike had programmed the task so that a *zoom effect* occurred after an approach or avoid movement: if you pulled the joystick toward you, the picture size on the computer screen increased, and if you pushed the joystick away from yourself, it shrunk in size. The first test of the strength of action tendencies was done in students with varying degrees of fear of spiders. Participants generally found it easier to push spiders away than to pull them toward them, and this was more strongly the case in participants who were afraid of spiders.

I suggested trying a similar test with respect to alcohol and changing the assessment a bit, namely not to instruct people in one block of the task to pull spiders toward them and in another block to push them away, but to do so on the basis of a characteristic unrelated to the content of the picture: the format. The reason to propose these more indirect instructions was to be able to measure a more automatic action tendency. It may sound complicated, but the participants' task was simple: they had to push away all landscape pictures and pull all portrait pictures toward them, no matter what was on them (or the reverse instruction in the other half of participants). We had them practice this with gray pictures of blocks in portrait or landscape format, so that the response to the shape of the picture became more automatic. This was followed by the pictures we were interested in, those of alcohol and of soft drinks, which came either in portrait or landscape format. In addition, we had added general pictures from a standard picture collection, both positive (e.g., a sweet looking puppy) and negative (e.g., a fiercely barking dog), all in one of the two formats (one to be pulled, the other to be pushed). What would happen in heavy and light drinkers?

We found, as expected, that heavy drinkers found it easier to pull alcohol pictures than to push them away (that means they were faster and made less errors).[60] Interestingly, this was not true for the general positive or negative pictures (puppy versus dangerous dog); we found no reliable differences between these categories for pulling versus pushing. That may seem surprising, but was consistent with the result of previous emotion research: emotional pictures evoke an action tendency (approaching positive things and avoiding negative things) only when people are asked to categorize the pictures as positive or negative, and not, when indirect instructions are used and they have to pay attention to something else (as in our case, the shape of the picture).[61] So for the tendency to approach alcohol, the action tendency was found *despite* these indirect instruction, which shows a relatively automatic approach tendency for alcohol cues in heavy drinkers only. This approach-tendency was particularly strong in heavy drinkers who had a risk version of a gene we encountered earlier (OPRM1) related to craving and salivating in response to a favorite drink.[62,63] Hence, we had found a way to measure an automatically activated approach bias, and its presence was later demonstrated for a variety of other addictive substances, such as cigarettes in smokers (but not in ex-smokers, as my second cousin Corinde Wiers had shown),[64] for cannabis pictures in cannabis addicted people[65] and for gambling pictures in gamblers, although the latter finding did not replicate in a recent study, making it questionable to what extent an approach bias is also found for non-substance addictions.[66,67] It should be noted that the measurement is more reliable when you ask participants to categorize the pictures during the test (i.e., pull alcohol and push non-alcoholic drinks in one block, reverse instructions in another block), so my nice idea to use more indirect instructions was actually not a good idea for measurement, but it did open up the road to developing a training variety of the task.[68]

The next question, of course, was whether we could also influence this relatively automatic approach tendency to alcohol as we had done with the attentional bias and if that could likewise have an effect on addiction. I still have a vivid memory of when I first had this thought and began to elaborate it in my head. It was at a meeting of the European Association of Cognitive and Behavior Therapy in 2005, in Thessaloniki, Greece. I was attending a talk that just wouldn't captivate, but sat in the middle of the audience and it was too awkward to get up and walk out, as I knew the presenter. *Trapped.* I decided to stop listening and let my thoughts run wild.

We had just finished the first study of attention training in heavy drinking college students and had just started measuring action tendencies with the alcohol version of the joystick task. Would we be able to manipulate that *bias* as well, as we had done with attention training? We could offer pictures of alcohol and soft drinks, as in the measurement task, and then half in the format that was to be pushed (e.g., landscape) and half in the format that was to be pulled (e.g., portrait). Then we could change this contingency over time, so that after a while, one group would pull alcohol all the time (and push soft drinks away), while the other group would push alcohol away all the time (and pull soft drinks towards them), and see what would happen with their motivation to drink alcohol. The cool thing was that we could start with the measurement task (react to the format of the picture; half of the alcohol pictures pushed and half pulled, same for soft drinks), and change into a manipulation task, without any further instructions (they would keep on responding to the format of the pictures). Would this affect how much they would feel like drinking alcohol afterwards and how much they would actually drink? That same night, I discussed the idea with Mike, who agreed it was worth the try.

Back in the lab, with a German intern, we selected socially drinking students, who were randomly assigned to one of two conditions: after a brief measurement phase, one group would pull alcohol pictures (and push soft drink pictures) and a second group would push away alcohol pictures (and pull soft drink pictures). After this, they did a would-be "taste test", in which they rated three types of beer and three types of cola, guessed the brand, and responded to some taste questions (how bitter/sweet, etc.). What we were concerned with was how much they would drink of the beer and whether that would be affected by the manipulation of their action tendencies (pulling or pushing alcohol). One sip per drink was required to complete the taste-questionnaires, but more was allowed.

Study participants sat in a cubicle for 10 minutes with three glasses of beer and three glasses of cola and a number of questionnaires. What did they do? Light drinkers were not affected by the manipulation. In the somewhat heavier social drinkers, the training did show an effect: those who had pulled the joystick in response to alcohol pictures, drank almost all the beer (almost the entire three glasses), while those who had pushed alcohol away drank as little as the light drinkers (some sips of each).[69] We also found other signs of generalization: the approach tendency changed for untrained pictures, and we even found an effect on the Implicit Association Test, a sorting task with words (Figure 1.1), in which alcohol and soft drink words had to be categorized with approach or avoidance words: after having pushed alcohol pictures away, it became easier to sort alcohol words with avoidance words, and after having pulled alcohol, it became easier to sort alcohol words with approach words. This is a strong generalization because the training worked with pictures and this effect occurred in a task involving words. And as we saw, even their drinking behavior was affected, which was an important generalization. We were enthusiastic about the results, but of course this was a *proof of principle study*, with healthy students who did not participate in the study to change their drinking, but who had come for the reward or the prospect of a free beer tasting (which was mentioned in the recruitment poster to warn participants that they would be getting alcohol, which probably helped recruitment).

Cognitive bias modification: clinical studies

As we saw, the next question in the experimental medicine approach to intervention development is whether the intervention also has clinical effects. We investigated this in a new collaboration with a large German clinic. In our first clinical trial on attention training, three Dutch addiction clinics participated, but in the end, only 43 alcohol-addicted patients participated after 2.5 years.[56] Eni Becker knew the director of a large addiction clinic in Lindow, Germany (about an hour from Berlin), Johannes Lindenmeyer. Could we perhaps try this new method there? Johannes was immediately enthusiastic and so began a wonderful collaboration that has continued for more than a decade now. Because the initial results in healthy volunteers of changing action tendencies were stronger than for attentional bias, we decided that this training would be most promising to test with the patients, as an addition to their regular treatment. Hundreds of patients could participate, so we decided to create four experimental groups. Two experimental groups would consistently push alcohol away and pull non-alcoholic drinks toward them, for four sessions. The difference was that one group responded to the shape of the picture during training (as in the student study), while the other group was explicitly instructed to push alcohol away. The remaining patients were divided into two control groups: one that continued to pull and push away pictures of alcohol and soft drinks equally often (extended assessment or placebo training) and one that received no training at all.

The results were clear: both training groups (with or without instruction) changed their dominant action tendency from approaching alcohol to avoiding alcohol, while those in the control groups still showed an approach tendency to alcohol pictures. And there was generalization: we found the effect of the training also for pictures that were not included in the training. We further found a corresponding effect on the word sorting task (the IAT; see Figure 1.1): before training, most participants were faster to sort alcohol with approach words, and that changed only in the group that had received the real training, who now sorted alcohol words faster with avoidance words. So very nice results again in terms of generalization of effects, but the most important question remained to be answered: would it also help patients to remain abstinent after they left the clinic?

The training took place in the first week of the inpatient stay (four consecutive days of about 20 minutes of training), and then the patients would stay for an average of three more months, during which they received primarily cognitive behavioral therapy for addiction and, in addition, other therapies (for example, aggression regulation training for those to which this was relevant or a program to eat healthier or quit smoking). After about three months they left the clinic, and a year after that a standard survey was done to see how they were doing: were they still abstinent or had they relapsed into their old drinking patterns?[vi] Could one still expect anything from four days training for some 20 minutes each time, on outcomes some 15 months later? The results were surprising, if not *mind-blowing*: the training group showed 13% less relapse in the year after treatment. Of the participants who had received placebo training or no training in addition to treatment, more than half had relapsed (59%); of the group that had received real training, it was 46%. Wow! The article was published in *Psychological Science*, where it attracted considerable attention and was discussed, among other things, in a piece on cognitive bias modification (CBM) in *The Economist.*[vii]

A follow-up question was how long we could best train people. For that, we set up a study in which one group trained for 12 sessions and another group did not train at all (because there was no difference between the active control group and the group that did nothing in the first study, we chose a passive control group here). More than five hundred alcohol-dependent patients participated, half of whom were trained and half of whom were not, again in addition to the regular treatment, which everyone received. The trained group was 9% less likely to have relapsed a year after treatment discharge.[70] This effect was related to the decrease in their approach tendency to alcohol (so-called "statistical mediation"). The training was most effective in patients who had a strong tendency to approach alcohol before the training. What was the optimal amount of training? We analyzed the learning curves and found that there were lots of differences between participants: some were no longer improving after two sessions, while others were still learning at the twelfth session.[71] After six sessions most people reached their plateau in learning, so that became the new standard, although it is clear that longer training is desirable when there is more brain damage,

vi Interesting detail: that standard assessment of one-year outcomes is required in Germany by the insurance company paying for the treatment, in this case the pension insurance company. After all, when people drop out around 45 (the average age) because of alcohol addiction, it costs the pension funds a lot of money. They invest in treatment, and want the outcomes measured properly. This does not happen in many other countries.

vii Issue 3 March 2011. The title, *therapist-free therapy*, was misleading because we found effects of training as an adjunct to therapy. Thus, the treatment was not "therapist-free", and this title caused some unnecessary resistance from some therapists.

such as in patients suffering from Korsakoff syndrome.[72] This shows that targeted cognitive training may also be of benefit to addicted people with brain damage.

In a large follow-up study at the same clinic, we wanted to compare the effects of the two forms of cognitive bias modification discussed so far: attention training and action tendency training. We randomly assigned patients to one of seven groups, three training groups, three groups with variants of placebo training, and one group that received no training at all. The training groups received either six sessions of action-tendency training (always pushing in response to alcohol pictures), or six sessions of attention training (training attention "away" from the alcohol), or three sessions of each. The placebo training groups received corresponding placebo training.[viii] It was the largest clinical CBM study so far; more than 1,400 alcohol-addicted patients participated.[58] How did this training benefit recovery from alcohol addiction? The groups that had received some form of training did better than the control groups. At the standard measurement one year after treatment discharge, they were 8.4% less likely to have relapsed. Unlike the previous study, we did not find that this clinical outcome was associated with the change in cognitive bias, which was small. This likely had to do with the fact that the training data were often missing, which was a consequence of mandatory strict, privacy protection measures.[ix]

Meanwhile, a group in Australia had become excited by our work, and under the leadership of Victoria Manning investigated the effect of action tendency training during detoxification. In a first relatively small study (across 83 patients divided into two groups), promising results were found: four consecutive days of training reduced the chance of relapse in the two weeks after *detox* by 22%, and in the group that had done all the training (real or placebo), that difference was 30%. That's a great result, but because this was a small group and a short period of time, it was important that it was replicated. That happened in a large clinical trial with three hundred alcohol-addicted patients, who trained again during detox—either with real training or placebo training. The findings were recently published. Again, a beneficial effect of CBM training was found: people who had undergone the real training relapsed 12% less often than those who had

viii Either only action-tendency training, only attention training, or three sessions of both, but always in the version in which they trained toward alcohol as often as away from it (continued assessment).

ix All computers are emptied by default at the end of the day for privacy reasons, so training data that was not pulled off that same day was lost.

done the placebo training, but this was again about the short-term effect after two weeks. Meanwhile, its long-term effects have also been studied, showing that real training leads to a later relapse and a greater likelihood of remaining abstinent. This remained statistically significant until three months after training; it was no longer significant after 6, 9 and 12 months.[73]

Finally, in a recent study from the Lindow clinic in Germany, we examined whether training would also work for alcohol-dependent patients who had a diagnosis of anxiety or depression, in addition to their alcohol problem.[74] A previous small study of people with an alcohol problem and social anxiety had shown no effects in this group for attention training,[75] but in that study, only 86 participants were divided among four groups, which made the groups so small that the chances of finding a positive effect were tiny.[x] Furthermore, participants in that study received no treatment in addition to attention training (which is why the study is not listed in Table 8.1 below). In our study, over seven hundred alcohol-addicted patients were randomly assigned either to a group that received real action-tendency training or placebo training in addition to regular therapy. The training yielded a reduction in the probability of relapse, one year after treatment discharge, of 10%, which is about the average of the outcome of studies in Germany (ranging from 8.4% to 13%). The interesting finding in this study was that this effect was *stronger* for alcohol-addicted patients who diagnosed with comorbid anxiety or depression. This is important because several studies have shown that this combination makes for a poor prognosis for treatment outcome.[76,77] Thus, especially for this category of addicted people, it seems a good idea to add training to treatment.

One clinical study has been published so far in which no positive effects have been found in a clinical group.[78] In that study, a new gamified version of attention training was added to the treatment of addiction to alcohol or cannabis. In the treatment (in the Netherlands), participants decided their own treatment goal: abstinence or reduction. The fact that participants differed both in the substance to which they were addicted (alcohol or marijuana as primary drug) and in their treatment goal (abstinence or reduction), makes interpretation of the results difficult: it could be that the training works less well for cannabis than for alcohol, or it may be

x In technical terms, the study had low statistical power. That is, the probability of finding the effect, if it is actually there, is small, because of the low number of people tested. That's why researchers like to have enough participants in their experiments, but that's not always possible.

Table 8.1 Review of published, controlled studies (with control group) in which cognitive training was added to the clinical treatment of alcohol dependence

Study	*Number of patients*	*Type CBM*	*Effect on relapse*	*Other effects/comments*
Schoenmakers et al. 2010[56]	43	attention bias	later relapse	effect on attention bias with generalization
Wiers et al. 2011[79]	214	approach bias	13% less years later	effect on approach bias with generalization
Eberl et al. 2013[70]	509	approach bias	9% less years later	effect on approach bias partly explains clinical effect (mediation)
Manning et al. 2016[80]	83	approach bias	22% less 2 weeks later	promising effect in small group during detox
Rinck et al. 2018[58]	1405	attention and/or approach bias	8.5% less years later	both attention training and action tendency training had small positive effect
Heitman et al. 2021[78]	169	attention	—	part alcohol, part cannabis, part focused on abstinence, part focused on reduction, no effects
Manning et al. 2021[73], 2022[81]	300	approach bias	12% less 2 weeks later, difference significant up to 3 months	approach bias training during detox helps against rapid relapse.
Salemink et al. 2021[74]	729	approach bias	10% less relapse	stronger effect in patients with anxiety or depression in addition to alcohol dependence

that the treatment goal of total abstinence is a crucial background ingredient (which was the treatment goal in all studies where an effect was found; see Table 8.1).

In the countries where the large clinical controlled studies took place (Germany and Australia), the consistent positive results regarding relapse of adding approach bias training led to a clinical recommendation to add this form of training to the treatment of alcohol addiction.[82,83] In other countries, this is not (yet) the case. What could play a role here is an early meta-analysis by the team that also published the first critical meta-analysis of the effects of this type of training in anxiety and depression.[84]

The authors concluded that CBM appeared to have an effect on *bias*, but not on clinical outcomes. The reason for this was that most of the studies included in their analyses were studies from the first stage of intervention development: proof-of-principle studies in healthy volunteers (usually students), who did not participate in the study to stop drinking, but to get course credit, a reward or free beer. In that group, it makes little sense to examine "clinical" effects. As we saw, the purpose of this type of study is to determine causality: if you temporarily increase the bias in volunteers, are they more likely to drink than if you temporarily weaken the same bias? Once that is confirmed, the next phase of the experimental medicine approach to intervention development can be started, and the method can be tested in patients.[41,85] Taking these different kinds of studies together in a single meta-analysis comes down to comparing apples to oranges.[86] You assess clinical effectiveness based on studies in which people have a clinically relevant problem that they want to do something about. Not based on studies in healthy volunteers.

In addition to a conceptual form of critique, in which we pointed out the essential difference between experimental proof of principle studies in healthy volunteers and clinical studies in patients,[86] and showed that the clinical studies almost all yielded positive results (at least for the excessive consumption of alcohol—see Table 8.1; for smoking, results are less clear), we did a meta-analysis in which we included only clinical studies; those in which the goal of the researchers and participants was to change substance use by participating in a training.[87] This showed that CBM-training changed the targeted bias and produced a small clinical effect (about as small as for current medication; you need 10 to 15 patients to cure one patient), and that more data are needed to properly understand why the intervention sometimes works and sometimes does not.

We can conclude that while there is strong evidence that cognitive training can be supportive in treating alcohol dependence (almost exclusively positive clinical studies, see Table 8.1),[xi] the same is not true of training offered via the Internet. As with anxiety, the logical idea was that a computerized intervention might as well be done at home. The studies on Internet versions of training also showed a consistent picture, but a different one from the clinical studies: everyone improved and reduced their alcohol use in the process (*Everybody has won, and all must have prizes*). That may sound nice, but it means that no difference in the reduction in drinking was found between the real training and the placebo training.[88–92] What probably played an important role here was the goal of the participants. In clinical treatment, that is almost always abstinence, whereas online volunteers participated to control their drinking and to drink less. And they succeed in doing so, no matter whether they received real or placebo training. It appears that the combination with treatment is crucial to the effect of this type of training in dealing with alcohol addiction, perhaps combined with an abstinence goal. This might explain the aforementioned negative exception in terms of effectiveness in clinical studies, since some of the alcohol- or cannabis-addicted participants did not want to quit, but only to reduce.

Furthermore, the beneficial effect of the training for smoking seems to be less evident than for alcohol use, which may have to do with the fact that most studies did not offer the training as part of a therapy-supported quit attempt, but as a stand-alone intervention, often via the Internet. One study on the effect of attention training in smoking cessation, did show a beneficial effect, although the training was delivered via the Internet.[93] An important detail of that study was that participants who were interested in participating in the training were called to find out if they were really planning a quit attempt, and if so, when? Only when they planned an actual quit attempt, they could participate. The majority of interested potential participants still indicated they wanted to quit, but not just yet. Among the heavier smokers who actually made a quit attempt, the percentage who were still

xi There is one as-yet unpublished negative Belgian study in which either approach bias modification or attentional bias modification was added to treatment as usual, in 247 alcohol-dependent patients with an abstinence goal.[174] One possible reason for this null-finding was the way the training was designed: in the successful clinical studies in Germany, a brief assessment phase (pulling and pushing alcohol pictures equally often) was followed by a long training phase, in which alcohol pictures were always pushed, which led to reduced relapse a year later. In the Australian trial, during the training, 95% of the alcohol pictures were pushed, and this led to significantly less relapse up to 3 months, but not longer. In the negative Belgian study, 87,5% of alcohol pictures were pushed or avoided, and no effects were found regarding relapse, even an indication of more relapse after alcohol avoidance training. This suggests that effective training needs to be consistent (consistent positive results for training in which alcohol is always pushed away).

abstinent six months after the training doubled (47%, compared to 22% for the placebo training). Among light smokers, the training had no effect. This study represents a positive exception (at least for the heavy smokers) among a number of other studies on adding CBM to smoking addiction treatment that showed no effect for smoking cessation.[94,95] All in all, the effects of CBM appear to be weaker in smoking cessation than as an add-on to abstinence-oriented treatment for alcoholism. One possible reason for this difference is that there is no universal alternative to smoking, as there is to alcohol (non-alcoholic drinks), to which people can be trained. In the training studies in smoking, typically a visually similar picture is used, for example, where a smoking-related picture would show a hand holding a cigarette, the control picture was the same hand holding a pen. But is that an alternative to smoking? As we will see later, a new kind of cognitive training has been developed in which participants are trained to personally relevant alternatives. Perhaps that will yield better results for smoking cessation; we are testing that now.

Thus, the clinical effects of this form of cognitive training are positive as an add-on in the treatment of alcohol addiction, with a statistically small effect, of the order of magnitude of effective medication in addiction.[96] The context of these effects does seem to be different: as we saw in the previous chapter, it is not the case that talk therapy and medication always reinforce each other. In contrast, CBM has been found to have positive effects *only* when combined with therapy. Finally, two more studies combined attention training and action-tendency training in alcohol-dependent patients with direct brain stimulation (the barely perceptible weak current, tDCS, described in the previous chapter).[97,98] The combination of tDCS with approach-bias training seemed to produce slightly less relapse[xii] and participants learned to push alcohol away faster during training. It is not clear to what extent this is clinically relevant, as ultimately everyone learns this in training and no additional effects were found on relapse.

Brain effects of cognitive training in addiction

About ten years ago I was called by a colleague from England with an unexpected question: whether my name was common in the Netherlands. I could deny that. Wiers is an obscure family name from the north of the Netherlands (Groningen), but whence the question? She had a visiting student, Corinde Wiers, and she also wanted to do addiction research! Corinde did not know me, studied at the University of Amsterdam

xii An effect at so-called statistical-trend level. It can be understood as a slight indication that there may be an added effect of brain stimulation, but it needs replication.

before I returned from Maastricht and Nijmegen, but after some inquiries we turned out to be second cousins: our grandfathers were brothers. She was interested in neurocognitive mechanisms in addiction: what changes in the brain when someone becomes addicted? After she finished her internship in Brighton, we met in Amsterdam, and she was looking for a PhD position, which she found in Berlin, in a renowned center for brain research in addiction. The clinic where we had done most of our studies on the clinical effects of CBM is about an hour's drive from Berlin. Maybe we could do a study together! We fantasized that one day, we should write a Wiers & Wiers publication (which we eventually did).[99]

Corinde tested the brain correlates of a series of tasks in the scanner, including the assessment of the approach tendency for alcohol with a special joystick without metal (metal is out of the question in the magnetic MRI scanner).[100] She found the approach tendency for alcohol in the alcohol-dependent patients and not in the control subjects, which is less trivial than it might seem, because people lie on their back in the scanner, in a noisy sealed capsule, which makes the conditions for finding an effect in a relatively small number of participants suboptimal (small groups of participants are often used in fMRI research given the high costs). She further found that this difference was related to specific activity in brain areas related to reward and motivation: the nucleus accumbens and medial prefrontal cortex. The latter plays a role in making trade-offs between alternatives when there is something to choose from, and has been related to the "common currency" discussed in Chapter 5.

The follow-up question was what the CBM training would change in these brain responses to alcohol pictures, compared to placebo training (in both cases again in addition to regular treatment). When the alcohol-addicted patients looked at alcohol pictures (compared to non-alcohol pictures), their brains showed the characteristic pattern of a brain response to something relevant and rewarding (a neural circuit was active including the amygdala and nucleus accumbens). This disappeared in those patients who had received CBM training, but not in those who had received placebo training with the same alcohol pictures.[101] Moreover, the response in the same circuit increased to pictures of non-alcoholic drinks, which likely indicates a stronger motivational salience of the alternative.

The approach tendency to alcohol decreased in the group that had received real training,[102] which was related to a stronger decrease in activation in the medial prefrontal cortex and to reduced craving for alcohol. One might tentatively conclude that training made the relevant decision-making easier—you don't have to think about it anymore, you know you're going to avoid alcohol—but basing psychological interpretations on brain patterns is dangerous, because one can easily fall into the trap of circular reasoning.[103] Nevertheless, the interpretation is consistent with what a patient told in a TV interview about our training: after he had left the clinic and was cruising behind his cart in a supermarket, he was pulled toward the big beer section, and as soon as he became aware of this, he immediately steered his cart in the other direction.[xiii] We can conclude that the training affects the brain's response to alcohol in addicted people, which likely contributes to their reduced chance of relapse after leaving the clinic. To complete Corinde's story, after her PhD she became a postdoc in Nora Volkow's lab at NIDA and now works at the University of Pennsylvania.

Cognitive mechanisms of action: changing associations or inferences?

In addition to research into the effects of CBM training on the brain, there has also been research into cognitive mechanisms: how exactly does this training affects our thinking? Much of this research has been conducted by Pieter van Dessel, researcher at Ghent University, in collaboration with Jan de Houwer, who has done much groundbreaking research over the past twenty years on cognitive processes underlying our (health-related) actions. The background to this research is that the cognitive training programs described above were originally developed based on dual process models, as discussed earlier. The idea was that cognitive training could influence automatic, sometimes unconscious processes, which would not be easily achieved by talk therapy alone. Talk therapy is also important from this perspective, especially to determine long-term goals, but automatic processes could be influenced more efficiently by targeted cognitive training.[55] According to dual process models, evolutionarily ancient motivational processes can determine behavior automatically, without interference from conscious thought processes, just as we immediately pull our hand away when touching a hot stove, without first having to devote thoughts about it that take extra time and cause extra damage. The question is the extent to which the same is true of reactions to addictive substances: are some parts of the addicted brain hijacked so badly that there is no more influence of conscious considerations, no more choice? As we saw in Chapter 4, most addicted people can still make a choice other than taking the drug and the evidence for compulsive automatic responses in addiction is thin at best.

Jan de Houwer has developed a research program based on the idea that human behavior is determined by propositional processes, even

xiii In an episode of the popular science program *Labyrinth* about addiction.

seemingly automatic behavior (except reflexes), related to the currently dominant predictive brain account of our thinking. Reflexes are triggered by simple associative processes in the peripheral nervous system, allowing us to save our hand from being burned. In this case, the response is driven from the spine and the reaction has already occurred by the time the information reaches the brain. But conditioned responses are brain-mediated, therefore the question is to what extent associative responses can explain them, or whether propositional representations of the predictive brain best account for the observed behavior. These are predictions of the type: if I drink beer now, I will feel relaxed after. A characteristic of propositions is that they have a direction: John loves Mary means something different from Mary loves John. De Houwer and colleagues argue that conditioning effects rely on propositional representations in the brain, perhaps even in Pavlov's dog.[104] A proposition may or may not be true (bell → meat: food follows the sound of the bell), which is not true of an association, because it only indicates that two things occur together frequently: bell ↔ meat (without direction or order). Conditioning research shows that order is crucial to find an effect. For example, if the meat is presented first, before the bell rings, conditioning is less likely to occur than if the bell is followed by the meat.[104] Furthermore, learning a predictive relationship requires attention, which is no longer necessary once the predictive relationship is learned.

According to De Houwer and colleagues, propositional representations determine our behavior. People need not be aware of these predictions from their continuously predicting brain, but our behavior is driven by them. Hence, this is fundamentally different from dual process models that argue that we have two different thinking systems in our heads: one with fast associative responses and one with slow propositional responses.[105–107] For those interested in further details of this interesting but rather technical discussion, I refer to a number of "target articles", to which experts from different disciplines have responded, followed by a response from the authors.[104,108]

Importantly, the claim by De Houwer and colleagues that behavior is driven by propositional predictions applies to healthy people. The question is whether this also holds for people with psychological disorders, for example, for severely addicted people. Perhaps there are cases where associative processes can indeed directly elicit behavior, irrespective of the expected outcome.[109] That could be a feature of addiction as a (rare) chronic brain disease: when behavior is no longer driven by expectations, but occurs when provoked by a cue, regardless of the consequences.

Back to cognitive training. As mentioned, our original idea behind cognitive training in addiction was that the training would affect automatic processes.[110] According to the alternative propositional approach, conscious attention is required for learning and thus for training effects. De Houwer and colleagues had already shown that conscious attention is necessary in humans to find conditioning effects.[104] How would that relate to cognitive training of approach and avoidance tendencies, which we had shown to help alcohol-addicted people as an adjunct to treatment? Van Dessel and colleagues found across several experiments with healthy volunteers that awareness of the relationship between a category (e.g., alcohol) and an action (e.g., pushing away) was necessary to obtain training effects.[111,112] This actually matches the account of the trained patient, who explained that he now knew what to do, when approaching the beer section.

From the idea that cognitive training is about learning propositions, one might expect that it could also work by instruction only, by only explaining the principle to people rather than actual training. Would that indeed be the case? Van Dessel and colleagues conducted a series of experiments that indeed showed that training effects can occur purely as a result of instruction, without any actual training.[113–115] Importantly, these were *proof of principle* studies with healthy volunteers. The question is whether this also holds true for addicted people. A group of German researchers tried to figure this out in people who wanted to quit smoking, and found some evidence of training effects by only having people imagine throwing away their cigarette instead of bringing it to their mouths.[116,117] In any case, it can be concluded that the results in healthy people are more consistent with the propositional model than with the dual process model, in which training would uniquely affect associative processes.

From that, a logical next step was to add a consequence of the trained action to the training. While the original training taught people to push alcohol away and to pull other drinks toward them, this new training variation involved an action that was always followed by a consequence: for example, a picture referring to a distal goal (e.g., feeling better the next day) after approaching non-alcoholic drinks or avoiding alcoholic drinks. Van Dessel and colleagues tested this new version in healthy volunteers and found better effects than for the original action-tendency training in the domain of eating.[118]

Based on these new insights and a motivational model of addiction,[119] developed by Catalina Köpetz from Wayne State University, we joined forces and developed a new form of cognitive training: ABC training.[120] ABC stands for three concepts: Antecedents (the context of situation that elicits a desire to use), Behavioral alternatives and Consequences of the behavioral choice. Addictive behavior in many cases is triggered by a situation or an internal antecedent (a feeling), which is something that is examined in therapy. For example, you tend to drink (or smoke) when you come home from work tired, in order to relax. Then there is a choice: you can engage in your favorite addictive behavior or do something else to relax. Hence, it is important to think of good alternatives for the situation beforehand, which meet your need to relax in a different way. Maybe you could go for a walk instead. Or go swim or meditate or have some herbal tea.

We already saw that the effects of training are clearest when the training is added to abstinence-oriented therapy for alcohol addiction and that effects are less clear for smoking (in other addictions, cognitive training has hardly been tested yet). We argued in an earlier study that this may have to do with the lack of a universally relevant alternative in other addictions. With alcohol, there is a general alternative: non-alcoholic drinks. But "not smoking" is not a clear category. And it is not motivating to be trained toward visually matching pictures (someone holding a pen instead of a cigarette). Perhaps the effects could be improved if people were allowed to choose their own alternatives for smoking. Not smoking can be drinking a special tea for one person, walking for the next and playing computer games for someone else.[121,122] That is the B (the personally relevant *Behavioral alternative* in the risk situation).

Finally, there is the Consequence of the choice, which Pieter van Dessel had already shown to enhance training effects in healthy volunteers. In the example, it would amount to a person choosing between smoking or a relevant alternative (say walking) and, after the choice is made, the consequence is made visible regarding effects on a personally relevant goals (for example, health or saving money). The new ABC-training fits well with the latest findings on the psychological mechanisms of action of training (changing propositions rather than associations) and has shown promising results in an initial study in healthy volunteers.[123]

In a recent as-yet unpublished series of studies in healthy volunteers participating in the dry January abstinence challenge, we found that ABC-training better helped people to remain abstinent than standard approach-bias modification or sham-training.[124] The big remaining question, of course, is if this new training also works better for people with addiction, which in turn relates to the question to what extent the general model of biased choice holds true for addicted people. We certainly intend to investigate this further, but, as is often the case in the Netherlands, research funding is a problem.

The new ABC training is closer to cognitive behavioral therapy for addiction than the original cognitive bias modification (CBM): risk situations (As) are also identified in therapy, as are possible ways to deal with them (Bs). Consequences have to do with why the client wants to change, which is crucial at the beginning of therapy (elicited with the motivational interviewing, discussed earlier).[125] So the ABC training is closely linked to therapy, and can be seen as targeted practice to make better choices in view of one's own goals. This is an important advantage, because research has shown that some forms of CBM (especially the original attention training) were sometimes experienced as pointless and boring.[126] To illustrate, in the first controlled clinical trial of attention training for alcohol addiction,[56] we had clients guess afterwards whether they thought they had received real or placebo training. Almost all patients thought they had received placebo training. This is good from an experimental perspective (because there is little chance that the effects found are placebo effects), but not from a clinical perspective: the training is experienced as useless. Note that this was not the case with approach-bias training and that more engaging versions of attentional training have been developed, for example, a version where one's favorite music plays when the participant looks at the target pictures but stops when the non-target pictures are looked at.[127]

ABC training is also conceptually related to so-called implementation intentions. These are specific plans that can help people change habits.[128,129] Suppose you typically smoke marijuana when you come home tired and you want to change that, you can make a specific plan for an alternative action in that situation. Implementation intentions do this in a specific if → then format, for example: if I come home tired, then I go for a walk. These are the kinds of combinations that are also trained in ABC training, adding an effect on the relevant goal (consequence). Implementation intentions can help people change habits, only this simple method does not work as well when the habit is stronger, as in addiction.[130] In this regard, ABC training might do more by adding practice, but research has yet to test this.

An important ingredient is motivation: you will only commit to developing implementation intentions or doing ABC training if you are imbued with the need to change your behavior. For this purpose, a short intervention has been developed by Gabriele Oettingen, from NY University, with the acronym WOOP.[131,132] This is a method by which you first identify your desire to change (*Wish*) and what positive outcomes it will ultimately bring (*Outcomes*), a minimal version of the film script intervention we saw earlier. The next O represents an obstacle to achieving the goal, and for that you then create a plan (the P) using implementation intentions (concrete plans in the if → then format). With this method, the implementation intention is linked to the motivation to overcome an obstacle. This method is simple and can be used for free via an automated online site.[xiv]

xiv www.woopmylife.org.

We can conclude that cognitive training helps as an addition to the treatment of alcohol addiction and that research into the underlying mechanisms has provided new ideas for improving training. An important question here is whether this can also strengthen the effectiveness of training in alcohol addicted people. Also, the new trainings create possibilities to tackle other addictions for which no natural alternative exists. It is important to do further research on this (said the researcher).

A Clockwork Orange

To end this discussion of cognitive training in addiction, I briefly mention two other varieties of cognitive training: evaluative conditioning and selective inhibition. In evaluative conditioning, a category of stimuli (e.g., alcohol pictures) is consistently paired with a negative stimulus (e.g., a picture of someone vomiting). Volunteers who went through such a procedure subsequently had less desire to drink alcohol than volunteers in whom this connection was not made (control group).[133–135] To my knowledge, this form of training has not yet been applied to addicted patients, although a related method was studied in the 1960s and 1970s, that involved drinking alcohol followed by making someone nauseous, based on the pioneering taste-aversion work of John Garcia. This research had shown that rats who were given a drink with a certain taste and subsequently made nauseous would avoid that taste in the future.[xv]

The method of making people nauseous after drinking alcohol was also tried at that time (1970s) as an addition to the treatment of alcohol addiction. The problem was that the research was of poor quality; it was applied in an expensive private clinic, for example, and then the results were compared with outcomes from another, much less expensive clinic, where the prognosis was not as good anyway. So the conclusion of the early work on conditioned aversion was not that it did not work, but that we cannot tell really, because the studies were of too poor quality to draw firm conclusions.[136]

What did not help at the time was the similarity to the re-education of Alex, the protagonist in Anthony Burgess's novel *A Clockwork Orange*, which became a popular movie by Stanley Kubrick in the 1970s. In it, mad scientists in a dictatorial SF world tried to brainwash rebel Alex, with a variety of aversive conditioning. During the conditioning, they

xv I have lived experience with this method: as a student, I once became very sick after drinking ouzo (a Greek aperitif with strong flavor of anise). The following days I had no desire for alcohol, but that disappeared again. Only those particular aniseed drinks remained disgusting for years (but not anymore).

played Beethoven, which made him allergic to that music. Still, poor research is not a good reason to dismiss a method; good research should be done on the possible effectiveness of this almost forgotten method. Indeed, more recently, some promising effects have been reported of testing aversive conditioning in virtual reality, with reductions in craving (but no reported effects yet on improved treatment outcomes).[137,138]

I prefer to call the last form of cognitive training that I briefly discuss "selective inhibition", to distinguish it from training the general ability to stop (which amounts to training a general function, as in working memory training, discussed earlier).[26] In selective inhibition training, a stopping response is systematically trained in response to a particular category (e.g., alcohol). This method has been tested in a number of studies with healthy volunteers (college students), often finding a short-term effect; the trained group drank less in the week after training than the group that had received fake training.[139,140] The method has also shown promising results in other areas, such as unhealthy eating,[141] but all of those studies involved healthy volunteers, not clinical groups. Two studies tested this method as an online intervention in volunteers who wanted to drink less. Again, the same pattern was found as in other online studies: people in both groups started drinking less, whether they had received the real or fake training.[88,91]

Two recent studies tested a possible add-on effect of this type of training to abstinence-oriented treatment of alcoholism. In the first, no added effect was found, but it should be noted that this study was done in the German clinic where we had previously done the approach bias retraining studies, and there, after all the positive studies, approach bias retraining has become part of the standard treatment, with the argument that it would be unethical to withhold effective treatment from patients after three positive trials there. Hence, in this study, selective inhibition training was added to regular therapy with added approach bias modification, and no further added effect was found.[142] The second study tested an improved version of the training, in which the to be inhibited alcohol pictures were presented 25% of the time rather than 50% of the time, as has been done in previous selective inhibition training studies, and in this study a clinical effect was found compared to treatment without the active add-on training.[143] So this improved version of selective inhibition training deserves further exploration, to test if these effects replicate and perhaps if they can also be found to be of use in other addictions.

Mindfulness meditation

Please grab a mat and lie on your back. You can close your eyes if you like and concentrate on your breathing. Thoughts will probably come to you, that's normal. Don't condemn them, but bring your attention back to your breathing. Kindly but firmly. Indeed, thoughts come to mind. Thoughts like: What am I doing here, in the middle of a busy period, participating in a *mindful parenting* course? Is this one big placebo exercise or could this really help against stress? And against depression? And against addiction? *Too good to be true* ... But ... that's what some reviewers at first thought of our cognitive training. I wanted to experience it for myself, so experience it. Take an open attitude. And go back to your breathing.

American molecular biologist Jon Kabat-Zinn developed mindfulness training, which was based on centuries-old Buddhist meditation traditions, with a Western twist. The goal was to help people cope better with everyday stress. The basis of the method is to turn your attention inward to your stream of consciousness, let your thoughts flow and to become aware of the transient nature of thoughts. In this way, you better learn to see your thoughts for what they are (thoughts) and develop more freedom to ignore them, acting less on autopilot. You don't condemn your thoughts, but observe them, like passing clouds on a summer day. And since you train attentional processes, you could also think of mindfulness as a form of cognitive training.

The past decades, a number of specific mindfulness-based programs were developed to help people cope with stress and depression, followed by several programs to help people overcome their addictions. Furthermore, an exercise to deal with craving was incorporated into cognitive behavioral therapy, under the influence of the late clinical addiction researcher Alan Marlatt. He introduced the idea of "urge surfing": when you experience craving, you don't act but observe these waves of craving, as if you are surfing.[144] When the wave gets higher, you follow it and observe that the wave passes again, just like the craving.

Building on this, a mindfulness-based group intervention was developed to prevent relapse into addiction.[145] Specific mindfulness-based programs have also been put together for specific addictions, including a mindfulness-based smoking cessation program, a mindfulness-based recovery program, aimed at improving feeling and understanding your own emotions ("introception"), something addicted people often experience problems with.[146] Special variants were also developed for specific target groups, like women struggling with addiction.[147] Clearly a lot is happening in this field, what do we know about the effectiveness of these mindfulness-based interventions?

Initially, the effects of mindfulness were viewed with some suspicion from the scientific community, because positive effects attributed to mindfulness were often reported without comparison to active control groups in the study design. It is then possible that an effect is actually a placebo effect. For example, if people expect a lot from an intervention (which is likely with a popular intervention like mindfulness), then that positive expectancy alone may produce the effect. So that does not mean that there is no effect, but that you cannot attribute the observed effect to the method.

More recently, several studies have been published in which effects of mindfulness were compared with those of a proper active control group; for example, participants in the control group received relaxation exercises in the same pleasant environment, without the mindfulness-specific attention exercises. In many cases, this still yielded a better result for the mindfulness group compared to the active control group, although the difference was smaller in comparison to the earlier studies in which only a passive control group was included (people on a waiting list, for example).[148] Furthermore, mindfulness was found to work about as well as other proven effective therapies, such as cognitive behavioral therapy. The strongest and clearest effects were reported for depression, pain and addiction (especially for smoking cessation).[148] A recent review article described the effects of various mindfulness-based treatments for addiction. Here again, evidence was found that mindfulness works, although the number of well-controlled studies was still relatively small. Furthermore, it was found that the method appeared to be especially beneficial for people who suffer from anxiety and/or depression in addition to addiction,[147] the same group that profited most from cognitive bias modification, as add-on to regular therapy, as we saw earlier.[74]

A recent study by Eric Garland and colleagues, from the University of Utah, found strong effects for mindfulness in the treatment of people using opiates to manage their chronic pain, with most patients meeting criteria for addiction to the opiate medication. The control group received supportive psychotherapy, which was rated as positively as the mindfulness intervention. But in the mindfulness intervention group, many more participants had managed to get rid of their opiate addiction nine months later: 45% versus 24% in the active control group.[149] Remarkably, the difference *increased* during the post-measurements (three, six and nine months after the end of treatment), which contrasts with effects of other interventions (e.g., rewards[7] and cognitive bias modification[73]), which typically get smaller over time. The reason may be that when you succeed in teaching mindfulness exercises participants experience as beneficial, they continue to practice on their own after the treatment is over, which is typically not the case with other methods.

As with cognitive training, there have also been some studies on the underlying mechanisms of action of mindfulness. A few of them suggest that mindfulness exercises can affect cognitive biases, especially an attentional bias toward the addictive drug or in chronic pain.[150–152] So it could be that mindfulness has a similar effect as the much more specific attention training, discussed earlier. A direct comparison between these two rather different varieties of training has not yet been made, to the best of my knowledge. One study of heavy drinking college students did examine the effect of mindfulness training on automatically activated action tendencies, measured with the same test we used to find effects of action tendency training (the IAT; see Figure 1, in this case alcohol and soft drink words were again sorted with words of approach or avoidance). As discussed earlier, we found both in healthy students and in alcohol-dependent patients that cognitive training changed the tendency to sort alcohol more easily with approach to a stronger tendency to sort alcohol with avoidance.[69,153] What would mindfulness do to this action tendency? At first glance, the answer may be surprising: nothing at all.[154] However, while the strength of alcohol associations prior to the training predicted how much that person drank (the stronger the tendency to categorize alcohol with approach words, the more that person would drink), this relationship had disappeared after mindfulness training. This is consistent with the idea underlying mindfulness that you don't necessarily have to change your thoughts, but rather learn to stop acting on them, if they don't fit your goals. This suggests that mindfulness training might be considered as another road that may also lead to Rome: where CBM can change the tendency to approach alcohol, mindfulness helps to not put such a tendency to action.

In conclusion, despite initial hints of placebo effects, there is by now quite strong evidence that mindfulness can help to overcome addictions and other mental health problems (depression, chronic pain). It will still require large, well-controlled studies, as was also one of the conclusions of a recent review.[147] From the broader perspective of cognitive training, this is interesting because mindfulness is a more general training (like working memory training from the beginning of the chapter), where this has not been demonstrated. Its problem was generalization: people got better at the trained task, but did not know how to translate the gains into everyday life. In contrast, mindfulness provides tools that are immediately applicable, especially in high-risk situations, and also teaches how to deal with situations where the lure of the drug is strong. ("Concentrate on your breathing. This thought will pass even if you don't act on it.") In addition, mindfulness can help combat stress, which also plays a major role in substance abuse and relapse, and may help to create healthy habits (e.g., a quiet start of the day with some mindfulness exercises).[155]

It remains an interesting question how regular meditation, focusing on your breathing and observing your thoughts can help people with various problems, from depression to pain and addiction. Eric Garland

and colleagues, wrote an interesting piece on the question of what mindfulness does to mind and brain.[xvi] The authors argue that meditation in the original Buddhist tradition is related to meaning and experiencing life as meaningful.[156] When translated into Western practice, this characteristic had largely fallen out of the picture and the focus was mainly on the positive effects of mindfulness on negative experiences: it can help people who meditate to better cope with feelings of depression, pain, the tendency to take a drug when you don't want to, etc. In addition to these effects, there is emerging evidence that mindfulness (and meditation in general) can help to develop positive feelings, related to experiencing meaning in life. How does that work? Under the influence of stress and negative emotions people easily develop tunnel vision: you see negative things that have to be overcome and have little eye for positive things. In this way, you deprive yourself of the opportunity to experience new, positive things. People develop many habits to deal with negative feelings, such as using drugs, watching porn or gaming. Hence, meditation may not only help to see negative thoughts merely as thoughts (which you can observe without acting on them), but also to re-experience positive things, for example—despite all the misery—a beautiful sunset or the special smell of herbal tea. Meditation may help to bring back a broader view, allowing the meditator to regain new positive experiences from which meaning can be derived. And experiencing meaning in life is an important buffer against mental health problems, and it can also be trained, as my old friend Peter de Jong and colleagues recently demonstrated in a study with women with eating disorders.[157]

Ultimately, in recovery and behavioral change, it is important to dwell on the big questions in life: what is important to you, where do you want to go? The answer can be brought to the surface through meditation, but also through peer contact (AA) and through motivational interviewing. This often puts substance use in a different light, which can promote recovery. From this perspective, mindfulness in addiction could have a good impact both on meaning in life and on developing other habits that better align with one's long-term goals. So, while I initially viewed mindfulness somewhat skeptically, I now believe—based on the better research in recent years—that it is indeed a form of training that can help overcome addiction and perhaps other everyday akrasia problems, the topic of the next chapter. And perhaps it could be combined with targeted cognitive training to optimize effects, as we recently argued in a review paper on neurocognitive effects of

xvi Thanks to Tim Schoenmakers for pointing to this paper. He received his doctorate in research on the effects of attention training in alcohol addiction and is now researching effects of mindfulness and ACT (acceptance commitment therapy).

cognitive training and mindfulness.[158] It should be noted that this does not imply that mindfulness is a good intervention for everyone, as a recent large English study on mindfulness as universal school intervention in early adolescents showed: no positive effects were found and even negative effects in some.[159,160]

Conclusion and future

A variety of training programs have been developed to help people overcome addiction. The most basic idea is to reward alternative behavior, which can easily be applied in a treatment context (reward for a drug-free pee), but also in a broader social context, as in community reinforcement or in contingency management combined with a social program to quit smoking. Furthermore, various cognitive training programs have been developed. There are programs that train general functions, such as working memory—an important function for purposeful action. These training programs have shown consistent improvements on the trained function, but with limited generalization, and no effects on the addictive behavior. Nevertheless, there is evidence of improvements in other functions, such as the ability to act more purposefully on long-term outcomes and the ability to envision future steps in detail (episodic future thinking). Given the therapeutic relevance of this ability, recent promising efforts have been undertaken to directly train this ability. Another variety of general training that better succeeds in meaningful generalization is goal management training.

The second form of targeted training can be found in a family of training programs that train reactions to cues related to addiction, collectively called cognitive bias modification (CBM). In these programs, the tendency to direct attention or to move toward the substance is changed, which has proven successful in a specific application: as an add-on in the treatment of abstinence-focused alcohol addiction. In a large number of clinical studies, this provided a reduction in relapse of about 10% one year later, similar to the effects of medication. Results in smoking are less consistent, and CBM has no effect as a stand-alone intervention over the Internet (i.e., it helps reduce, but just as well as placebo training).

Based on research into the mechanisms of action, new forms of training are being developed that may work better, especially for other addictions where—unlike alcohol—there is no natural alternative to be trained toward (ABC training, for example). This still has to be tested with patients, but results in volunteers are promising. Finally, various forms of mindfulness meditation-based training have been developed for addictions and other mental health problems. There is now quite strong evidence that mindfulness training can help people with addictions.

Mindfulness can also help people have new, positive experiences that can help them find an alternative to addiction. In addition, it can help people develop new healthy habits, which can promote long-term recovery.

I think it would be wise to invest in further research on combining therapy with various forms of cognitive training. The trainings could be made more personally relevant based on conversations with a therapist, and perhaps also based on a person's own network of influencing factors (the network approach to mental problems discussed briefly earlier).[161–164] Participants measure the circumstances under which they take substances or perform their addictive behavior (where are you now? how are you feeling? have you used anything?) for several weeks using their cell phone, and then the patterns are interpreted with a therapist. That could be followed by personalized training, which should to develop new habits—more consistent with one's long-term goals.

Cognitive training has so far, in contrast to the clinical studies, proven not effective over the Internet. Here it is important to realize that this is unaccompanied training, without therapy alongside it, while that combination has proven effective in clinical groups. From this perspective, guided personalized training could hold promise. The potential of such supervised training is enormous (remember that less than 10% of addicted people receive treatment), but people will only (continue to) participate in it if they feel somewhat heard and have the idea of being helped by it. For that you don't necessarily need expensive therapists; it could probably be done with trained volunteers and maybe even partly automated using chatbots that have modern AI (artificial intelligence) behind them.[165] In this way you could reach many people with help tailored to their needs.

Finally, of course there is the brain side to this story. Addictions, as we have seen, affect the brain, with some functions recovering (or developing, according to Marc Lewis) after successful abstinence, but others not.[166] This is where targeted training could help. We already saw that CBM has effects on the brain; it causes addiction cues after training to no longer activate the neural network related to signaling personal relevance (salience).[101] Mindfulness also produces effects on this network, as well as on networks related to perceiving one's own sensations and feelings (introception). The aforementioned Paul Verschure and his team have developed a neurorehabilitation method based on the advancing insights about the brain as a self-organizing dynamic system, which successfully helps people recover after stroke.[167] Perhaps the brain problems that arise in (severely) addicted people can be improved in a similar way.[168] The advantage of the method is that it is tailored to the person and works with virtual reality, giving the participant the feeling of really reacting to situations, which works to motivate and promote recovery, at least after brain injury, perhaps also in recovery after addiction.[169,170]

In conclusion, effective therapy should provide perspective: what are my long-term goals, what values are important to me? Once this is clear, the path toward it can be mapped out and practiced, whether with personalized training, mindfulness or other techniques. An advantage of including training is that it promotes the feeling that you actively work toward change and leave your problems behind. And that applies not only to people struggling with addiction, but to all of us, which is the bridge to the next chapter.

References

1. Higgins ST, Budney AJ, Bickel WK, Hughes JR, Foerg F, Badger G. Achieving cocaine abstinence with a behavioral approach. Am J Psychiatry. 1993;150:763–9.
2. McKay JR, Lynch KG, Coviello D, Morrison R, Cary MS, Skalina L, et al. Randomized trial of continuing care enhancements for cocaine-dependent patients following initial engagement. J Consult Clin Psychol. 2010;78:111–20.
3. Schierenberg A, van Amsterdam J, van den Brink W, Goudriaan AE. Efficacy of contingency management for cocaine dependence treatment: a review of the evidence. Curr Drug Abuse Rev. 2012;5:320–31.
4. Emmelkamp PMG, Merkx M, de Fuentes-Merillas L. Contingency management. Gedragstherapie. 2015;48(2):153–70.
5. Petry NM. Contingency management for substance abuse treatment: a guide to implementing evidence-based practice. NY: Routledge; 2012.
6. Petry NM, Alessi SM, Olmstead TA, Rash CJ, Zajac K. Contingency management treatment for substance use disorders: how far has it come, and where does it need to go? Psychol Addict Behav. 2017;31:897–906.
7. Benishek LA, Dugosh KL, Kirby KC, Matejkowski J, Clements NT, Seymour BL, et al. Prize-based contingency management for the treatment of substance abusers: a meta-analysis. Addiction. 2014;109:1426–36.
8. Brand FA Van Den, Nagelhout GE, Winkens B, Chavannes NH, Schayck OCP Van. Effect of a workplace-based group training programme combined with financial incentives on smoking cessation: a cluster-randomised controlled trial. Lancet Public Heal [Internet]. 2018;2667. Available from: 10.1016/S2468-2667(18)30185-3
9. Kelly JF, Magill M, Stout RL. How do people recover from alcohol dependence? A systematic review of the research on mechanisms of behavior change in Alcoholics Anonymous. Addict Res Theory. 2009; 17:236–59.
10. Roozen HG, Boulogne JJ, Van Tulder MW, Van Den Brink W, De Jong CAJ, Kerkhof AJFM. A systematic review of the effectiveness of the community reinforcement approach in alcohol, cocaine and opioid addiction. Drug Alcohol Depend. 2004;74:1–13.
11. Alexander BK, Coambs RB, Hadaway PF The effect of housing and gender on morphine self-administration in rats. Psychopharmacology (Berl). 1978;58:175–9.
12. Venniro M, Zhang M, Caprioli D, Hoots JK, Golden SA, Heins C, et al. Addiction in rat models. Nat Neurosci [Internet]. 2018;21. Available from: 10.1038/s41593-018-0246-6
13. Diamond A, Lee K. Interventions shown to aid executive function development in children 4 to 12 years old. Science (80–) [Internet]. 2011;333:959–64.

Available from: www.pubmedcentral.nih.gov/articlerender.fcgi?artid=3159917&tool=pmcentrez&rendertype=abstract
14. van Lier PAC, Huizink A, Crijnen A. Impact of a preventive intervention targeting childhood disruptive behavior problems on tobacco and alcohol initiation from age 10 to 13 years. Drug Alcohol Depend. 2009;100:228–33.
15. Pihl RO, Peterson J, Finn PR. Inherited predisposition to alcoholism: characteristics of sons of male alcoholics. J Abnorm Psychol. 1990;99:291.
16. Wiers RW, Gunning WBW, Sergeant JAJ. Is a mild deficit in executive functions in boys related to childhood ADHD or to parental multigenerational alcoholism? J Abnorm Child … [Internet]. 1998 [cited 2013 Apr 5];26:415–30. Available from: http://link.springer.com/article/10.1023/A:1022643617017
17. Nigg JT. On inhibition/disinhibition in developmental psychopathology: views from cognitive and personality psychology and a working inhibition taxonomy. Psychol Bull. 2000;126:220.
18. Bickel WK, Yi R, Landes RD, Hill PF, Baxter C. Remember the future: working memory training decreases delay discounting among stimulant addicts. Biol Psychiatry. 2011;69:260–5.
19. Bickel WK, Moody L, Quisenberry A. Computerized working-memory training as a candidate adjunctive treatment for addiction. Alcohol Res Curr Rev. 2014;36:123–6.
20. Snider SE, Deshpande HU, Lisinski JM, Koffarnus MN, LaConte SM, Bickel WK. Working memory training improves alcohol users' episodic future thinking: a rate dependent analysis. Biol Psychiatry Cogn Neurosci Neuroimaging [Internet]. 2018;3:160–7. Available from: 10.1016/j.bpsc.2017.11.002
21. Wanmaker S, Leijdesdorff SMJ, Geraerts E, van de Wetering BJM, Renkema PJ, Franken IHA. The efficacy of a working memory training in substance use patients: a randomized double-blind placebo-controlled clinical trial. J Clin Exp Neuropsychol [Internet]. 2017;00:1–14. Available from: www.tandfonline.com/doi/full/10.1080/13803395.2017.1372367
22. Sonuga-Barke EJS, Brandeis D, Cortese S, Daley D, Ferrin M, Holtmann M, et al. Nonpharmacological interventions for ADHD: systematic review and meta-analyses of randomized controlled trials of dietary and psychological treatments. Am J Psychiatry [Internet]. 2013;170:275–89. Available from: http://journals.psychiatryonline.org/article.aspx?articleID=1566975
23. Bickel WK, Jarmolowicz DP, Mueller ET, Gatchalian KM. The behavioral economics and neuroeconomics of reinforcer pathologies: implications for etiology and treatment of addiction. Curr Psychiatry Rep. 2011;13:406–15.
24. Sonuga-Barke EJS, Taylor E, Sembi S, Smith J. Hyperactivity and delay aversion—I. The effect of delay on choice. J Child Psychol Psychiatry. 1992;33:387–98.
25. Marco R, Miranda A, Schlotz W, Melia A, Mulligan A, Müller U, et al. Delay and reward choice in ADHD: an experimental test of the role of delay aversion. Neuropsychology. 2009;23:367–80.
26. Wiers RW. Cognitive training in addiction: does it have clinical potential? Biol Psychiatry Cogn Neurosci Neuroimaging. 2018;3.
27. Houben K, Wiers RW, Jansen A. Getting a grip on drinking behavior: training working memory to reduce alcohol abuse. Psychol Sci [Internet]. 2011 [cited 2013 Mar 8];22:968–75. Available from: www.ncbi.nlm.nih.gov/pubmed/21685380
28. Bickel WK, Freitas R, Jeremy L, Quddos F, Fontes RM, Barbosa B, et al. Episodic future thinking as a promising intervention for substance use

disorders: a reinforcer pathology perspective. Curr Addict Reports [Internet]. 2023; Available from: https://doi.org/10.1007/s40429-023-00498-z

29. Alfonso JP, Caracuel A, Delgado-pastor LC, Verdejo-García A. Combined goal management training and mindfulness meditation improve executive functions and decision-making performance in abstinent polysubstance abusers. 2011;117:78–81.
30. Valls-Serrano C, Caracuel A, Verdejo-Garcia A. Goal management training and mindfulness meditation improve executive functions and transfer to ecological tasks of daily life in polysubstance users enrolled in therapeutic community treatment. Drug Alcohol Depend [Internet]. 2016;165:9–14. Available from: 10.1016/j.drugalcdep.2016.04.040
31. Bates ME, Buckman JF, Nguyen TT. A role for cognitive rehabilitation in increasing the effectiveness of treatment for alcohol use disorders. Neuropsychol Rev. 2013;23:27–47.
32. Silveira H, Moraes H, Oliveira N, Coutinho ESF, Laks J, Deslandes A. Physical exercise and clinically depressed patients: a systematic review and meta-analysis. Neuropsychobiology. 2013;67:61–8.
33. Lynch WJ, Peterson AB, Sanchez V, Abel J, Smith MA. Exercise as a novel treatment for drug addiction: a neurobiological and stage-dependent hypothesis. Neurosci Biobehav Rev [Internet]. 2013;37:1622–44. Available from: 10.1016/j.neubiorev.2013.06.011
34. Robinson TE, Berridge KC. Addiction. Annu Rev Psychol. 2003;54:25–53.
35. Klein AM, de Voogd L, Wiers RW, Salemink E. Biases in attention and interpretation in adolescents with varying levels of anxiety and depression. Cogn Emot. 2018;32(7):1478–86.
36. Field M, Cox WM. Attentional bias in addictive behaviors: a review of its development, causes, and consequences. Drug Alcohol Depend. 2008; 97:1–20.
37. Ataya AF, Adams S, Mullings E, Cooper RM, Attwood AS, Munafò MR. Internal reliability of measures of substance-related cognitive bias. Drug Alcohol Depend [Internet]. 2012;121:148–51. Available from: 10.1016/j.drugalcdep.2011.08.023
38. Grafton B, Teng S, MacLeod C. Two probes and better than one: development of a psychometrically reliable variant of the attentional probe task. Behav Res Ther [Internet]. 2021;138:103805. Available from: 10.1016/j.brat.2021.103805
39. Wiechert S, Grafton B, MacLeod C, Wiers RW. When alcohol-adverts catch the eye: a psychometrically reliable dual-probe measure of attentional bias. Int J Environ Res Public Health. 2021;18:13263.
40. MacLeod C, Rutherford E, Campbell L, Ebsworthy G, Holker L. Selective attention and emotional vulnerability: assessing the causal basis of their association through the experimental manipulation of attentional bias. J Abnorm Psychol. 2002;111:107–23.
41. Sheeran P, Klein WMPP, Rothman AJ. Health behavior change: moving from observation to intervention. Annu Rev Psychol. 2017;68:573–600.
42. See J, MacLeod C, Bridle R. The reduction of anxiety vulnerability through the modification of attentional bias: a real-world study using a home-based cognitive bias modification procedure. J Abnorm Psychol. 2009;118:65–75.
43. Amir N, Beard C, Burns M, Bomyea J. Attention modification program in individuals with generalized anxiety disorder. J Abnorm Psychol [Internet]. 2009 [cited 2013 Aug 15];118:28–33. Available from: www.ncbi.nlm.nih.gov/pubmed/19222311%0Awww.pubmedcentral.nih.gov/articlerender.fcgi?artid=PMC2645540

44. Schmidt NB, Richey JA, Buckner JD, Timpano KR. Attention training for generalized social anxiety disorder. J Abnorm Psychol [Internet]. 2009 [cited 2013 Aug 8];118:5–14. Available from: www.ncbi.nlm.nih.gov/pubmed/19222309
45. Carlbring P, Apelstrand M, Sehlin H, Amir N, Rousseau A, Hofmann S, et al. Internet-delivered attention bias modification training in individuals with social. BMC Psychiatry. 2012;12:1–9.
46. Boettcher J, Leek L, Matson L, Holmes EA, Browning M, MacLeod C, et al. Internet-based attention bias modification for social anxiety: a randomised controlled comparison of training towards negative and training towards positive cues. PLoS One. 2013;8.
47. Cristea IA, Kok RN, Cuijpers P. Efficacy of cognitive bias modification interventions in anxiety and depression: meta-analysis. Br J Psychiatry. 2015;206:7–16.
48. MacLeod C, Grafton B. Anxiety-linked attentional bias and its modification: illustrating the importance of distinguishing processes and procedures in experimental psychopathology research. Behav Res Ther [Internet]. 2016;86:68–86. Available from: http://linkinghub.elsevier.com/retrieve/pii/S0005796716301164
49. Linetzky M, Pergamin-Hight L, Pine DS, Bar-Haim Y. Quantitative evaluation of the clinical efficacy of attention bias modification treatment for anxiety disorders. Depress Anxiety. 2015;32:383–91.
50. Fodor LA, Georgescu R, Cuijpers P, Szamoskozi Ş, David D, Furukawa TA, et al. Efficacy of cognitive bias modification interventions in anxiety and depressive disorders: a systematic review and network meta-analysis. The Lancet Psychiatry. 2020;7:506–14.
51. Blackwell SE. Clinical efficacy of cognitive bias modification interventions. The Lancet Psychiatry. 2020;7:465–7.
52. Field M, Eastwood B. Experimental manipulation of attentional bias increases the motivation to drink alcohol. Psychopharmacology (Berl). 2005;183:350–7.
53.. Field M, Duka T, Eastwood B, Child R, Santarcangelo M, Gayton M. Experimental manipulation of attentional biases in heavy drinkers: do the effects generalise? Psychopharmacology (Berl). 2007;192:593–608.
54. Schoenmakers TM, Wiers RW, Jones BT, Bruce G, Jansen ATM. Attentional re-training decreases attentional bias in heavy drinkers without generalization. Addiction [Internet]. 2007 [cited 2013 Mar 12];102:399–405. Available from: www.ncbi.nlm.nih.gov/pubmed/17298647
55. Wiers RW, Schoenmakers T, Houben K, Thush C, Fadardi JS, Cox WM. Can problematic alcohol use be trained away? 2008;187–208.
56. Schoenmakers TM, de Bruin M, Lux IFM, Goertz AG, Van Kerkhof DH a T, Wiers RW. Clinical effectiveness of attentional bias modification training in abstinent alcoholic patients. Drug Alcohol Depend [Internet]. 2010 [cited 2013 Mar 25];109:30–6. Available from: www.ncbi.nlm.nih.gov/pubmed/20064698
57. Cox WM, Hogan LM, Kristian MR, Race JH. Alcohol attentional bias as a predictor of alcohol abusers' treatment outcome. Drug Alcohol Depend. 2002;68:237–43.
58. Rinck M, Wiers RW, Becker ES, Lindenmeyer J. Relapse prevention in abstinent alcoholics by cognitive bias modification: clinical effects of combining approach bias modification and attention bias modification. J Consult Clin Psychol. 2018;86:1005–16.

59. Rinck M, Becker ES. Approach and avoidance in fear of spiders. J Behav Ther Exp Psychiatry. 2007;38:105–20.
60. Wiers RW, Rinck M, Dictus M, Van Den Wildenberg E. Relatively strong automatic appetitive action-tendencies in male carriers of the OPRM1 G-allele. Genes, Brain Behav [Internet]. 2009 [cited 2013 Mar 9];8:101–6. Available from: www.ncbi.nlm.nih.gov/pubmed/19016889
61. Rotteveel M, Phaf RH. Automatic affective evaluation does not automatically predispose for arm flexion and extension. Emotion. 2004;4:156–72.
62. Van Den Wildenberg E, Wiers RW, Dessers J, Janssen RGJH, Lambrichs EH, Smeets HJM, et al. A functional polymorphism of the μ-opioid receptor gene (OPRM1) influences cue-induced craving for alcohol in male heavy drinkers. Alcohol Clin Exp Res [Internet]. 2007 [cited 2013 Mar 11];31:1–10. Available from: www.ncbi.nlm.nih.gov/pubmed/17207095
63. Filbey FM, Ray L, Smolen A, Claus ED, Audette A, Hutchison KE. Differential neural response to alcohol priming and alcohol taste cues is associated with DRD4 VNTR and OPRM1 genotypes. Alcohol Clin Exp Res. 2008;32:1113–23.
64. Wiers CE, Kühn S, Javadi AH, Korucuoglu O, Wiers RW, Walter H, et al. Automatic approach bias towards smoking cues is present in smokers but not in ex-smokers. Psychopharmacology (Berl). 2013;229.
65. Cousijn J, Goudriaan AE, Wiers RW. Reaching out towards cannabis: approach-bias in heavy cannabis users predicts changes in cannabis use. Addiction [Internet]. 2011 [cited 2013 Mar 5];106:1667–74. Available from: www.pubmedcentral.nih.gov/articlerender.fcgi?artid=3178782&tool=pmcentrez&rendertype=abstract
66. Boffo M, Smits R, Salmon JP, Cowie ME, de Jong DTHA, Salemink E, et al. Luck, come here! Automatic approach tendencies toward gambling cues in moderate-to-high risk gamblers. Addiction [Internet]. 2017;289–98. Available from: http://doi.wiley.com/10.1111/add.14071
67. Galvin HR, Boffo M, Snippe L, Collins P, Pronk T, Salemink E, et al. Losing sight of luck: automatic approach tendencies toward gambling cues in Canadian moderate-to high-risk gamblers-a replication study. Addict Behav. 2023;107778.
68. Field M, Caren R, Fernie G, De Houwer J. Alcohol approach tendencies in heavy drinkers: comparison of effects in a relevant stimulus-response compatibility task and an approach/avoidance Simon task. Psychol Addict Behav. 2011;25:697–701.
69. Wiers RW, Rinck M, Kordts R, Houben K, Strack F. Retraining automatic action-tendencies to approach alcohol in hazardous drinkers. Addiction. 2010;105:279–87.
70. Eberl C, Wiers RW, Pawelczack S, Rinck M, Becker ES, Lindenmeyer J. Approach bias modification in alcohol dependence: do clinical effects replicate and for whom does it work best? Dev Cogn Neurosci [Internet]. 2013 [cited 2013 Mar 23];4:38–51. Available from: www.ncbi.nlm.nih.gov/pubmed/23218805
71. Eberl C, Wiers RW, Pawelczack S, Rinck M, Becker ES, Lindenmeyer J. Implementation of approach bias re-training in alcoholism: how many sessions are needed? Alcohol Clin Exp Res [Internet]. 2014 [cited 2014 Aug 19];38:587–94. Available from: www.ncbi.nlm.nih.gov/pubmed/24164417
72. Loijen A, Rinck M, Walvoort SJW, Kessels RPC, Becker ES, Egger JIM. Modification of automatic alcohol-approach tendencies in alcohol-dependent patients with mild or major neurocognitive disorder. Alcohol Clin Exp Res. 2018;42:153–61.

73. Manning V, Garfield JBB, Reynolds J, Staiger PK, Piercy H, Bonomo Y, et al. Alcohol use in the year following approach bias modification during inpatient withdrawal: secondary outcomes from a double-blind, multi-site randomized controlled trial. Addiction. 2022;1–10.
74. Salemink E, Rinck M, Becker E, Wiers RW, Lindenmeyer J. Does comorbid anxiety or depression moderate effects of approach bias modification in the treatment of alcohol use disorders? Psychol Addict Behav. 2021;36(5):547–54.
75. Clerkin EM, Magee JC, Wells TT, Beard C, Barnett NP. Randomized controlled trial of attention bias modification in a racially diverse, socially anxious, alcohol dependent sample. Behav Res Ther [Internet]. 2016; 87:58–69. Available from: 10.1016/j.brat.2016.08.010
76. Stapinski LA, Rapee RM, Sannibale C, Teesson M, Haber PS, Baillie AJ. The clinical and theoretical basis for integrated cognitive behavioral treatment of comorbid social anxiety and alcohol use disorders. Cogn Behav Pract. 2015;22:504–21.
77. Sliedrecht W, de Waart R, Witkiewitz K, Roozen HG. Alcohol use disorder relapse factors: a systematic review. Psychiatry Res [Internet]. 2019;278:97–115. Available from: 10.1016/j.psychres.2019.05.038
78. Heitmann J, Van Hemel-Ruiter ME, Huisman M, Ostafin BD, Wiers RW, MacLeod C, et al. Effectiveness of attentional bias modification training as add-on to regular treatment in alcohol and cannabis use disorder: a multicenter randomized control trial. PLoS One. 2021;16.
79. Wiers RW, Eberl C, Rinck M, Becker ES, Lindenmeyer J. Retraining automatic action tendencies changes alcoholic patients' approach bias for alcohol and improves treatment outcome. Psychol Sci [Internet]. 2011 [cited 2013 Feb 27];22:490–7. Available from: www.ncbi.nlm.nih.gov/pubmed/21389338
80. Manning V, Staiger PK, Hall K, Garfield JBB, Flaks G, Leung D, et al. Cognitive bias modification training during inpatient alcohol detoxification reduces early relapse: a randomized controlled trial. Alcohol Clin Exp Res. 2016;40:2011–9.
81. Manning V, Garfield JBB, Staiger PK, Lubman DI, Lum JAG, Reynolds J, et al. Effect of cognitive bias modification on early relapse among adults undergoing inpatient alcohol withdrawal treatment: a randomized clinical trial. JAMA Psychiatry. 2021;78:133–40.
82. Kiefer F, Batra A, Bischof G, Funke W, Lindenmeyer J, Mueller S, et al. S3-Leitlinie "Screening, Diagnose und Behandlung alkoholbezogener Störungen". Sucht. 2021. Available from: https://econtent.hogrefe.com/doi/full/10.1024/0939-5911/a000704.
83. Haber PS, Riordan BC, Winter DT, Barrett L, Saunders J, Hides L, et al. New Australian guidelines for the treatment of alcohol problems: an overview of recommendations. Med J Aust. 2021;215:S3–S32.
84. Cristea IA, Kok RN, Cuijpers P. The effectiveness of cognitive bias modification interventions for substance addictions: a meta-analysis. PLoS One. 2016;11:e0162226.
85. Wiers RW, Boffo M, Field M. What's in a trial? The authors respond: persistent mixing of apples and oranges, or carefully synthesizing and designing the next steps in research on cognitive bias modification in addiction. J Stud Alcohol Drugs. 2018;79:348–9.
86. Wiers RW, Boffo M, Field M. What's in a trial? On the importance of distinguishing between experimental lab studies and randomized controlled

trials: the case of cognitive bias modification and alcohol use disorders. J Stud Alcohol Drugs. 2018;79:333–43.
87. Boffo M, Zerhouni O, Gronau QF, van Beek RJJ, Nikolaou K, Marsman M, et al. Cognitive bias modification for behavior change in alcohol and smoking addiction: Bayesian meta-analysis of individual participant data. Neuropsychol Rev. 2019;29:52–78.
88. Van Deursen DS. Where is the bias? Measuring and retraining cognitive biases in problem drinkers. University of Amsterdam; 2019.
89. Wittekind CE, Lüdecke D, Cludius B. Web-based approach bias modification in smokers: a randomized-controlled study. Behav Res Ther. 2019;116:52–60.
90. Wen S, Larsen H, Boffo M, Grasman RPPP, Pronk T, Van Wijngaarden JBG, et al. Combining web-based attentional bias modification and approach bias modification as a self-help smoking intervention for adult smokers seeking online help: double-blind randomized controlled trial. JMIR Ment Heal. 2020;7.
91. Jones A, McGrath E, Robinson E, Houben K, Nederkoorn C, Field M. A randomised controlled trial of inhibitory control training for the reduction of alcohol consumption in problem drinkers. J Consult Clin Psychol. 2018;86:991–1004.
92. Wiers RW, Houben K, Fadardi JS, van Beek P, Rhemtulla M, Cox WM. Alcohol cognitive bias modification training for problem drinkers over the web. Addict Behav [Internet]. 2015;40:21–6. Available from: 10.1016/j.addbeh.2014.08.010
93. Elfeddali I, de Vries H, Bolman C, Pronk T, Wiers RW. A randomized controlled trial of web-based attentional bias modification to help smokers quit. Health Psychol. 2016;35.
94. Wittekind CE, Reibert E, Takano K, Ehring T, Pogarell O, Rüther T. Approach-avoidance modification as an add-on in smoking cessation: a randomized-controlled study. Behav Res Ther [Internet]. 2019;114:35–43. Available from: 10.1016/j.brat.2018.12.004
95. Wittekind CE, Lüdecke D, Cludius B. Web-based approach bias modification in smokers: a randomized-controlled study. Behav Res Ther. 2019; 116:52–60.
96. Jonas DE, Amick HR, Feltner C, Bobashev G, Thomas K, Wines R, et al. Pharmacotherapy for adults with alcohol use disorders in outpatient settings: a systematic review and meta-analysis. JAMA—J Am Med Assoc. 2014;311:1889–900.
97. den Uyl TE, Gladwin TE, Rinck M, Lindenmeyer J, Wiers RW. A clinical trial with combined transcranial direct current stimulation and alcohol approach bias retraining. Addict Biol. 2017;22:1–9.
98. den Uyl TE, Gladwin TE, Lindenmeyer J, Wiers RW. A clinical trial with combined transcranial direct current stimulation and alcohol attentional retraining. Alcohol Clin Exp Res. 2018;in press.
99. Wiers CE, Wiers RW. Imaging the neural effects of cognitive bias modification training. Neuroimage. 2017;151:81–91.
100. Wiers CE, Stelzel C, Park SQ, Gawron CK, Ludwig VU, Gutwinski S, et al. Neural correlates of alcohol-approach bias in alcohol addiction: the spirit is willing but the flesh is weak for spirits. Neuropsychopharmacology. 2014;39.
101. Wiers CE, Stelzel C, Gladwin TETE, Park SQSQ, Pawelczack S, Gawron CKCK, et al. Effects of cognitivebias modification training on neural alcohol cue reactivity in alcohol dependence. Am J Psychiatry. 2015;172:335–43.

102. Wiers CE, Ludwig VU, Gladwin TE, Park SQ, Heinz A, Wiers RW, et al. Effects of cognitive bias modification training on neural signatures of alcohol approach tendencies in male alcohol-dependent patients. Addict Biol. 2015;20:990–9.
103. Vul E, Harris C, Winkielman P, Pashler H. Voodoo correlations in social neuroscience. Perspect Psychol Sci. 2009;4:274–90.
104. Mitchell CJ, Houwer J, Lovibond PF. The propositional nature of human associative learning: the behavioral and brain sciences. 2009;32:183–98; discussion 198–246. Available from: www.ncbi.nlm.nih.gov/pubmed/19386174
105. Gawronski B, Bodenhausen G V. Associative and propositional processes in evaluation: Conceptual, empirical, and metatheoretical issues: reply to Albarracín, Hart, and McCulloch (2006), Kruglanski and Dechesne (2006), and Petty and Briñol (2006). Psychol Bull. 2006;132:745–50.
106. Deutsch R, Gawronski B, Strack F. At the boundaries of automaticity: negation as reflective operation. J Pers Soc Psychol [Internet]. 2006;91:385–405. Available from: www.ncbi.nlm.nih.gov/pubmed/16938026
107. Strack F, Deutsch R. Reflective and impulsive determinants of social behavior. Personal Soc Psychol Rev. 2004;8:220–47.
108. Evans JSBT, Stanovich KE. Dual-process theories of higher cognition: advancing the debate. Perspect Psychol Sci. 2013;8:223–41.
109. Moors A, Boddez Y, De Houwer J. The power of goal-directed processes in the causation of emotional and other actions. Emot Rev. 2017;9:310–8.
110. Stacy AW, Wiers RW. Implicit cognition and addiction: a tool for explaining paradoxical behavior. Annu Rev Clin Psychol [Internet]. 2010 [cited 2013 Mar 13];6:551–75. Available from: www.pubmedcentral.nih.gov/articlerender.fcgi?artid=3423976&tool=pmcentrez&rendertype=abstract
111. Van Dessel P, De Houwer J, Gast A. Approach-avoidance training effects are moderated by awareness of stimulus–action contingencies. Personal Soc Psychol Bull. 2016;42:81–93.
112. Dessel P Van, De Houwer J, Roets A, Gast A. Failures to change stimulus evaluations by means of subliminal approach and avoidance training. J Pers Soc Psychol. 2016;110:e1–e15.
113. Van Dessel P, De Houwer J, Gast A, Smith CT. Instruction-based approach-avoidance effects. Exp Psychol. 2015;62(3):161–9.
114. Van Dessel P, De Houwer J, Gast A, Smith CT, De Schryver M. Instructing implicit processes: when instructions to approach or avoid influence implicit but not explicit evaluation. J Exp Soc Psychol [Internet]. 2016;63:1–9. Available from: 10.1016/j.jesp.2015.11.002
115. Van Dessel P, De Houwer J, Gast A, Roets A, Smith CT. On the effectiveness of approach-avoidance instructions and training for changing evaluations of social groups. J Pers Soc Psychol. 2020;119:e1–e14.
116. Moritz S, Paulus AM, Hottenrott B, Weierstall R, Gallinat J, Kühn S. Imaginal retraining reduces alcohol craving in problem drinkers: a randomized controlled trial. J Behav Ther Exp Psychiatry [Internet]. 2019;64:158–66. Available from: 10.1016/j.jbtep.2019.04.001
117. Gehlenborg J, Göritz AS, Moritz S, Lüdtke T, Kühn S. Imaginal retraining reduces craving for tobacco in 1-year controlled follow-up study. Eur Addict Res. 2022;28(1):68–79.
118. Van Dessel P, Hughes S, De Houwer J. Consequence-based approach-avoidance training: a new and improved method for changing behavior. Psychol Sci. 2018;29:1899–910.

119. Köpetz CE, Lejuez CW, Wiers RW, Kruglanski AW. Motivation and self-regulation in addiction: a call for convergence. Perspect Psychol Sci [Internet]. 2013 [cited 2013 Mar 2];8:3–24. Available from: http://pps.sagepub.com/lookup/doi/10.1177/1745691612457575
120. Wiers RW, Van Dessel P, Köpetz C. ABC training: a new theory-based form of cognitive-bias modification to foster automatization of alternative choices in the treatment of addiction and related disorders. Curr Dir Psychol Sci. 2020;29:499–505.
121. Kopetz C, MacPherson L, Mitchell AD, Houston-Ludlam AN, Wiers RW. A novel training approach to activate alternative behaviors for smoking in depressed smokers. Exp Clin Psychopharmacol. 2017;25:50–60.
122. Wen S, Larsen H, Wiers RW. A pilot study on approach bias modification in smoking cessation: activating personalized alternative activities for smoking in the context of increased craving. Int J Behav Med. 2021;1–14.
123. Dessel P Van, Cummins J, Wiers RW. ABC-training as a new intervention for hazardous alcohol drinking: a proof-of-principle study. Addiction. 2023;118(11):2141–55.
124. Pan T, Szpak V, Laverman J, van Dessel P, Bovens R, Larsen H, et al. A novel improvement in cognitive bias modification: ABC-training for alcohol use during a voluntary abstinence challenge. Unpubl MS. 2023.
125. Merkx MJM. Individuele cognitieve gedragstherapie bij middelengebruik en gokken. In: GM Schippers, AM Smeerdijk, MJM Merkx (Eds.). Handboek cognitieve gedragstherapie bij middelengebruik en gokken. Amersfoort: Resultaten Scoren; 2014. pp. 105–264.
126. Beard C, Weisberg RB, Primack J. Socially anxious primary care patients' attitudes toward cognitive bias modification (CBM): a qualitative study. Behav Cogn Psychother [Internet]. 2012;40:618–33. Available from: http://search.ebscohost.com/login.aspx?direct=true&db=psyh&AN=2012-24762-009&site=ehost-live%5Cncourtney_beard@brown.edu%5Cnhttp://search.ebscohost.com/login.aspx?direct=true%7B&%7Ddb=psyh%7B&%7DAN=2012-24762-009%7B&%7Dsite=ehost-live%5Cncourtney%7B_%7Dbe
127. Lazarov A, Pine DS, Bar-Haim Y. Gaze-contingent music reward therapy for social anxiety disorder: a randomized controlled trial. Am J Psychiatry. 2017;174:649–56.
128. Gollwitzer PM. Implementation intentions: strong effects of simple plans. Am Psychol. 1999;54:493.
129. Gollwitzer PM, Sheeran P. Implementation intentions and goal achievement: a meta-analysis of effects and processes. In: Advances in experimental social psychology. Academic Press; 2006. pp. 69–119.
130. Webb TL, Sheeran P, Luszczynska A. Planning to break unwanted habits: habit strength moderates implementation intention effects on behaviour change. Br J Soc Psychol. 2009;48:507–23.
131. Oettingen G, Reininger KM. The power of prospection: mental contrasting and behavior change. Soc Personal Psychol Compass. 2016;10:591–604.
132. Oettingen G. Future thought and behaviour change. Eur Rev Soc Psychol. 2012;23:1–63.
133. Houben K, Schoenmakers TM, Wiers RW. I didn't feel like drinking but I don't know why: the effects of evaluative conditioning on alcohol-related attitudes, craving and behavior. Addict Behav [Internet]. 2010 [cited 2013 Mar 12];35:1161–3. Available from: www.ncbi.nlm.nih.gov/pubmed/20810220
134. Houben K, Havermans RC, Wiers RW. Learning to dislike alcohol: conditioning negative implicit attitudes toward alcohol and its effect on

drinking behavior. Psychopharmacology (Berl) [Internet]. 2010 [cited 2013 Apr 3];211:79–86. Available from: www.pubmedcentral.nih.gov/articlerender.fcgi?artid=2885295&tool=pmcentrez&rendertype=abstract
135. Zerhouni O, Houben K, El Methni J, Rutte N, Werkman E, Wiers RW. I didn't feel like drinking, but I guess why: evaluative conditioning changes on explicit attitudes toward alcohol and healthy foods depends on contingency awareness. Learn Motiv. 2019;66.
136. Wilson GT. Chemical aversion conditioning in the treatment of alcoholism: further comments. Behav Res Ther. 1991;29:415–9.
137. Lee SH, Han DH, Oh S, Lyoo IK, Lee YS, Renshaw PF, et al. Quantitative electroencephalographic (qEEG) correlates of craving during virtual reality therapy in alcohol-dependent patients. Pharmacol Biochem Behav [Internet]. 2009;91:393–7. Available from: 10.1016/j.pbb.2008.08.014
138. Wang Y guang, Liu M hui, Shen Z hua. A virtual reality counterconditioning procedure to reduce methamphetamine cue-induced craving. J Psychiatr Res [Internet]. 2019;116:88–94. Available from: 10.1016/j.jpsychires.2019.06.007
139. Houben K, Nederkoorn C, Wiers RW, Jansen A. Resisting temptation: decreasing alcohol-related affect and drinking behavior by training response inhibition. Drug Alcohol Depend [Internet]. 2011 [cited 2013 Feb 28];116:132–6. Available from: www.ncbi.nlm.nih.gov/pubmed/21288663
140. Houben K, Havermans RC, Nederkoorn C, Jansen A. Beer?? No-go: learning to stop responding to alcohol cues reduces alcohol intake via reduced affective associations rather than increased response inhibition. Addiction. 2012;107:1280–7.
141. Allom V, Mullan B, Hagger M. Does inhibitory control training improve health behaviour? A meta-analysis. Health Psychol Rev [Internet]. 2015;7199:1–38. Available from: www.tandfonline.com/doi/full/10.1080/17437199.2015.1051078
142. Schenkel EJ, Schöneck R, Wiers RW, Veling H, Becker ES, Lindenmeyer J, et al. Does selective inhibition training reduce relapse rates when added to standard treatment of alcohol use disorder? A randomized controlled trial. Alcohol Clin Exp Res. 2023;47:963–74.
143. Verdejo-Garcia A, Rezapour T, Giddens E, Khojasteh Zonoozi A, Rafei P, Berry J, et al. Cognitive training and remediation interventions for substance use disorders: a Delphi consensus study. Addiction. 2023;118:935–51.
144. Ostafin BD, Marlatt GA. Surfing the urge: experiential acceptance moderates the relation between automatic alcohol motivation and hazardous drinking. J Soc Clin Psychol [Internet]. 2008;27:404–18. Available from: http://guilfordjournals.com/doi/10.1521/jscp.2008.27.4.404
145. Bowen S, Witkiewitz K, Clifasefi SL, Grow J, Chawla N, Hsu SH, et al. Relative efficacy of mindfulness-based relapse prevention, standard relapse prevention, and treatment as usual for substance use disorders. JAMA Psychiatry. 2014;71:547–56.
146. Paulus MP, Stewart JL. Interoception and drug addiction. Neuropharmacology [Internet]. 2014;76:342–50. Available from: 10.1016/j.neuropharm.2013.07.002
147. Korecki JR, Schwebel FJ, Votaw VR, Witkiewitz K. Mindfulness-based programs for substance use disorders: a systematic review of manualized treatments. Subst Abus Treat Prev Policy. 2020;15.
148. Goldberg SB, Tucker RP, Greene PA, Davidson RJ, Wampold BE, Kearney DJ, et al. Mindfulness-based interventions for psychiatric

disorders: a systematic review and meta-analysis. Clin Psychol Rev [Internet]. 2018;59:52–60. Available from: 10.1016/j.cpr.2017.10.011
149. Garland EL, Hanley AW, Nakamura Y, Barrett JW, Baker AK, Reese SE, et al. Mindfulness-oriented recovery enhancement vs supportive group therapy for co-occurring opioid misuse and chronic pain in primary care: a randomized clinical trial. JAMA Intern Med. 2022;84112:407–17.
150. Garland EL, Baker AK, Howard MO. Mindfulness-oriented recovery enhancement reduces opioid attentional bias among prescription opioid-treated chronic pain patients. J Soc Social Work Res. 2017;8:493–509.
151. Garland EL, Gaylord SA, Boettiger CA, Howard MO. Mindfulness training modifies cognitive, affective, and physiological mechanisms implicated in alcohol dependence: results of a randomized controlled pilot trial. J Psychoactive Drugs. 2010;42:177–92.
152. Garland EL, Howard MO. Mindfulness-oriented recovery enhancement reduces pain attentional bias in chronic pain patients. Psychother Psychosom. 2013;82:311–8.
153. Eberl C, Wiers RW, Pawelczack S, Rinck M, Becker ES, Lindenmeyer J. Approach bias modification in alcohol dependence: do clinical effects replicate and for whom does it work best? Dev Cogn Neurosci [Internet]. 2013 [cited 2013 Mar 23];4:38–51. Available from: www.ncbi.nlm.nih.gov/pubmed/23218805
154. Palfai TP, Ostafin BD. Alcohol-related motivational tendencies in hazardous drinkers: assessing implicit response tendencies using the modified-IAT. Behav Res Ther. 2003;41:1149–62.
155. Sinha R. Chronic stress, drug use, and vulnerability to addiction. Ann N Y Acad Sci. 2008;1141:105–30.
156. Garland EL, Farb NA, R. Goldin P, Fredrickson BL. Mindfulness broadens awareness and builds eudaimonic meaning: a process model of mindful positive emotion regulation. Psychol Inq. 2015;26:293–314.
157. van Doornik SFW, Glashouwer KA, Ostafin BD, de Jong PJ. The effects of a meaning-centered intervention on meaning in life and eating disorder symptoms in undergraduate women with high weight and shape concerns: a randomized controlled trial. Behav Ther [Internet]. 2023; Available from: 10.1016/j.beth.2023.05.012
158. Larsen JK, Hollands GJ, Garland EL, Evers AWM, Wiers RW. Be more mindful: targeting addictive responses by integrating mindfulness with cognitive bias modification or cue exposure interventions. Neurosci Biobehav Rev [Internet]. 2023;153:105408. Available from: 10.1016/j.neubiorev.2023.105408
159. Ford T, Degli Esposti M, Crane C, Taylor L, Montero-Marín J, Blakemore SJ, et al. The role of schools in early adolescents' mental health: findings from the MYRIAD study. J Am Acad Child Adolesc Psychiatry. 2021;60:1467–78.
160. Montero-Marin J, Allwood M, Ball S, Crane C, De Wilde K, Hinze V, et al. School-based mindfulness training in early adolescence: what works, for whom and how in the MYRIAD trial? Evid Based Ment Health. 2022;25:117–24.
161. Borsboom D. A network theory of mental disorders. World Psychiatry. 2017;16:5–13.
162. Bringmann LF, van der Veen DC, Wichers M, Riese H, Stulp G. ESMvis: a tool for visualizing individual experience sampling method (ESM) data. Qual Life Res [Internet]. 2021;30:3179–88. Available from: 10.1007/s11136-020-02701-4

163. Mansueto AC, Wiers RW, van Weert J, Schouten BC, Epskamp S. Investigating the feasibility of idiographic network models. Psychol Methods. 2022; 10.1037/met0000466.
164. Mansueto AC, Pan T, van Dessel P, Wiers RW. Ecological momentary assessment and personalized networks in cognitive bias modification studies on addiction: advances and challenges. J Exp Psychopathol. 2023;14:20438087231178124.
165. He L, Basar E, Wiers RW, Antheunis ML, Krahmer E. Can chatbots help to motivate smoking cessation? A study on the effectiveness of motivational interviewing on engagement and therapeutic alliance. BMC Public Health [Internet]. 2022;22:1–14. Available from: 10.1186/s12889-022-13115-x
166. Lewis M. Brain change in addiction as learning, not disease. N Engl J Med [Internet]. 2018;379:1551–60. Available from: www.nejm.org/doi/10.1056/NEJMra1602872
167. Grechuta K, Ballester BR, Espín Munne R, Molina Hervás B, Mohr B, Pulvermüller F, et al. Augmented sensorimotor dyadic therapy boosts recovery in patients with nonfluent aphasia: a randomised controlled trial. Stroke. 2019;50(5):1270–4.
168. Wiers RW, Verschure P. Curing the broken brain model of addiction: neurorehabilitation from a systems perspective. Addict Behav. 2020;106602.
169. Wiers RW, Verschure PFMJ. Curing the broken brain model of addiction: neurorehabilitation from a systems perspective. Addict Behav [Internet]. 2021;112:106602. Available from: 10.1016/j.addbeh.2020.106602
170. Malbos E, Borwell B, Einig-Iscain M, Korchia T, Cantalupi R, Boyer L, et al. Virtual reality cue exposure therapy for tobacco relapse prevention: a comparative study with standard intervention. Psychol Med. 2022;1–11.
171. Kazdin AE. Single-case experimental designs: evaluating interventions in research and clinical practice. Behav Res Ther [Internet]. 2019;117:3–17. Available from: 10.1016/j.brat.2018.11.015
172. Declercq L, Jamshidi L, Fernandez Castilla B, Moeyaert M, Beretvas SN, Ferron JM., Van den Noortgate W. Multilevel meta-analysis of individual participant data of single-case experimental designs: One-stage versus two-stage methods. Multivar. Behav. Res. 2022;57(2–3):298–317.
173. Fadardi JS, Cox WM. Reversing the sequence: reducing alcohol consumption by overcoming alcohol attentional bias. Drug Alcohol Depend. 2009;101:137–45.
174. Spruyt A, Laporte W, Boffo M, Herremans S, Impe P, Vercruysse I, et al. On the efficacy of cognitive bias modification training in alcohol-dependent inpatients: a double-blind, multi-site randomized control trial. Submitted.

9 Meat addiction?

Smartphones, fossil fuels and our future

My office phone calls. It is a documentary filmmaker. She introduces herself and then asks if I would like to participate in a documentary about her meat addiction. *Is this serious?*, I think. Definitely! She explains: she holds a firm belief that she should become vegan or at least vegetarian, because refraining from eating meat (and dairy) is one of the easiest things you can do to combat climate change. But it proved difficult in practice. For example, if she walks past the local butcher, and smells the chicken roasting on the spit her mouth waters and she is tempted to walk in to buy chicken. I recognized the problem, having been vegetarian myself for a while "without being too dogmatic", meaning that if I was invited to someone's house for dinner and they had meat on the menu, I wasn't going to make a fuss. Or, if I eat at a restaurant and really feel like eating meat, I'll have it and enjoy it. A friend summed up my version of vegetarianism as, "Reinout is vegetarian, except when he's eating."

I went over the criteria for addiction with the documentary maker and sure enough, she reported to have "meat cravings" (the title of the documentary later became *Craving for Meat*), but she wasn't socially dysfunctional because of her carnivorous tendencies, and she did not increasingly need more meat for the same effect. Thus, she did not pass the threshold for addiction by meeting two or more of the established criteria.

Could we scan her brain when she looked at meat? Sure, we could. And so, months later, I attended the premiere of *Craving for Meat* at an annual documentary festival, watching (with quite some embarrassment) my own laughing face on the giant screen. We were looking at the results of the documentary filmmaker's brain activity in response to meat versus other appetitive stimuli (our usual suspects, nice pictures of drinks, food, erotic couples). With a colleague, I was looking at the pretty colored fMRI pictures, and yes, the "reward centers" in her brain responded to pictures of meat—more strongly than to erotic pictures that more typically evoke this kind of brain response. But could we conclude that she was addicted to meat? No, it confirmed her craving for something she wanted to avoid, for

DOI: 10.4324/9781032634548-9

good reasons. After putting all the arguments together, which she did in the rest of the documentary, she had concluded that she did not want to eat meat anymore, and she was still craving it. That's not an addiction, that is a prototypical case of *akrasia*.

Meat addiction is not likely to be recognized as a real addiction, but what about "eating addiction"? That term has been used in recent years to explain the obesity crisis. There is no doubt there is one: in the US, the percentage of obese people has risen from 30% to over 40% in the past 20 years[1] (obesity is defined as a BMI over 30).[i] In the EU as a whole, this is about half the level of the US, with considerable differences between countries, with the Netherlands scoring relatively low at 13%.[2] However, also in this bike-country, as many as half of adults already score overweight (BMI higher than 25), including myself, and the majority of the rest of the middle aged population. Like our official addictions (smoking, alcohol, etc.), overweight and obesity carry huge health costs, including increased risk of cardiovascular disease, high blood pressure and type-2 diabetes. As with smoking, there is a clear link to difficult socioeconomic conditions (low education, poor neighborhood), in which both problems are relatively common, contributing strongly to the lower life expectancy of people in these conditions: in the Netherlands, someone with a low education lives on average six years shorter than someone with a high education, and the number of expected healthy life years is as much as 15 years shorter. Smoking is the main explanation for this difference and obesity and stress play an important role as well.

Should we therefore view excessive eating as an addiction? There are scientists who link eating addiction exclusively to a specific category of "ultra-processed foods" (highly manipulated foods with lots of artificial additives),[ii] which provide quick gratification in the short term and cravings in the longer term.[3] So while "meat addiction" is unlikely to become a common term, there are addiction-like aspects to snacking and eating junk food that likely play a role in the obesity crisis. Since obesity, like smoking, is common among poor people in the Western world, and especially in the US,[4] it is likely that it is also related to a lack of perspective, as with the aforementioned "deaths of despair" in the US, related to opiate addiction, depression, obesity and suicide.[4]

Obesity and related diseases are a major societal problem, like addictions, but that in itself does not prove that obesity is an addiction.

i BMI = body mass index = weight (in kg) ÷ height (in meters)^2.

ii Think of soft drinks, chocolate, candy, ice cream, processed meats, junk food and in more disguised forms in innocent-looking products with artificial sweeteners like some breads, yoghurts and so on.

Some proponents of the chronic brain disease model of addiction, including NIDA president Nora Volkow, have argued that this is justified because of similar changes in the brain in obese people compared to people with addictions to psychoactive substances.[5,6] This argument has subsequently also been used *against* the brain disease model of addiction, as previous neurobiological models of addiction that underpinned the brain disease model, indicated that addictive substances induce abnormally strong changes in specific brain mechanisms, much stronger than in more natural rewarders, such as sex and eating.[7] If this distinction is left, the question becomes what is special about addiction to substances, in comparison with engaging in other (short-term) rewarding activities, like eating, gambling and gaming. We can conclude that excessive eating has characteristics of addiction and of *akrasia*, without having to conclude that it is therefore a chronic brain disease.

One interesting finding in this comparison is that motivational interviewing, which has proven effective in addiction, is *not* effective in the treatment of obesity in adults,[8] nor in weight management in adolescents.[9] This suggests that in obesity, motivation is not the central problem, as is often the case in addictions to psychoactive substances, but acting in accordance with long-term goals is. Note that a more promising approach in young adolescents, discussed in Chapter 6, addressed core values of the adolescents and how they were manipulated by the junk food industry, for example by correcting the ads.[10]

What about other everyday behaviors? For example, does it make sense to talk about gaming, social media or smartphone addiction? The previous (fourth) edition of the American diagnostic determination guide of psychiatry, the *Diagnostic and Statistical Manual of Mental Disorders* (DSM), categorized addictions to psychoactive substances as "substance-related disorders", so gambling and other behavioral addictions could not be included. The DSM-5, introduced in 2013, moved gambling from impulse control disorders (in DSM-IV) to the category of "substance-related and addictive disorders". It was further recommended that more research be done on other non-drug-related addictive behaviors, such as excessive gaming and excessive sex, so that in the future it can be decided whether those behavioral problems can also be officially categorized as an addiction or not. Eating meat was not mentioned, but binge eating disorders are recognized under eating disorders in the DSM-5. In the alternative classification of the World Health Organization (WHO), the ICD-11 (*International Classification of Diseases*, 11th edition), gaming addiction is listed as the second non-commodity-related addiction (alongside gambling). The WHO committee ruled that there was sufficient evidence of negative effects of excessive gaming on other areas of life related to lack of exercise, poor sleep, and lack of real social contact outside the online world.

Relatedly, increasing discussions have been going on about smartphone addiction, especially in relation to excessive social media use. The smartphone, with access to the internet, can be used for a lot of behaviors that can get excessive, including gaming, gambling and watching porn. The difficulty is that the device is increasingly experienced as a necessary condition to navigate today's world, including literal navigation, one's agenda, notes, and other daily commodities. Therefore, when the use of one application becomes excessive (say a social media app), access is available every time one navigates, wants to make an appointment or order food. As the phone is so ubiquitous in today's life, we can become disorganized when our phone is gone; it has become a kind of extension of the body, maintaining contact with the outside world.[11] You can also endanger yourself and others by looking at your phone while in traffic: a quick message and BAM, an accident! In the case of the smartphone, it may make sense to speak of addiction, because excessive use can go at the expense of social contacts (but at the same time is also needed in many places for social contacts!), physical health, work, studies, hobbies—a similar list as can be made for excessive gaming, to which is added the direct danger to the person himself and to others when used in traffic. But does it make sense to talk about addiction to a multipurpose device, that is used by some primarily for social media, by others for navigation and oh yes, to call people. A comparison can be made to cigarette smoking: when cigarettes came on the market in the early twentieth century, as an easy and relatively cheap device to smoke tobacco, the prevalence of tobacco use disorders (and related diseases) went up quickly. Similarly, the availability of a handy portable device to use the internet on the go, makes for both handy applications (e.g., navigation, social contacts that extend into the offline world) and for applications with potential harms (gambling, passive social media use, games with addictive potential), available to large numbers of people, of whom some develop problematic use.

There is also evidence that intensive use of the phone changes our thinking: it makes us more restless and increasingly unable to concentrate on an activity, which is partly due to the constant switching that consumes a lot of mental energy. The journalist Johann Hari wrote a book about this topic, which is, like this one, probably too thick to read if you are constantly switching to reading messages on your phone in the meantime.[12] The author observed his godson Adam's inability to focus his attention because he was constantly on his phone. Hari figured it would be nice to get him out of this routine by doing something fun with him in the real world and he decided to take him to Graceland, the home of his godson's old love Elvis Presley. Upon arrival, they were given an iPad to accompany the tour, which meant they were once again looking at a screen, and, not surprisingly, Adam quickly preferred his own screen. Hari decided to write a book about the phenomenon, for which he interviewed experts around the world about attention in relation to phone use. He came to the conclusion that there is a crisis going on, an attention crisis; our attention is constantly being hijacked by the phone, and it takes us a lot of time and energy to bring that attention back to where we were when we take a quick look at some messages in between, which is accompanied by mentally exhausting switch-costs, making it difficult to concentrate on anything for long.

This conclusion in the context of this book raises a question: to what extent should these *smartphone-induced* changes in the brain be understood as a *chronic* brain disease or as a temporary problem that can be remedied by abstinence. Hari decided to put it to the test and did a "phone detox" for months, after which he noticed that his ability to concentrate improved again. A few months later, back in the "normal" world, his screen use quickly went back to its old level, with the additional negative effects on his attention.

Many adults still have something to long back to: I remember being engrossed in a book for whole days, being absorbed and forgetting the world around me, because I had moved to the world of the Three Musketeers, while reading. Hari had to think back to that time, when he spent some time in phone detox and was able to read long books again. This suggests a reversable mode of thinking that can be reversed with simple measures like switching back to a dumb phone without internet, as some hipsters and former Dutch prime minister Rutte did, or put the phone on silent or off if you want to work with concentration. Hari suggests a locker with a time lock, so you can't access your phone for a preset time. But will you do this when you do not have the previous experience of being absorbed in a book, to pine for?

At this point there is the risk of a one-sided gloomy perspective about youth in a digital world. Computer games require a lot of concentration and skill, and there is some evidence that they can have a positive effects on development.[13] The fantasy world of a game may be the current equivalent of wandering about in the parallel world of a novel or movie. For older folks like me, who did not experience this, the contemporary novel "tomorrow, tomorrow and tomorrow" by Gabrielle Zavin, provides a nice perspective on the creative and artistic side of gaming and game design. And maybe games can help us to envision how our choices now affect the future, as an aid in "episodic future thinking", which has shown to be a means against myopic choices in addiction,[14] with potential promise for other choices that affect the future, not only of the individual but also of mankind.

On a more general note, an important part of today's adolescents world is digital, which holds risks for mental health, especially excessive use of social media,[15,16] although it should be noted that this relationship is not strong, suggesting that excessive media use alone cannot be held responsible for the increase in mental health problems in youth.[17,18] The fact that most adolescents partly live in a digital world nowadays also creates opportunities for just-in-time interventions in adolescents and potentially to stimulate healthy trajectories for mental and physical health. One measure is to teach healthy engagement in social media, and more general preventive measures can be taken, such as helping to develop technology literacy and digital self-regulation skills during adolescence.[19] The optimal window of opportunity for creating healthy habits, both offline and online, appears to be early adolescence (around the onset of puberty), in which emerging adolescents become more tuned toward their peers, while at least sometimes still considering adult advise.[19,20] It also happens to be the period in which many adolescents get their first smartphone. It would appear wise to develop rules for use together with the emerging adolescent, for example, leaving the phone in the living room and not take it to the bedroom at night, because of the interference with sleep, which is very important in this developmental stage.[iii] Importantly, given the increased need for respect in adolescence, this should not be one-sided rule-setting, but rather respectfully helping the adolescent with their own goals (partnering rather than one-sided rule setting). Ideally, if this is coordinated through school and many families participate, the social norm is changed, because unplugging from social media becomes difficult when others are still (thought to be) online.

Akrasia and climate change

The most important global problem right now is arguably the climate crisis, assuming that mankind is smart enough to not cause a nuclear catastrophe. What does this have to do with *akrasia* and addiction? For one thing, it is sometimes stated that we are addicted to fossil fuels, which would be a similar case as the meat addiction of the documentary maker. I think both are better seen as cases of *akrasia*. There is no denying that the climate crisis is influenced by our everyday choices, such as flying and eating meat. Alarming reports follow one another in rapid succession. The latest, 6th Intergovernmental Panel on Climate Change (IPCC) report[21] addressed not only climate change, but also related

iii Unless an app is used that may help against sleep problems, as has been developed in the cognitive bias modification literature,[33] but it might be handier to use a non-digital interventions for this purpose, for example using cognitive behavioral and mindfulness techniques, including savoring positive moments of the day before falling asleep, that have been shown to be effective in improving adolescent sleep, without the phone.[34–36] human-caused scourges, such as rapidly deteriorating biodiversity: animal and plant species become extinct at an accelerating rate. In the report, scientific experts from all countries involved conclude that human-caused climate change is already underway and is causing extreme weather and loss of species around the globe.

Climate change also leads to the loss of human life, which for now is mostly in the southern hemisphere.[22] This is tragic, especially for the global south, because the vast majority of emissions that have given rise to climate change have been caused in the northern hemisphere (historically mostly by the US and Europe; in terms of current emissions, China tops the list), and the worst effects now hit the global South.[23] In Somalia, for example, great droughts occasionally occurred that, like storms in the US, were given names and caused so much misery that they stayed with people for a long time. The great drought is now so permanent that names are no longer given. Most of the livestock have died and farmers have fled the barren plains.

In Europe, extreme temperatures, drought, alternate with torrential rains and forest fires, have all been attributed to climate change. Warm areas can develop into deserts, such as the interior of Spain. More than half of the ice on Switzerland's glaciers has now melted away and all are expected to disappear in the course of this century. These effects occur at the current global temperature increase of approximately 1° Celsius. The effects at increases of 1.5° and 2° Celsius will be even more devastating, not only for areas in the global South, but also for coastal cities worldwide, threating Amsterdam and "New Amsterdam" (New York) alike.

I live close to the coast myself, but nothing in the area indicates an impending disaster, even though much of the area is barely above sea level. The urgency to confront it seems to be hardly felt, if at all. After two years of COVID misery, we were again "entitled" to fly to warmer climates, even though most people know that flying is an activity that contributes greatly to the climate crisis, not only because of the exhausted CO_2, but even more so because they are emitted at high altitudes in vulnerable parts of the atmosphere. This is a typical case of *akrasia*: when we put all arguments together, it is clear that we should not fly, and yet we do it. One difficulty is that relevant choices are made in a social context. When you are convinced that you should not fly because of environmental impacts, but all the people around you do, what do you do? Tellingly, at the moment flying is not so much perceived as a problem, as the fact that it is so crowded at airports.

Because the climate is a complex system, feedback mechanisms can amplify changes and "points of no return" can be reached, after which, for example, the melting of the ice caps becomes unstoppable, even in the unlikely event that we are successful in reducing CO_2 emissions rapidly (so far, they have only grown). An example of such a feedback mechanism can now be seen in Siberia and northern Canada, where thawing permafrost areas are causing methane emissions, which have an even stronger greenhouse gas effect than CO_2. This causes additional warming, which in turn will release more methane. Much of the heat is still absorbed by oceans, making them more acidic, which leads to coral degradation and mass mortality of marine animals. At a certain level of acidity, heat absorption reaches its maximum, after which temperature rise will accelerate, and the summer of 2023 has witnessed signs of this, with ocean temperatures going "off the charts" (no longer in the range of normal variability).[24] Human responses to rising temperatures can also cause a further rise: it is estimated that increasing use of air conditioning (omnipresent already in the US and middle east, increasingly so in heating-up Europe) will cause an additional half-degree rise in temperature.[25] Clearly, we are in the midst of a global crisis where the question is whether it can still be redirected, or whether we will see the "doomed-to-extinction solution" of the Fermi paradox (from Chapter 2) play out before our eyes: we won't find intelligent life on other planets because always one species will evolve that will dominate the rest, leading to mass extinction. Is there anything more we can do to avert this fate?

What can we do?

Akrasia and our daily choices are thus relevant not only in relation to addiction, but also for our future. What can we do? On a daily basis, we all face *akrasia* issues. As individuals, we make choices that often come down to short-term pleasure versus alternative choices that come with less immediate pleasure, but provide better outcomes in the longer term, for ourselves, our children and grandchildren, and for the planet: whether it's Martin's cigarette, eating meat, taking a sun vacation by plane versus the relevant alternatives like eating a carrot with hummus or do a bike holiday. If we all continue to consume more and more, we will make our earth uninhabitable for ourselves, making the scientific name of our species, *homo sapiens*, ironic.

Like the addict, we have to become aware of our akrasia problems and make wiser choices for the future. As for the addict, the way out of the treadmill of overconsumption is to pause and consider the long-term consequences: where do we want to go, what do we consider important in the long run? Such considerations require concentration, which should not be interrupted by digital distractions. Perhaps meditation can help, not only in overcoming addiction but also in choosing solutions in our daily decisions that are consistent with our long-term goals.

The good news is that we can indeed do something about these threats ourselves, and as we do it with several people at once, it has a substantially greater effect. Let's start with the daily business of eating.

The scientific journal *Lancet* had a scientific team of top international researchers from various disciplines determine the optimal diet both for the health of the individual and for the planet.[26] Briefly, the diet boils down to a mostly vegan diet, with occasional dairy and meat or fish if desired, and few *ultra-processed* foods. Basically, just cook like grandma did (indeed, my grandma made everything herself, including a wonderful mayonnaise, and categorically refused to eat anything from a jar). This diet is not complicated: as with alcohol, you can opt for total abstinence and become vegetarian or vegan, or for moderation and eat meat or fish only occasionally during the weekend, for example, which made this diet far more palatable in my own family than total vegetarianism. We have been following this rule for several years now, which has reduced our meat consumption by more than half, compared to the years before. The nice thing is that the diet is not dogmatic—if you still like to eat meat or fish occasionally, fine, but no more than once a week—and meanwhile you contribute to a better future for the planet and for yourself (this diet is healthier than eating meat every day, as the Lancet experts made clear). Furthermore, there is also something nice about making the eating of meat a special exception, as it was during most of our history: it used to be something for special occasions, rather than daily fare.

The same goes for alcohol and other drugs: get out the habit and apply a simple rule to it that is easy to follow, for example, not to drink during weekdays (or smoke marijuana, or whatever you do when you know you really shouldn't do it if you put all the arguments together). Many people benefit from participating in challenges like "Dry January" (voluntary abstinence for a month) or "Stoptober", a campaign to quit smoking in October. While most heavy drinkers can cut down their drinking in January or more in general, using simple rules, this appears to be harder for cigarette smoking: few people are able to smoke from time to time without escalating. A recent study on "stable intermediate states" (use without becoming addicted) for various substances showed that for smoking, the vast majority ends up in either tobacco addiction or quitting altogether.[27] And the *smartphone*? Because we use the device for so many things, total abstinence becomes difficult (if not impossible) in today's world, and controlled use is probably the best option for most. At least don't use it in traffic and if possible don't have a phone nearby if you want to work with concentration.

Parents I would recommend setting clear rules, but at the same time discuss underlying values, especially in (emerging) adolescence. As we saw, this has a positive effect on alcohol consumption: setting a clear rule that no alcohol can be drunk before a certain age has a protective effect, but only if this is done before the children have started drinking and the reason is explained. The difficulty is again the social context: our rule of not getting a phone before secondary education (in the Netherlands at age 12) worked fine for the oldest two, but proved to be a dead end for our youngest at age 9, when she turned out to be the only child without a smartphone, which excluded her from her peers, because all appointments were organized with WhatsApp. We provided her with my old phone (great excuse to buy a new one), with rules about usage, like not taking a phone upstairs at night. See for further guidelines a recent handbook of adolescent digital media use and mental health.[28]

As mentioned, the alcohol research also yielded another interesting finding, related to *akrasia*: if you impose rules on children, such as not drinking until a certain age, it was shown to have a positive effect on the development of their self-control. Importantly, that was only the case in the combined condition, where the children themselves had also learned about the reasons to not start drinking at an early age, not in the parent-only intervention, when the adolescents would possibly regard the rule-setting by the parents as disrespectful. When adolescent and parent agree on the need for certain rules, it may help them to later also set rules for themselves that are in line with their long-term goals. This has been related to predictable circumstances being positive for the development of self-control and goal-directed action.[29] In a predictable environment, the predictive brain can develop optimally. That can help them later to deal with *akrasia problems*, whether it's not eating meat during the week (even though it smells so good!), not flying—unless strictly necessary—or not smoking and not drinking alcohol during the week, in view of long-term goals.

Growth and change

The things we can do ourselves, as outlined above, are important, but of course we are part of a larger system. When it comes to saving the planet as a habitable place for humans, experts agree that a systems change is necessary, along with individuals changing, and the two can reinforce each other.[22] There are two visions of how to achieve this: *degrowth* and *low-carbon growth.* Jason Hickel wrote the interesting book *Less Is More: How Degrowth Will Save the World.*[23] He described the capitalist model of economic growth as the fundamental cause of the climate crisis, an analysis endorsed not only by climate activists, but also several influential economists.[iv] The point is that growth leads to exponential

iv For example, by Herman Daly, former World Bank economist and winner of the Right Livelihood Award, and by Abhijit Banerjee and Esther Duflo, who won the "Nobel Prize" in economics ("the Sveriges Riksbank Prize in Economic Sciences in Memory of Alfred Nobel"). Note that this perspective echoes some older perspectives, from the 1970s and 1980s, including the limits of growth from the Club of Rome (1972), "small is beautiful" from Schumacher (1973) and the *Turning Point* by Fritjof Capra (1982).

increases in use of resources and greenhouse gas emissions, in addition to the self-reinforcing effects that the initiated climate crisis has on the complex system. A model assuming 3% economic growth per year sounds perfectly reasonable, if not on the modest side. What we easily forget is that this is exponential growth (growth upon growth), which means that the size of the economy doubles in 23 years. In short, it is all too human to underestimate exponential growth.

Hickel tells an old fable from India, about a king who wanted to reward a sage who had defeated him at chess. The king asked what the sage would like as a reward. I am a modest man, the sage replied, one grain of rice on the first square of the chessboard is enough, and then double on the next square and so on, until the chessboard is full. Sounds reasonable, doesn't it? The king laughed and agreed. At the end of the first row, there were less than two hundred grains on the board, not yet enough for a meal. But after that, the king's laughter wore off and the exponential growth made itself felt, because halfway through the plate, there had to be more than 2 trillion grains of rice, which would bankrupt him. By the 64th square, it would be enough rice to cover all of India with a meter of rice.

The current exponential growth is starting to get out of control, as we are now seeing in the climate crisis. When I became aware of environmental issues in the 1980s, at a global level we were just at a level of consumption that could be sustainable, where of course the distribution was totally uneven and inhabitants of the Western world were already way above that level. Now we are at double that level. In the fable of the chessboard, this is the doubling that already requires more rice than the kingdom has. Yet we continue to assume "healthy" economic growth, which begs the question: is this sustainable?

In poor countries it is obvious: the prosperity and well-being of the inhabitants then increase, but this relationship ends very quickly. In richer countries the same relationship does not exist; indeed, it seems that further growth in the economy will actually come at the expense of the well-being of the vast majority of the world's population. Life expectancy and perceived happiness are greater today in Costa Rica and Portugal than in the US, where per capita income is much higher: in the US, average income has doubled since 1970. Has that improved the lives of Americans? No, at the population level, the opposite has happened: more people live below the poverty line and average wages have lagged behind inflation, so many people have to work multiple jobs to survive. Profits have gone mostly to the very richest 1% of the population, and among that group there is no relationship between wealth and life happiness (this relationship holds only in the poor). Thus, economic growth in America has gone hand in hand with an average *decline* in residents' well-being. An important factor here is perceived injustice: the greater the inequality in wealth in a country, the greater the mental problems, such as depression, addiction and deaths of despair.

The solution is clear (from the *degrowth perspective*): when we leave behind the dogma of economic growth, invest in general services and reduce inequality, the result is greater well-being and preservation of the planet. Costa Rica has shown that this can be done: there, welfare and average lifespan increased in the 1980s, without economic growth. What did it do to achieve this? Invest in health care and education during that time. Unfortunately, in some countries—such as the Netherlands and the US—environmentalism is associated with liberal politics, while the preservation of a livable planet should be of paramount importance to all. In politics, it is often difficult to get the necessary things done, as these often imply economic offers (or less growth) in the short run, while gains in terms of welfare often come later, well beyond the next election. An alternative is to force governments to take the necessary actions through the law. For example, the Dutch state was successfully sued by the legal Urgenda foundation because it endorsed international agreements to limit greenhouse gas emissions, without taking sufficient action (as many countries do). The court concluded that this negligence puts residents at risk and forced the government to take action, and this showcase has been followed in other European countries and Brazil. A related legal strategy can be to recognize natural areas as legal entities, as New Zealand has done. More countries are trying to secure the rights of nature in this way, against the relentless expansionism of growth-driven economics.

The other side in this debate argues that *degrowth* is a fiction because humans have a natural tendency to want to grow, hence degrowth would imply a return to communism, which has been shown to fail. However, economic growth so far has often been at the expense of the earth, and this must change; low-carbon varieties of growth must be developed stimulated.[30] This also requires changing the human diet (in line with the aforementioned *Lancet diet*) and investing in technological alternatives, from cultured meat to shared cars—according to Diederik Samson, former *de-growther*, who is now supporting the European Commission in the EU's green transition, the "Green Deal".[30] A discussion of these positions revealed that many of the proposed measures (reducing meat consumption, taxing kerosine to reduce flying, reusing more and throwing away less) are espoused by both sides of the debate. The point of dispute is whether the necessary changes can also be achieved in the context of economic growth.

According to Hickel, it is a utopia to continue to grow economically and still avert the doom of our future on earth. Furthermore, it is extremely risky to tie our fate to technological innovation that promise to lead to decreases in greenhouse gases in the future. The problem is that it is likely that a point of no return has been reached before, after which further changes cannot be stopped, even if a technological solution would work. As I am finishing this book, the Greenland ice sheet has been reported to perhaps already have reached such a *point of no return*. If that is true, it implies that even in the unlikely case that we stop emitting greenhouse gases today, the melting of Greenland's glaciers will continue, which will result in a sea level rise of at least 28 centimeters. This is peanuts compared with the "Doomsday glacier" in Antarctica, Thwaites (the size of Florida), that appears to be close to reaching that point, but is still "hanging on by its fingernails". When that glacier reaches the point of *no return*, its nickname will make sense: for now, it still forms a buffer between the huge ice sheet of western Antarctica and the warmer seas, which after melting could cause a seawater rise of meters.

Climate scientists have been warning for years that it is 2 to 12; the problem is that the urgency has not yet dawned on us in everyday life. We don't see the seawater rise as we walk along the beach and hope it will be okay. Much like the smoker who realizes smoking jeopardizes future health, but is not quite ready for action yet. Others embrace fake news that denies or trivializes the climate crisis, symbolized by stickers I saw the other day on my way to the beach affixed to two water-scooters on a trailer behind a gas-guzzling hummer: *F*ck Greta*. However, on a more positive note, research shows that most people do care about climate change, and would be willing to take action, if that is facilitated.[22]

Assuming this analysis is correct, how can we achieve this? In a democracy, parties affected by the measures (such as currently farmers in the Netherlands) will resist, supported by populist parties. Do we need a dictator to put an end to the dogma of unbridled growth? Or can it be achieved democratically? Maybe science can teach us something here: an experiment published in *Nature* examined how people make decisions about limited natural resources when asked to consider future generations. Most people (about two-thirds) took future generations into account in their decisions, even if it meant less spending space in the short term. But a sizeable minority did not, which ultimately still resulted in depletion of limited resources and undermining the motivation of the majority. A key finding of this study was that this problem disappeared when participants engaged in democratic deliberation about how to conserve resources for future generations.[31] Under these circumstances, restrictions on extraction were implemented with almost unanimous support. This is encouraging and is consistent with Plato's views on *akrasia*, as described in Chapter 2: people eventually agree on what is the right thing to do, when well informed, and are then willing to act upon it.

This was an academic experiment, would this also work in the real world? In France a citizens' forum was set up as a real-life experiment, including 150 "ordinary" people, chosen by lot with some stratification, to make sure different social classes and regions were represented. Their task was to consider environmental problems and possible measures. While in France about a third of the electorate tends to vote for radical right-wing parties, which generally have little interest in environmental measures, the citizens' forum unanimously came up with a whole palette of such measures, such as lowering the speed limit on highways from 130 to 110 km per hour and the end of the combustion engine by 2025. Unfortunately, after the report had been presented to the president and parliament, these considered the agreed upon measures as *suggestions* and largely overruled them. This is considered as a one of the reasons why the margin between President Macron and his far right opponent Le Pen was significantly smaller, in his second election: ignoring the citizens' forum's proposals on the environment was perceived by many as a slap in the face of democracy.

In the Netherlands, Wilders's right extremist party has become the biggest in the most recent elections, in November 2023, with some 25% of the votes, but his anti-environmental and anti-immigration stances will be watered down through the necessary process of coalition formation. And the Netherlands are a relatively small player internationally. A major political threat for climate change at the time of writing concerns the next American election, where climate change sceptic and anti-democrat Trump could be reelected and undo the positive climate actions initiated by President Biden.

Nevertheless, both the academic and the French experiment on citizen's forums (and a successful Irish one as well) can give us some hope: when you talk to people about the future of the planet, and that of our children and grandchildren, the vast majority are prepared to take measures, even if they are unpleasant in the short term (eating limited amounts of meat, not flying unless absolutely necessary, etc.). Citizens' forums can play a role in the necessary changes, but then the results must be taken seriously, otherwise it is counterproductive and the outcome undermines trust in democracy.[32] As a final note of hope, in January 2024, heiress Marlene Engelhorn, a descendant of the founder of German chemical company BASF, inherited 25 millions and did not agree with the lack of taxation of her acquired fortune. She decided to give it all away and to install a committee of 50 random Austrians to decide the best purposes for the money.

Look at the future and act on it

When you give an addicted person a choice between a clean future or continuing the addiction, the vast majority will choose the clean future—perhaps with occasional use of their favorite poison, if possible—but surely an ending of the yoke of addiction. We also know that this is not easy: kicking the habit, finding alternative rewards, building a different life. But it is possible, because we are capable of imagining another life and allowing our behavior to be influenced to some extent by our imagination, even when temptations are at our fingertips. In those difficult situations, it helps if we know what to do to hold on to the clean picture of the future.

Hence, this is our situation: it is clear that we must change our behavior if we want to preserve a livable earth for the future. We ourselves can make important choices with an eye to the future, and we can get politicians to do so, by implementing effective measures: think (electric) shared cars, forcing manufacturers to make sustainable products (the growth model rewards manufacturing cheap products with a short lifespan, but you could change this by obliging manufacturers by law to repair broken products), banning advertisements that create artificial needs that are not congruent with our goals as people who want to preserve a livable planet (e.g., ban advertisements for airplane holidays like those for cigarettes). Because we can imagine a future other than one in which we ruin ourselves, and because we can adjust our behavior based on such a depiction, there is hope.

Perhaps surprisingly, "hope" was one of the *plagues* that escaped from Pandora's box from Greek mythology. Hope is often considered as a positive quality, of course, but sometimes hope for normality (everything stays the same), or for a magical solution in the future, can get in the way of acting appropriately while this is still possible. Hence, hope needs to be accompanied by action, not by fantasies that everything will be all right without taking action. In doing so, we have to give future generations and young people an important voice so that the discussion is in the perspective of actions for the future. That is the only way to overcome our *akrasia* problems and survive.

References

1. Hales CM, Carroll MD, Fryar CD, Ogden CL. Prevalence of obesity and severe obesity among adults: United States, 2017–2018. NCHS Data Brief. 2020;1–8.
2. Eurostat. Overweight and obesity: BMI characteristics [Internet]. 2020. Available from: https://ec.europa.eu/eurostat/statistics-explained/index.php?title=Overweight_and_obesity_-_BMI_statistics#Obesity_in_the_EU:_gender_differences
3. Schulte EM, Chao AM, Allison KC. Advances in the neurobiology of food addiction. Curr Behav Neurosci Reports. 2021;8:103–12.
4. Sterling P, Platt ML. Why deaths of despair are increasing in the US and not other industrial nations—insights from neuroscience and anthropology. JAMA Psychiatry. 2022;79(4):368–74.

5. Volkow ND, Wang GJ, Tomasi D, Baler RD. Obesity and addiction: neurobiological overlaps. Obes Rev. 2013;14:2–18.
6. Volkow ND, Baler RD. NOW vs LATER brain circuits: implications for obesity and addiction. Trends Neurosci [Internet]. 2015;38:345–52. Available from: 10.1016/j.tins.2015.04.002
7. Heather N, Best D, Kawalek A, Field M, Lewis M, Rotgers F, et al. Challenging the brain disease model of addiction: European launch of the addiction theory network. Addict Res Theory [Internet]. 2018;26:249–55. Available from: 10.1080/16066359.2017.1399659
8. Makin H, Chisholm A, Fallon V, Goodwin L. Use of motivational interviewing in behavioural interventions among adults with obesity: a systematic review and meta-analysis. Clin Obes. 2021;11.
9. Amiri P, Mansouri-Tehrani MM, Khalili-Chelik A, Karimi M, Jalali-Farahani S, Amouzegar A, et al. Does motivational interviewing improve the weight management process in adolescents? A systematic review and meta-analysis. Int J Behav Med [Internet]. 2022;29:78–103. Available from: 10.1007/s12529-021-09994-w
10. Bryan CJ, Yeager DS, Hinojosa CP. A values-alignment intervention protects adolescents from the effects of food marketing. Nat Hum Behav [Internet]. 2019;3:596–603. Available from: 10.1038/s41562-019-0586-6
11. Larsen H, Wiers RW, Su S, Cousijn J. Excessive smartphone use and addiction: when harms start outweighing benefits. Addiction. 2023;118:586–8.
12. Hari J. Stolen focus: why you can't pay attention. London: Bloomsbury; 2022. Extract available from: www.theguardian.com/science/2022/jan/02/attention-span-focus-screens-apps-smartphones-social-media
13. Granic I, Lobel A, Engels RCME. The benefits of playing video games. 2014;69:66–78.
14. Bickel WK, Freitas R, Jeremy L, Quddos F, Fontes RM, Barbosa B, et al. Episodic future thinking as a promising intervention for substance use disorders: a reinforcer pathology perspective. Curr Addict Reports [Internet]. 2023; Available from: 10.1007/s40429-023-00498-z
15. Bollen J, Gonçalves B, van de Leemput I, Ruan G. The happiness paradox: your friends are happier than you. EPJ Data Sci [Internet]. 2017;6:1–10. Available from: 10.1140/epjds/s13688-017-0100-1
16. Su S, Larsen H, Cousijn J, Wiers RW, Van Den Eijnden RJJM. Problematic smartphone use and the quantity and quality of peer engagement among adolescents: a longitudinal study. Comput Human Behav [Internet]. 2022;126:107025. Available from: 10.1016/j.chb.2021.107025
17. Orben A, Przybylski AK. The association between adolescent well-being and digital technology use. Nat Hum Behav [Internet]. 2019;3:173–82. Available from: 10.1038/s41562-018-0506-1
18. Rodriguez M, Aalbers G, McNally RJ. Idiographic network models of social media use and depression symptoms. Cognit Ther Res [Internet]. 2022;46:124–32. Available from: 10.1007/s10608-021-10236-2
19. Giovanelli A, Ozer EM, Dahl RE. Leveraging technology to improve health in adolescence: a developmental science perspective. J Adolesc Heal [Internet]. 2020;67:S7–S13. Available from: 10.1016/j.jadohealth.2020.02.020
20. Dahl RE, Allen NB, Wilbrecht L, Suleiman AB. Importance of investing in adolescence from a developmental science perspective. Nature [Internet]. 2018;554:441–50. Available from: 10.1038/nature25770

21. Pörtner HO, Roberts DC, Adams H, Adler C, Aldunce P, Ali E, et al. Climate change 2022: impacts, adaptation and vulnerability [Internet]. IPCC; 2022. Available from: www.ipcc.ch/report/ar6/wg2/
22. Steg L. Psychology of climate change. Annu Rev Psychol. 2023;74:391–421.
23. Hickel J. Less is more: how degrowth will save the world. Dublin: Penguin Random House; 2020.
24. Institute CC. Climate reanalyzer [Internet]. 2023 [cited 2023 Oct 2]. Available from: https://climatereanalyzer.org/clim/sst_daily/
25. Luttikhuis P. Airco's zijn blinde vlekken in het energiedebat. Men schaft ze aan, maar ze dragen bij aan het probleem. NRC [Internet]. 2022; Available from: www.nrc.nl/nieuws/2022/07/15/de-wereld-kan-niet-meer-zonder-aircos-straks-zijn-er-45-miljard-a4136553
26. Willett W, Rockström J, Loken B, Springmann M, Lang T, Vermeulen S, et al. Food in the Anthropocene: the EAT–Lancet Commission on healthy diets from sustainable food systems. 2019;6736:1–47.
27. Epskamp S, Maas HLJ Van Der, Peterson RE, Van HM, Aggen SH, Kendler KS. Intermediate stable states in substance use. Addict Behav [Internet]. 2022;107252. Available from: 10.1016/j.addbeh.2022.107252
28. Nesi J, Telzer EH, Prinstein MJ. Handbook of adolescent digital media use and mental health. Cambridge University Press; 2022.
29. Munakata Y, Placido D, Zhuang W. What's next? Advances and challenges in understanding how environmental predictability shapes the development of cognitive control. Curr Dir Psychol Sci. 2023;32(6). 10.1177/09637214231199102
30. Stellinga M. Wordt het krimpen voor het klimaat, of groen groeien? 2022. Available from: www.nrc.nl/nieuws/2022/06/24/wordt-het-krimpen-voor-het-klimaat-of-groen-groeien-a4134587
31. Hauser OP, Rand DG, Peysakhovich A, Nowak MA. Cooperating with the future. Nature [Internet]. 2014;511:220–3. Available from: 10.1038/nature13530
32. Rovers E. Nu is het aan ons. De Correspondent, editor. Amsterdam; 2022.
33. Clarke PJF, Bedford K, Notebaert L, Bucks RS, Rudaizky D, Milkins BC, et al. Assessing the therapeutic potential of targeted attentional bias modification for insomnia using smartphone delivery. Psychother Psychosom. 2016; 85:187–9.
34. Blake M, Waloszek JM, Schwartz O, Raniti M, Simmons JG, Blake L, et al. The SENSE study: post intervention effects of a randomized controlled trial of a cognitive-behavioral and mindfulness-based group sleep improvement intervention among at-risk adolescents. J Consult Clin Psychol. 2016; 84:1039–51.
35. McMakin DL, Ricketts EJ, Forbes EE, Silk JS, Ladouceur CD, Siegle GJ, et al. Anxiety treatment and targeted sleep enhancement to address sleep disturbance in pre/early adolescents with anxiety. J Clin Child Adolesc Psychol [Internet]. 2019;48:S284–97. Available from: 10.1080/15374416.2018.1463534
36. Blake MJ, Sheeber LB, Youssef GJ, Raniti MB, Allen NB. Systematic review and meta-analysis of adolescent cognitive–behavioral sleep interventions. Clin Child Fam Psychol Rev. 2017;20:227–49.

10 Conclusions and lessons

Akrasia is a concept from classical Greek philosophy that stands for making a choice against better judgment. You consider all pros and cons of different choices and subsequently do *not* pick the optimal choice. Plato introduced *akrasia* and concluded that it is not possible to choose against your own well considered preferences. The corollary of this view is that addiction does not exist: the chronic drunk drinks because of a strong liking of liquor, which was the general opinion until the early nineteenth century. This corresponds to the moral model of addiction: the drunk chooses to drink too much and is therefore solely responsible for the consequences.

In the early nineteenth century, the concept of addiction was introduced, related to the disease model: after frequent excessive use, people could lose control over their drinking or drug use (opium eating, for example, at the time). Addiction thus became a disease, a disease of the will. The only cure was total abstinence. This vision is at the roots of the AA self-help movement and the current biomedical perspective on addiction as a chronic *brain* disease, which was the latest variety of the disease model, that developed in the decade of the brain.

In recent years, there has been increasing criticism of the idea that addiction should be seen as a chronic brain disease. This is because most people get over their addiction, and most do so without help, which is not true of progressive brain diseases such as dementia or Parkinson's. Further, the fact that there are brain changes associated with addiction in itself does not prove that it is a brain disease: this is always the case when we learn new motivationally salient things. The evidence that the brain permanently changes and that those changes cause addiction to persist is based primarily on research in laboratory animals, of which the value for understanding addiction in humans has been questioned. One reason is that when laboratory animals have a social alternative, the large majority prefers that to an addictive drug, even when they have been made drug-dependent. Furthermore, people can radically change course based on a

DOI: 10.4324/9781032634548-10

vision of the future, which appears to be an essential feature that cannot be captured well in animal models.

This is not to say that the brain does not change in addiction or that these neuroadaptations are not important. They are true and explain important aspects of addictions, such as continuing despite good reasons to quit, in which a sensitized responses to cues predicting the opportunity to engage in the addictive behavior play an important role, which become motivational magnets and induce craving. In addition, escaping from negative aftereffects of the addictive behavior often plays a role, as does habit formation. These motivational mechanisms are shared with many other animals and clearly play a role in addiction, but they are not the whole story in addiction in humans.

In addition to the question of the extent to which the model of addiction as a chronic brain disease is supported by science (which can be debated), there is the question of its effect on the people it affects: the person who is addicted, loved ones and treatment providers. The contention was that the disease model would result in treatment rather than incarceration, as the result of the changed perspective from a morally evil person who chooses to be addicted, to a patient suffering from a chronic brain disease. However, research has shown that the effect of this change in perspective is not only positive: when people adhere to the brain disease model, addicted people are indeed blamed less for their addiction, but they are also stigmatized more, and seen as fundamentally different from normal people, even more than people with other psychiatric disorders, from whom it is also better to stay away. This attitude also undermines confidence in the outcome of treatment (once addicted is always addicted), both on the side of the addicted people themselves and by the people treating them.

The perspective of addiction as a chronic brain disease may hold true for a small group of severely addicted people who, despite repeated attempts, are unable to discontinue their addiction. This was the rationale behind the medical heroin dispensing project, which reduced use as well as stress in the chronically addicted participants, and improved their lives. In these exceptional cases it may also help to accept the diagnosis of a chronic addiction rather than despair about it, but for the vast majority of addicted people the image of people with chronic brain disease is neither justified nor useful.

An alternative has been developed in recent years, which amounts to addiction being characterized by *biased choice*. According to this perspective, we make decisions based on predictions of the consequences of our actions ("whatever's next"), and this process can be influenced by therapy and by varieties of cognitive training, either computerized or in the form of mindfulness meditation.

This view recognizes that it makes sense to acknowledge (some degree of) free will, unlike what some neuroscientists have led us to believe in recent years. With our imagination, generated by our brain (the ultimate VR prediction machine), we influence our decisions. This fragile and energy-guzzling system gave evolutionary advantage (at least in the short term), which is hard to imagine for a system that only makes up reasons for previous unconscious choices in hindsight.

"Free will" is an important concept at the psychological level, just like money and love. It cannot be reduced one-to-one to underlying processes, which does not detract from reality at the psychological level. To say that free will is only brain-functioning and therefore does not exist can be compared to saying that money is only paper or love is only biochemistry.

Free will can be compared to sailing. We experience that we can steer as in a motorboat, turning the rudder all the way around at will and even moving backwards, but this turns out to be untrue: free will has limitations; sometimes other factors determine our behavior. Nor is it the case that free will is merely the vane that indicates where we are sailing, with no effect on the actual course (the neuro-reductionist view). We can focus on a point on the horizon and head for it, if we have learned how to sail. This implies that sometimes you cannot go straight to your goal, but must cross to reach it and that is something you need to learn.

The fact that we can resist temptations and make choices that are beneficial in the longer term, while in the short-term leading to less pleasure or more pain, is a sign of free will, made possible by our imagination.

Language has added a rich dimension to our ability to imagine, allowing us to color our VR world, for better or for worse. For example, under the influence of propaganda, we can learn to view certain groups of people as vermin, as the Nazis have shown in history. The other side of the same coin is that these abilities also enable us to imagine ourselves in a different future and act accordingly, for example, when we want to stop an addiction or radically change our behavior to save the earth.

Regarding addiction, change begins with an image of a different future, which provides motivation to change. This can come about in a variety of ways: through a dramatic event (the smoking father who sees his children standing in the rain in his rearview mirror as he drives off to get cigarettes), with the help of motivational interviewing, through seeing divine light (like Bill Wilson, before he founded AA), through mindfulness meditation, or perhaps a psychedelic drug. Once people are motivated to change, there are a variety of techniques that can be helpful in enacting the change, such as cognitive behavioral therapy, self-help groups, medication and meditation.

Furthermore, rewards can help, especially when used in a social context, and various cognitive training programs have been developed that reduce the likelihood of relapse when added to abstinence-oriented treatment of alcohol addiction. Interventions such as these increase the addict's freedom of choice.

While there are new entry points to treat addictions, prevention is always better. There are interventions for all ages that can contribute to this, from developing self-control in children with games and rules in the classroom, combined parent-and-child interventions in junior high school, and in adolescents through targeted interventions in at-risk groups, where respect for the young person is important.

Children must be protected from early substance use, as it is a strong predictor of later addiction problems. Setting rules can help, and has the added benefit that, perhaps counterintuitively, it reinforces the development of self-control, just like an orderly and predictable environment does. In (emerging) adolescents, it is crucial that the rule-setting is done collaboratively, in line with the increased need for respect at this age.

What some neuroscientists consider the "naive" idea that we can influence our own destiny with our consciousness seems to be a crucial factor in the positive development that resilient children can experience. Thus, from this idea, they can "trump their genes" and avoid developing addiction, for example, despite a genetic vulnerability or a difficult start.

Akrasia is relevant not only to understand and encourage change in addiction, but also in our everyday choices that negatively affect the future of our planet, such as eating meat and flying. It is better for our own health and that of the planet to eat meat at most once a week, despite possible meat cravings. And we shouldn't fly either because of climate change, but it is so nice to be in a different environment in *no time* and get away from it all, just like our friends. With everyday *akrasia problems,* it is important to be aware of the long-term effects. Do we want a world in which the last glaciers in the Alps and Rockies have melted, sea levels rise faster and faster, threatening coastal areas with floods and inland areas becoming deserts? Or a world in which temperature rise and related consequences are halted in time? If we want the latter, we must act accordingly—in essence no different from the addict, who must radically modify behavior, and find strategies to overcome temptations.

Change is difficult when you are alone, as the addict will attest. We should therefore organize ourselves if we want to save the planet. Social connection and joint action is crucial to save us from despair and to develop positive motivation to change. Civic forums could be a tool, assuming that Plato was right and we all ultimately want the same thing: to leave behind a healthy planet.

Person Index

Subject Index